SO-CDR-011

Medical Technology Examination Review

A comprehensive examination review to assist students of clinical medicine and laboratory practitioners

SECOND EDITION

Lorraine D. Doucet, CSC, PhD
Professor of Biology and
Director of Allied Health Programs
Notre Dame College, Manchester, NH and

Albert E. Packard, M.S., MT (ASCP)
Assistant Professor of Biology
Notre Dame College, Manchester, NH

J.B. Lippincott Company
Philadelphia
London   Mexico City   New York
St. Louis   São Paulo   Sydney

SECOND EDITION

Copyright © 1984, by J. B. Lippincott Company
Copyright © 1979, by J. B. Lippincott Company

This book is fully protected by copyright and, with
the exception of brief excerpts for review, no part
of it may be reproduced in any form, by print, photo-
print, microfilm, or any other means, without written
permission from the publisher.

ISBN 0-397-54486-3

Library of Congress Catalog Card Number 84-4378

Printed in the United States of America

3 5 6 4 2

_____

Library of Congress Cataloging in Publication Data

Doucet, Lorraine D.
    Medical technology examination review.

    Includes bibliographies.
    1. Medical technology--Examinations, questions, etc.
I. Packard, Albert E. II. Title.   [DNLM: 1. Technology,
Medical--Examination questions. QY 18 D728m]
RB37.D68 1984   610'.28   84-4378
ISBN 0-397-54486-3

Contributors/Advisors

Barry Corriveau, B.S., MT(ASCP)
Program Director
Medical Technology Program
Westbrook College
Portland, Maine

Joyce DiCenso, MT(ASCP)
Blood Bank Supervisor
Instructor of Immunohematology
Central Maine Medical Center
Lewiston, Maine

Karol LaCroix, MT(ASCP) M.O.E.
Chairman, Associate Professor
Medical Technology Program
University of New Hampshire
Durham, New Hampshire

Normand R. Martel, MS, MT(ASCP)
Medical Technology Program Director
Central Maine Medical Center
Lewiston, Maine

Joyce M. Cuff, Ph.D.
Assistant Professor of Biology
Thiel College
Greensville, Pennsylvania

Doris J. Gagne, MT(ASCP), SH
Hematology Supervisor
Catholic Medical Center
Manchester, New Hampshire

Elaine M. Larock, MT(ASCP)
Blood Bank Technologist
Concord Hospital
Concord, New Hampshire

James J. Vaillancourt, MT(ASCP)
Supervisor, Clinical Chemistry
Concord Hospital
Concord, New Hampshire

Preface

The first and second editions of this book have been designed to assist students of medical technology, as well as practicing clinical laboratory scientists, who wish to prepare themselves for taking lengthy multidisciplinary registry and certification examinations. We feel, however, that this book need not be restricted to this purpose. The field of laboratory science has been, and continues to be, a rapidly changing area of study. It would be virtually impossible for the laboratory scientists to keep abreast of all the changes occurring in the field. Consequently, many laboratory scientists have become "specialists". This era of specialization has caused many people in laboratory science to feel "boxed in" or obsolete. One of the remedies for obsolescence, though definitely not a panacea, is a good program of self-assessment and self-development. It is our hope that this book will serve the dual purpose of preparing students for taking examinations and for helping practicing clinical laboratory scientists refresh their memories in those areas in which they may feel deficient.

This book would not have been possible without:

the encouragement and support of Jeannette Vezeau, CSC, and all the other outstanding religious women at Notre Dame College; and my very special friends BES, GRH and RMH.

L. D.

and

the understanding of Nancy, David and Lynn for the many hours they spent minus a husband and father respectively.

A. P.

We also wish to express our gratitude to Kathleen Scanlon and Marsha Glance for their availability, efficiency and tolerance in typing and retyping this manuscript; and also Kathleen Richmond for her clear and precise scientific illustrations; and also we wish to express our sincere appreciation to Susan Nay for typing the second edition of our book and for being able to tolerate our hieroglyphics and "strange words".

Contents

8 Contents

CHAPTER 1

Introduction

In this, the second edition of the Medical Technology Examination Review, we have retained our original purpose of attempting to help the student of clinical laboratory science and the clinical laboratory scientist in their preparation for taking registry or certification examinations. Specifically, we hope to aid the students taking the American Society of Clinical Pathologists registry examination, the American Medical Technologists Registry Examination, the National Certification Agency for Medical Laboratory Personnel Certification Examination and the International Society for Clinical Laboratory Technology Registry Examination. Additionally, we hope to be of assistance to those laboratory practitioners who will be sitting the Health and Human Services Proficiency Examination. This text has a self diagnostic test, composed of 200 questions, which is designed to help individuals assess their strong and weak points. Following the diagnostic test are chapters of questions designed to assist individuals in strengthening their weak points by allowing them to answer the questions and after answering, review their answers with respect to the explained answers found at the end of each chapter. The review chapters include: Procedures in Microbiology, Bacteriology, Mycology, Parasitology, Virology, Immunology/Serology, Immunohematology, Hematology, Nuclear Medicine, Clinical Chemistry, Toxicology, Endocrinology, Urinalysis, Body Fluid Analysis, Cytogenetics/Cytology, and Quality Control/Laboratory Safety/Laboratory Management. We have attempted to present questions that are applicable to the every day operation of the clinical laboratory.

In this second edition, we have utilized a total of seven multiple choice formats in our questions, with the majority of the questions being the standard multiple choice format. The questions in each vary in number with specific emphasis on the areas of Clinical Chemistry, Microbiology, Hematology, and Immunology/Immunohematology. We have made improvements and revisions in all of the major areas. We have increased the number of questions from just over 1,100 to a little more than 1,500 which represents an overall increase of approximately 35%. The diagnostic test is entirely new and reflects the changing technology, particularly with reference to the Immunology and Therapeutic Drug monitoring questions.

Along with the questions in each chapter, we have included explanatory answers and a listing of our bibliographies and recommended readings. Additionally, there are, at the end of the book, answer sheets for each of the chapters.

Once again, we would like to add the following strategies, suggestions and hints relative to test taking and we hope that they will be of value to each of the individuals utilizing this test.

Test-Taking Strategy. The 200 diagnostic test questions should familiarize you with the types of questions and the level of difficulty encountered in the various clinical areas. One suggestion is that you work all 200 questions during the recommended time period and score your answers before you study the Examination Review book. This will give you a pretest score. Then you can study the Examination Review book, other bibliographic materials and recommended readings. Later, when you feel you are adequately prepared, take the 200 diagnostic test questions again to see how your performance has changed. This will be your post test score. At the end of the diagnostic test there are instructions on how to score your performance. For self assessment purposes, follow those instructions carefully to determine your percentile ranking.

General Test Taking Suggestions. This review book was developed and designed to test your knowledge and skills in several clinically related areas. There are no "trick" or "catch" questions in either the diagnostic or practice tests. Each question is straight-forward and based directly upon the seven formats presented in this Review book.

To score high in the diagnostic test and the practice tests, we suggest the following:

1. Read each test direction and test question carefully and completely. Be certain that you know what each question is looking for.
2. Answer as many test questions as possible. For each wrong answer in the diagnostic test you will lose ¼ of a point from the corresponding number of correct answers. For example if you have 160 correct answers and 40 incorrect answer your raw score will be determined as follows:

          200 questions - 40 incorrect answers = 160 correct answers
          160 correct answers minus ¼ point for each incorrect answer = minus 10 points
          160 correct answers - 10 points = 150 raw score.

Having established your raw score, you can refer to the table on page 40 to determine your percentile ranking.
3. Read through the entire test first. Answer those questions which are most familiar to you and then return to the questions you have left unanswered. It is advisable to leave the most difficult questions until last. This will allow you to make the most efficient use of the time allotted for the examination.
4. The recommended time allotted for the diagnostic test is four hours. This is based on the fact that most registry or certification examinations do not exceed four hours. Keep this in mind in the diagnostic test, which can serve to simulate an actual examination, to determine the pace at which you must work. Establish a work pace in the practice test areas. This should help you improve your diagnostic post test score and help you to work more efficiently during an actual examination.
5. Be certain that the answer space you mark on the answer sheet corresponds with the question number in the practice tests. Do not be concerned if there are more answer spaces on the answer sheet than test questions.

Analyzing Test Questions.
1. Do not <u>read</u> <u>into</u> questions. By this we mean do not include in your thought process an "all", "every", "always", or "never" that is not in the question which may cause you to select the wrong answer. Furthermore, do not unconsciously add qualifying phrases which are not contained in the question. This too may cause erroneous answer selections.

2. Do not <u>leave</u> <u>out</u> or overlook qualifying phrases which are in a question.
Answer the question asked, not the question that you think is asked. You cannot
overlook such modifiers as "generally", "sometimes", "usually", "in part" or "not".
To do so may also cause you to select the wrong answer.

3. Beware of the meaning of negatives: "No one is always contracting this
disease" does not mean "someone is always contracting this disease."

MEDICAL TECHNOLOGY EXAMINATION

ANSWER PRE-TEST FORM

1 A B C D E	11 A B C D E	21 A B C D E	31 A B C D E	41 A B C D E
2 A B C D E	12 A B C D E	22 A B C D E	32 A B C D E	42 A B C D E
3 A B C D E	13 A B C D E	23 A B C D E	33 A B C D E	43 A B C D E
4 A B C D E	14 A B C D E	24 A B C D E	34 A B C D E	44 A B C D E
5 A B C D E	15 A B C D E	25 A B C D E	35 A B C D E	45 A B C D E
6 A B C D E	16 A B C D E	26 A B C D E	36 A B C D E	46 A B C D E
7 A B C D E	17 A B C D E	27 A B C D E	37 A B C D E	47 A B C D E
8 A B C D E	18 A B C D E	28 A B C D E	38 A B C D E	48 A B C D E
9 A B C D E	19 A B C D E	29 A B C D E	39 A B C D E	49 A B C D E
10 A B C D E	20 A B C D E	30 A B C D E	40 A B C D E	50 A B C D E
51 A B C D E	61 A B C D E	71 A B C D E	81 A B C D E	91 A B C D E
52 A B C D E	62 A B C D E	72 A B C D E	82 A B C D E	92 A B C D E
53 A B C D E	63 A B C D E	73 A B C D E	83 A B C D E	93 A B C D E
54 A B C D E	64 A B C D E	74 A B C D E	84 A B C D E	94 A B C D E
55 A B C D E	65 A B C D E	75 A B C D E	85 A B C D E	95 A B C D E
56 A B C D E	66 A B C D E	76 A B C D E	86 A B C D E	96 A B C D E
57 A B C D E	67 A B C D E	77 A B C D E	87 A B C D E	97 A B C D E
58 A B C D E	68 A B C D E	78 A B C D E	88 A B C D E	98 A B C D E
59 A B C D E	69 A B C D E	79 A B C D E	89 A B C D E	99 A B C D E
60 A B C D E	70 A B C D E	80 A B C D E	90 A B C D E	100 A B C D E
101 A B C D E	111 A B C D E	121 A B C D E	131 A B C D E	141 A B C D E
102 A B C D E	112 A B C D E	122 A B C D E	132 A B C D E	142 A B C D E
103 A B C D E	113 A B C D E	123 A B C D E	133 A B C D E	143 A B C D E
104 A B C D E	114 A B C D E	124 A B C D E	134 A B C D E	144 A B C D E
105 A B C D E	115 A B C D E	125 A B C D E	135 A B C D E	145 A B C D E
106 A B C D E	116 A B C D E	126 A B C D E	136 A B C D E	146 A B C D E
107 A B C D E	117 A B C D E	127 A B C D E	137 A B C D E	147 A B C D E
108 A B C D E	118 A B C D E	128 A B C D E	138 A B C D E	148 A B C D E
109 A B C D E	119 A B C D E	129 A B C D E	139 A B C D E	149 A B C D E
110 A B C D E	120 A B C D E	130 A B C D E	140 A B C D E	150 A B C D E
151 A B C D E	161 A B C D E	171 A B C D E	181 A B C D E	191 A B C D E
152 A B C D E	162 A B C D E	172 A B C D E	182 A B C D E	192 A B C D E
153 A B C D E	163 A B C D E	173 A B C D E	183 A B C D E	193 A B C D E
154 A B C D E	164 A B C D E	174 A B C D E	184 A B C D E	194 A B C D E
155 A B C D E	165 A B C D E	175 A B C D E	185 A B C D E	195 A B C D E
156 A B C D E	166 A B C D E	176 A B C D E	186 A B C D E	196 A B C D E
157 A B C D E	167 A B C D E	177 A B C D E	187 A B C D E	197 A B C D E
158 A B C D E	168 A B C D E	178 A B C D E	188 A B C D E	198 A B C D E
159 A B C D E	169 A B C D E	179 A B C D E	189 A B C D E	199 A B C D E
160 A B C D E	170 A B C D E	180 A B C D E	190 A B C D E	200 A B C D E

ANSWER POST-TEST FORM

Each item offers answer choices A B C D E.

1	11	21	31	41	101	111	121	131	141
2	12	22	32	42	102	112	122	132	142
3	13	23	33	43	103	113	123	133	143
4	14	24	34	44	104	114	124	134	144
5	15	25	35	45	105	115	125	135	145
6	16	26	36	46	106	116	126	136	146
7	17	27	37	47	107	117	127	137	147
8	18	28	38	48	108	118	128	138	148
9	19	29	39	49	109	119	129	139	149
10	20	30	40	50	110	120	130	140	150
51	61	71	81	91	151	161	171	181	191
52	62	72	82	92	152	162	172	182	192
53	63	73	83	93	153	163	173	183	193
54	64	74	84	94	154	164	174	184	194
55	65	75	85	95	155	165	175	185	195
56	66	76	86	96	156	166	176	186	196
57	67	77	87	97	157	167	177	187	197
58	68	78	88	98	158	168	178	188	198
59	69	79	89	99	159	169	179	189	199
60	70	80	90	100	160	170	180	190	200

CHAPTER 2

Medical Technology
Diagnostic Test

Time: 4 Hours

Directions. Select the one BEST answer for each of the following statements. Circle the appropriate response on the answer sheet.

1. Immunoglobulins (antibodies) are classified by:

    A. the type of heavy chains   C. the type of light chains
    B. their ability to fix complement D. none of the above

2. The major histocompatibility complex is located on which of the following chromosomes?

    A. somatic chromosome 1   C. somatic chromosome 6
    B. somatic chromosome 12   D. the X chromosome

3. Quality control programs are used to determine or check which of the following?

    A. precision and accuracy of results
    B. technical performance of laboratory personnel
    C. performance of laboratory equipment
    D. performance of reagents
    E. all of the above

Questions 4-18

Directions. For each of the numbered items select the appropriate lettered response. Do not use the same letter more than once.

4. periodic acid-schiff (PAS)   A. iron stain
5. sudan black B   B. glycogen
6. new methylene blue   C. supravital stain
7. prussian blue   D. lipids

8. LSD   A. phencylclidine
9. PCP   B. thioridizine
10. mellaril   C. lysergic acid diethylamine
11. elavil   D. amitriptyline
                 E. diazepam

12. energy requiring
13. substrate level phosphorylation
14. can cause aplastic anemia
15. NADH

A. passive diffusion
B. active transtort
C. 3 ATP's
D. GDP
E. chloramphenicol

16. multiple myeloma
17. urinary casts
18. normally found in urine

A. amylase
B. Tamm-Horsfall mucoprotein
C. Bence-Jones protein
D. beta-lipoprotein

Questions 19-28

Directions. The column on the left contains 3 scientifically related categories while the column on the right contains 4 items which may illustrate a scientific phenomenon or process. Three of the items in the column on the right relate to only one of the categories on the left. First, indicate the category in which the 3 processes or phenomena belong. Second, indicate the one process or phenomenon which is not related to the category.

Category

Phenomenon

19. A. IgG
    B. IgA
    C. IgM

20. A. anti-Fy^a
    B. anti-E
    C. anti-M
    D. anti-Kell

21. A. Kidd
    B. Duffy
    C. Kell

22. A. Penney
    B. Cartwright
    C. Sutter
    D. Matthew

23. A. Listeria
    B. Corynebacteria
    C. Brucella

24. A. meningitis
    B. "tumbling motility."
    C. cold enrichment
    D. gram positive coccus

25. A. Clostridium
    B. Bacillus
    C. Francisella

26. A. spore former
    B. aerobic
    C. gram negative
    D. Woolsorter's disease

27. A. Rickettsia
    B. Brucella
    C. Chlamydia

28. A. intracellular
    B. insect vector
    C. psittacosis
    D. tsutsugamushi

Questions 29-44

Directions. Select the one BEST answer for each of the following statements. Circle the appropriate response on the answer sheet.

29. Which of the following concentrations of serum salicylate would be considered the therapeutic range for arthritic patients on salicylate therapy?

    A. 5 - 10 mg/dl   C. 15 - 30 mg/dl
    B. 10 - 20 mg/dl   D. 40 - 60 mg/dl

30. In the Trinder reaction for the determination of serum salicylate levels, which of the following is true?

    A. a violet colored complex is formed between the ferric ions and the carboxyl group of the salicylic acid
    B. a violet colored complex is formed between the ferric ions and the phenol group of the salicylic acid
    C. a violet colored complex is formed between the mercuric salt and the carboxyl group of the salicylic acid
    D. a violet colored complex is formed between the mercuric salt and the phenol group of the salicylic acid

31. Which of the following drugs is used, therapeutically, in the management of asthma?

    A. phenytoin   C. primidone
    B. phenobarbital   D. theophylline

32. Hepatotoxicity due to overdosage of acetaminophen is determined by:

    A. the dose ingested   C. the plasma half-life
    B. the plasma concentration   D. all of the above

33. Which of the following drugs is measured to assess adequate control of an epileptic patient receiving anti-epileptic therapy?

    A. salicylate   C. theophylline
    B. acetaminophen   D. phenytoin

34. The drug phenytoin has a half-life of approximately:

    A. 6 hours   C. 24 hours
    B. 12 hours   D. 48 hours

35. Which of the following statements concerning lead poisoning is NOT true?

    A. gastrointestinal absorption is greater in adults than in children
    B. one of the mechanisms of lead intoxication involves the inhibition of heme synthetase
    C. exposure to lead may be due to contact with paints, glazed pottery and storage batteries
    D. lead intoxication in children may lead to growth retardation and impaired mental function

36. The chemical determination of which of the following sugars could be used to assess germinal cell activity in the production of spermatazoa?

    A. glucose   C. sucrose
    B. fructose   D. lactose

37. Which of the following statements concerning the differentiation between transudates and exudates is NOT true?

    A. there is no clot formation in transudates
    B. transudates are noninflammatory serous fluids
    C. exudates are inflammatory serous fluids
    D. the total protein concentration is usually higher in transudates than in exudates

38. Serologic surveys show, that adults in the general population, do not usually contract hepatitis B infections. However, certain members of the population may be risks. Which of the following could be considered risks?

    A. nurses   C. hospital cooks
    B. hospital custodians   D. immunohematologists

39. Male carriers or male patients suffering with an acute hepatitis B infection would be found to have the highest HBV concentration in their:

    A. urine   C. semen
    B. saliva   D. blood

40. Piroplasmosis is also known as:

    A. babesiosis   C. toxoplasmosis
    B. malaria   D. echinococcosis

41. In the life cycle of Paragonimus westermani, which of the following stages of development infects the fresh water crab?

    A. ova   C. cercaria
    B. miracidium   D. metacercaria

42. In the life cycle of Paragonimus westermani, which of the following stages of development infects humans?

    A. ova   C. cercaria
    B. miracidium   D. metacercaria

43. Down's syndrome is the result of trisomy 21. Consequently the somatic cells of individuals with Down's syndrome have 47 chromosomes instead of 46. Down's syndrome is then the result of:

    A. crossing over   D. translocation
    B. chromosome deletion   E. nondisjunction
    C. chromosome inversion

44. Which of the following methods is used for the determination of urinary corticosteroids?

    A. Zimmerman reaction   C. both A and B
    B. Porter-Silber method   D. neither A nor B

Questions 45-54

Directions. One, some, or all of the responses for each of the following statements may be correct. Indicate your response as follows:

A. if items 1 and 3 are correct
B. if items 2 and 4 are correct
C. if three of the items are correct
D. if all of the items are correct
E. if only one of the items is correct

45. ^{131}I taken orally may be expected to appear in:

1. hydroiodic acid in the stomach   3. saliva
2. urine   4. hydroxyapatite

46. ^{131}I-albumin is used to assay plasma volume because:

1. it is measurable in small quantities
2. it has a beta which is optimal for counting
3. it leaves the blood slowly
4. one only needs to fast for 6 hours prior to the test

47. Which of the following are considered to be suitable for alcohol analysis?

1. capillary blood by fingerstick   3. venous whole blood
2. venous serum   4. urine

48. Besides the toxicity of a drug, which of the following is considered to be a life-threatening drug reaction?

1. syncope   3. anaphylaxis
2. allergy   4. urticaria

49. A hemolytic anemia would be characterized by the following laboratory findings:

1. increased reticulocyte   3. decreased haptoglobin level
2. decreased hgb values   4. increased bilirubin

50. Disseminated intravascular coagulation (DIC) can be presumptuously diagnosed by using the following laboratory tests:

1. platelet count   3. activated partial thromboplastin time
2. prothrombin time   4. fibrinogen degradation

51. Which of the following organisms may involve the liver during some stage of development?

1. Echnicoccus granulosus   3. Fasciola hepatica
2. Plasmodium vivax   4. Opistorchis sinensis

52. Which of the following is/are most likely to be acquired from the ingestion of improperly cooked beef?

    1. Trichinella spiralis
    2. Toxoplasma gondi
    3. Taenia solium
    4. Taenia saginata

53. Which of the following substances will produce positive results with the Clini-test method for glucose determination?

    1. sucrose
    2. fructose
    3. strong oxidants
    4. ascorbic acid

54. Which of the following urine volumes would be considered oliguric?

    1. a 24 hour volume of 1000 ml
    2. a 24 hour volume of 1500 ml
    3. a 24 hour volume of 2500 ml
    4. a 24 hour volume of 600 ml

Questions 55-59

Directions. For each of the numbered words or phrases listed below, select the appropriate response as follows:

A. if the item is associated with A only
B. if the item is associated with B only
C. if the item is associated with both A and B
D. if the item is associated with neither A nor B

    A. asexual spore production
    B. sexual spore production

55. Actinomyces israelii
56. Candida albicans
57. Cladosporium carrionii
58. Absidia corymbifera
59. Sporothrix schenkii

Questions 60-91

Directions. Select the one BEST answer for each of the following statements. Circle the appropriate response on the answer sheet.

60. The direct antiglobulin test is utilized for the detection of:

    A. circulating antibody
    B. cell bound antibody
    C. circulating antibody-complement complexes
    D. IgM antibodies

61. Which of the following lymphokines is NOT heat stable at 56°C?

    A. migration inhibitory factor
    B. lymphotoxin
    C. chemotactic factor
    D. transfer factor

62. Which of the following is considered to be the major chemotactic factor?

    A. C3a   C. C5a
    B. C4a   D. C9

63. In a typical example of atopic sensitization, cytotropic antibody (IgE) is bound to which of the following cells?

    A. polymorphonuclear cells   C. B-lymphocytes
    B. mast cells   D. reticuloendothelial cells

64. In anaphylactic reactions, chemical mediators are released from mast cells. Which of the following chemical mediators does NOT act by increasing capillary permeability?

    A. histamine   C. heparin
    B. bradykinnin   D. slow reacting substance A

65. The mobilities obtained on hemoglobin electrophoresis at pH 8.6 show:

    A. HbS moves faster than HbA
    B. HbC moves faster than HbA
    C. HbA moves slower than HbC or HbS
    D. HbS moves faster than HbC but more slowly than HbA

66. Schumm's test is used to identify:

    A. methemoglobin   C. oxyhemoglobin
    B. sulfhemoglobin   D. methemalbumin

67. Which of the following would give a reliable hematocrit determination?

    A. collect 1 ml of blood in a 5 ml EDTA tube
    B. perform fingerstick and squeeze finger to fill the capillary tube
    C. omit the buffy coat from the measurement of the cell column height
    D. centrifuge the hematocrit until you think the RBC are well packed

68. Which of the following needles has the largest berul?

    A. 18 gauge   C. 21 gauge
    B. 20 gauge   D. 22 gauge

69. Erythropoietin is produced in man primarily in the:

    A. pancreas   C. kidney
    B. small intestine   D. pituitary

70. Which of the following is NOT considered to be a cestode?

    A. Hymenolepsis diminuta   C. Taenia saginata
    B. Schistosoma mansoni   D. Echniococcus granulosus

71. Which of the following lumen dwelling organisms is most likely to be the largest?

   A. Entamoeba hartmani   C. Iodamoeba butschlii
   B. Entamoeba histolytica   D. Balantidium coli

72. Which of the following ectoparasites is the vector for endemic typhus?

   A. Tunga penetrans   C. Sarcoptes scabei
   B. Pediculus humanus   D. Phlebotomus spp.

73. Blood components prepared in an open system have an outdate of:

   A. 21 days   C. 2 hours
   B. 6 hours   D. 24 hours

74. A person who inherits the genes A,B,hh,Le,se will have the following antigens present in their saliva:

   A. H,A,B   C. H,A,B,Le^a,Le^b
   B. H,A,B,Le^a D. Le^a

75. In the process of identifying an antibody, the technologist observes a 2+ reaction with 3 of the 8 cells in the identification panel after immediate spin saline phase. These reactions disappear following incubation at 37°C and after the anti-human globulin phase. The antibody most likely to be responsible for these findings is:

   A. anti-M   C. anti-C
   B. anti-Fy^a D. anti-D

76. The most significant test in the investigation of autoimmune hemolytic anemia is:

   A. Donath-Landsteiner test   C. Kleihauer-Betke test
   B. direct antiglobulin test   D. ABO test

77. Two weeks after the transfusion of fifteen units of blood, a patient has a 3gm drop in hemoglobin and jaundice. No evidence of bleeding is found. Which of the following should be performed on a fresh specimen?

   A. direct antiglobulin test
   B. antigen screen for Rh-hr, Kell and Duffy
   C. screen serum for unexpected antigen
   D. test the serum for cold agglutinins

78. A sputum is submitted to the laboratory for gram stain, culture and sensitivity. Examination of the gram stain reveals: P.M.N.'s=0; many epithelial cells; moderate gram negative diplococci; diphtheroids; many gram positive cocci in clusters and small chains. Based on these findings the physician is informed that the specimen is unsatisfactory for culture. Why?

   A. the results indicate the specimen was collected in a non-sterile container
   B. the results are consistent with a specimen which has been standing too long at room temperature
   C. the results are consistent with normal oral flora and the specimen is more likely saliva than sputum
   D. sputums are not cultured if more than one type of organism is seen on the gram stain

79. Referring to the above question: The physician asks the technologist how best to avoid this problem in the future. Of the following, which would be the best approach.

    A. instruct the patient to thoroughly cleanse his mouth with mouthwash prior to collection
    B. submit a specimen collected at branchoscopy
    C. have the patient expetorate from deep within the lungs
    D. collect the specimen by transtracheal aspiration

80. The laboratory receives a call from the charge nurse in the surgical unit. She wishes to know how to handle a urine for culture and sensitivity and states that the urine cannot be transported to the laboratory for a few hours. She should be informed to:

    A. leave the urine at the desk until it can be transported to the laboratory
    B. place the urine in a refrigerator until ready for transport
    C. add a few drops of merthiolate to the specimen for preservation
    D. collect another specimen when it can be transported immediately

81. A urine specimen, collected by suprapubic aspiration, is submitted for a colony count, identification and sensitivity. Upon reading the requisition, the techno-logist in charge of bacteriology notices that the specimen has been in transit 4 hours since its collection. The best course of action would be:

    A. discard the specimen and request a fresh specimen
    B. hold the specimen in the refrigerator, notify the physician and wait for his/her instructions
    C. immediately streak the specimen onto the appropriate media
    D. perform a semi-quantitative gram-stain and discard the specimen, if more than one organism per oil immersion field is observed

82. Pleural transudative effusions are associated with all of the following except:

    A. cardiac insufficiency   C. actinomycosis
    B. hypoalbuminemia   D. obstruction to venous flow

83. Low cerebrospinal fluid glucose levels are associated with all of the following except:

    A. hypoglycemia   C. toxoplasmosis
    B. hyperglycemia   D. fungal meningitis

84. The measurement of glucose, has traditionally been expressed in terms of mg/dl. The SI recommendation is that it be reported in terms of mmol/liter. Therefore, a plasma concentration of 70 mg/dl would be reported in which of the following SI terms?

    A. 0.7 mmol/L   C. 0.388 mmol/L
    B. 7.0 mmol/L   D. 3.88 mmol/l

85. Which of the following statements is TRUE with respect to uncompensated metabolic alkalosis?

    A. pH will be elevated without an elevation of the pCO_2
    B. pH will be elevated with an elevation of pCO_2
    C. pH will be elevated with a decrease in pCO_2
    D. none of the above

86. Which of the following is TRUE of a fully compensated metabolic acidosis?

    A. pH will be decreased without a decrease in pCO_2
    B. pH will be decreased with a decrease in pCO_2
    C. pH will be decreased with an increase in pCO_2
    D. none of the above

87. Which of the following enzymes is NOT used to determine liver dysfunction?

    A. aldolase   C. gamma-glutamyl transpeptidase
    B. alkaline phosphatase   D. 5'-nucleopeptidase

88. Which of the following enzymes is used for the detection of exposure to organo-phosphate insecticides?

    A. gamma-glutamyl transpeptidase   C. pseudocholinesterase
    B. guanine deaminase   D. ornithine-carbamoyl transferase

89. According to the National Diabetes Data Group recommendations, which of the following statements is TRUE with regards to the following findings?

        Fasting glucose 130 mg/dl   2 hour post prandial glucose 210 mg/dl

    A. the patient may be diagnosed as having diabetes mellitus
    B. the patient is diagnosed as having impaired glucose tolerance
    C. the patient is diagnosed as having diabetes insipidous
    D. the patient is normal

90. Microscopic morphology of Yersinia pestis reveals:

    A. colonies with a drop-like appearance
    B. gram positive bacilli
    C. gram negative bacilli with a tendency toward bi-polar staining
    D. gram positive bacilli with a tendency toward bi-polar staining

91. Klebsiella pneumoniae:

    A. is motile
    B. is methyl red positive
    C. causes about 3% of all acute bacterial pneumonias
    D. is not found in healty individuals

Questions 92-101

Directions. For each of the numbered items select the appropriate lettered response. Do not use the same letter more than once.

92.	plasmid	A.	erythromycins
93.	gram positive cell wall antigens	B.	beta lactamose
94.	inhibit protein synthesis	C.	teichoic acid
95.	oxygen	D.	fermentation
96.	pyruvate	E.	obligate aerobe

97.	leukemic reticuloendotheliosis	A.	gargoylism
98.	erythroleukemia	B.	hairy cell leukemia
99.	myelofibrosis	C.	agnogenic myeloid metaplasia
100.	Alder-Reilly	D.	DiGuglielmo's syndrome
101.	Cooley's anemia	E.	homozygous thalassemia

Questions 102-106

Directions. One, some or all of the responses for each of the following statements may be correct. Indicate your response as follows:

A. if items 1 and 3 are correct
B. if items 2 and 4 are correct
C. if three of the items are correct
D. if all of the items are correct
E. if only one of the items is correct

102. Patients receiving gentamycin therapy should have which of the following tests performed during the course of their therapy?

1. gentamycin level   3. creatinine
2. wound culture   4. alkaline phosphatase

103. It is important to use isotopes with short half-lives for clinical work because:

1. it decreases the radiation exposure to the patient
2. it increases the biological clearance rate of the compound
3. it decreases the interference with subsequent tests
4. it increases the effective half-life of the substance

104. Currently scintigraphic procedures are indicated in the determination of:

1. hypothyroidism   3. hyperthyroidism
2. thyroid tumor   4. ectopic thyroid tissue

105. Which of the following substances may be detected when utilizing the dipstick method for blood?

1. hemoglobin   3. myoglobin
2. red blood cells   4. bilirubin

106. Which of the following volumes would be considered to be classified as polyuria?

1. a 24 hour volume of 1000 ml   3. a 24 hour volume of 2500 ml
2. a 24 hour volume of 1500 ml   4. a 24 hour volume of 600 ml

Questions 107-136

Directions.   Select the one BEST answer for each of the following statements. Circle the appropriate response on the answer sheet.

107.   Hymenoptera venom (bee venom) is universally recognized as an antigen that is capable of producing an immune reaction. The antibody produced against this antigen is detectable in the blood for:

A.   up to 5 years   C.   up to 15 years
B.   up to 10 years   D.   up to 20 years

108.   Which of the following drugs are capable of producing a hemolytic drug reaction?

A.   aldomet   C.   quinidine
B.   penicillin   D.   all of the above

109.   Which of the following mediates various anti-viral activities?

A.   migration inhibitory factor   C.   macrophage activating factor
B.   interferon   D.   chemotactic factors

110.   Which of the following statements concerning IgA is NOT true?

A.   occurs in different polymeric forms
B.   has two subclasses
C.   fixes complement
D.   principle antibody of secretions

111.   Which of the following antibodies is most commonly associated with allergic reactions?

A.   IgA   C.   IgE
B.   IgD   D.   IgG

112.   Which of the following is NOT a requisite for immunogenicity?

A.   foreigness   C.   complexity of structure
B.   size   D.   contains DNA or RNA

113.   Which of the following endocrine glands is responsible for the production and excretion of glucagon?

A.   anterior pituitary gland
B.   alpha islet cells of the pancreas
C.   adrenal cortex
D.   beta islet cells of the pancreas

114.   A serum specimen is received in the laboratory and is found to have a "creamy layer over a turbid layer". Which of the following would most likely be responsible for the appearance of the serum?

A.   decreased serum cholesterol   C.   decreased chylomicrons
B.   increased serum triglycerides   D.   increased bilirubin content

115. Serum amylase converts starch to which of the following?

    A. glucose and dextrose   C. glucose and fructose
    B. glucose and maltose   D. fructose and maltose

116. The protein fraction that has the fastest mobility during electrophoresis is:

    A. albumin   C. beta globulin
    B. alpha globulin   D. gamma globulin

117. In an acute myocardial infarction, which of the following will be elevated?

    A. LD 1   C. CK-BB
    B. LD 5   D. all of the above

118. Hemolysis will affect which of the following results?

    A. CK   C. CK-BB
    B. Total LD   D. LD 1/Total LD ratio

119. A patient is admitted and diagnosed to have acute myocardial infarction. If, in fact, the patient has had an acute myocardial infarction, which of the following will be elevated on admission?

    A. Total LD   C. Total AST
    B. Total CK   D. Total ALT

120. A normal Free Thyroxin Index (FTI) is associated with which of the following?

    A. hyperthyroidism   C. euthyroidism
    B. hypothyroidism   D. none of the above

121. Which of the following are a requisite for the diagnosis of reactive hypoglycemia?

    A. glucose level below 50 mg/dl
    B. plasma cortisols increased at the time of the low glucose levels
    C. both of the above
    D. only A

122. Which of the following disorders would be the cause for a decrease in serum magnesium levels?

    A. vitamin D intoxication   C. acute pancreatitis
    B. uremia   D. treatment with human growth hormone

123. The Kleihauer-Betke test depends on the ability of fetal hemoglobin to resist elution by:

    A. alkaline solutions   C. neutral buffers
    B. acid solutions   D. ethanol

124. By history, a patient is known to have an anti-Fy^a antibody, which is no longer detectable by regular methods. In order to achieve a successful transfusion, which of the following statements are applicable?

    A.   enzyme treatment will aid the antibody detection
    B.   units found to be compatible by crossmatch can be used
    C.   as the antibody is not reactive at this time, it can be ignored
    D.   donors which are negative for the Fy^a antigen, and are compatible by cross-match, can be used

125. An $Rh_o(D)$ negative patient whose serum contains high titered IgG anti-D gave birth to a baby with a strongly positive direct antiglobulin test, but whose red cells are not agglutinated by saline anti-D antisera. The most likely explanation for this finding is that:

    A.   the baby is Rh-negative, and the positive direct antiglobulin test is due to another antibody produced by the mother
    B.   the baby is Rh-positive, but his/her Rh antigens are not sufficiently developed to react with saline anti-D
    C.   the baby is Rh-negative, and the positive direct antiglobulin test is due to in utero development of hemolytic anemia
    D.   the baby is Rh-positive, but the red cells are "coated" with anti-D, thereby blocking the reaction by saline anti-D

126. The terminal sugar which is added to the precursor chain to produce B substance is:

    A.   glucose   C.   fucose
    B.   galactose   D.   sucrose

127. If the cells of an individual agglutinate with A, lectin (Dolichos biflorus), the individual will be group:

    A.   A   C. A_2
    B. A_1 D. A_3

128. If a patient has an anti-hr' antibody, which of the following units may be transfused without an adverse reaction?

    A. R^1R^1 C. R^1r
    B. R^1R^2 D. $Rh_o(D)$ negative

129. Huntington's chorea is a disease of the nervous system. This disease is rare but fatal and the symptoms are not exhibited until middle age. This disease is inherited as an autosomal dominant trait. If an apparently normal man in his late twenties is informed that his father has been diagnosed as having Huntington's chorea, what are the chances of the son developing the disease himself?

    A.   100%   D.   25%
    B.   75%   E.   none at all
    C.   50%

130. A person is a sexual mosaic with sex chromosome constituents of XX/XXXY. How many Barr bodies would be found in that person's cells?

    A.   one or two   D.   only two
    B.   two or three   E.   only three
    C.   only one

131. In the assessment of fetal lung maturity through amniotic fluid analysis, which of the following statements is NOT true?

    A. the optical density of the amniotic fluid at 650 nm correlates well with the lecithin to sphingomyelin ratio
    B. an amniotic fluid creatinine concentration of 1.0 mg/dl is indicative of a pregnancy of over 35 weeks
    C. if the lecithin to sphingomyelin ratio is less than 1.2 the fetal lung is relatively immature
    D. if the lecithin to sphingomyelin ratio is greater than 2.0 the fetal lung is relatively mature

132. Children suffering with chickenpox or influenza-like infections are frequently treated with salicylate or medications containing salicylate. Prolonged salicylate usage possibly could cause an acute and serious syndrome which is characterized by lethargy and vomiting. The syndrome could also lead to delirium and coma. This syndrome is:

    A. Reye   C. Alder-Reilly
    B. Di Guglielmo   D. Guillain-Barre

133. Measles (rubeola) is frequently a severe disease which could lead to broncho-pneumonia. To be considered immune to measles, a person must have evidence of:

    A. laboratory proof of immunity
    B. a physician's statement of diagnosis of measles
    C. adequate immunization with live measles vaccine on or after the first birthday
    D. all of the above

134. Yellow fever, dengue fever, eastern and western equine encephalitis are arthropod-borne viruses which may ultimately infect individuals who come in contact with infected mosquitoes. The etiologic agents of these diseases are:

    A. poxviruses   D. arenaviruses
    B. echoviruses   E. none of the above
    C. togaviruses

135. Which of the following is the normal range for plasma levels of growth hormone in males?

    A. 0-8 ng/ml   C. 15-24 ng/ml
    B. 10-15 ng/ml   D. 18-30 ng/ml

136. Which of the following would NOT be considered an abnormal level for VMA (Vanilmandelic acid), in a 24 hour urine sample, for an infant?

    A. 75 ug/kg/day   C. 125 ug/kg/day
    B. 100 ug/kg/day   D. 150 ug/kg/day

Questions 137-150

Directions. One, some, or all of the responses for each of the following statements may be correct. Indicate your response as follows:

A. if items 1 and 3 are correct
B. if items 2 and 4 are correct
C. if three items are correct
D. if all of the items are correct
E. if only one of the items is correct

137. Which of the following is the least likely to be acquired by a strict vegetarian?

1. Fasciola hepatica
2. Schistosoma mansoni
3. Fasciolopsis buski
4. Taenia solium

138. Which of the following could be contracted from a family pet?

1. echinococcosis
2. toxoplasmosis
3. Toxocara infection
4. schistosomiasis

139. Which of the following are acquired from improperly cooked meats?

1. Taenia solium
2. Toxoplasma gondi
3. Taenia saginata
4. Trichinella spiralis

140. The harmful effects of radiation are dependent upon:

1. energy
2. penetrability
3. ionizing ability
4. half-life

141. ^{99m}Tc has a number of clinical usages because:

1. it has a short half-life
2. it emits a gamma which is optimal for counting
3. it is easily separated from its parent compound
4. it has a weak beta

142. Polycythemia vera is characterized by the following:

1. increased red cell mass
2. an increase in platelets and leukocytes
3. E.S.R. is increased
4. L.A.P. score is elevated

143. Macropolycytes are most commonly found in which disorder:

1. autoimmune hemolytic anemia
2. Pelger-Huet anomaly
3. paroxysmal nocturnal hemoglobinuria
4. folic acid and B12 deficiency

144. Thrombocytopenia may occur due to which of the following:

1. transfusion
2. drug ingestion
3. viral infections
4. cholecysthiasis

145. A cause of neutropenia could be:

    1. ingestion of certain drugs
    2. multiple myeloma
    3. hypersplenism
    4. malaria

146. Causes of thrombocytosis may include:

    1. iron deficiency anemia
    2. carcinoma
    3. splenectomy
    4. rheumatoid arthritis

147. What prominent type of red cell morphology would you expect to find on a smear from a patient with disseminated intravascular coagulation?

    1. schistocytes
    2. macrocytes
    3. spherocytes
    4. target cells

148. Which of the following substances may produce false elevations of the sulfosali-cylic acid test for urinary protein?

    1. tolbutamide
    2. penicillin
    3. para-aminoslicylic acid
    4. amylose

149. Which of the following methods of determining the solute concentration of urine will be affected by radiographic iodine preparations?

    1. the dipstick method
    2. refractometry
    3. osmolality
    4. urinometer determinations

150. Which of the following criteria are necessary for the formation of casts?

    1. acid pH
    2. high solute concentration
    3. Tamm-horsfall mucoprotein
    4. alkaline pH

Questions 151-173

Directions. Select the one BEST answer for each of the following statements. Circle the appropriate response on the answer sheet.

151. The metallochromic dye calgamite, is utilized in the determination of which of the following?

    A. zinc
    B. iron
    C. magnesium
    D. inorganic phosphorous

152. Which of the following is most frequently utilized for the diagnosis of malabsorption states?

    A. tolbutamide tolerance
    B. D-xylose tolerance
    C. fructose tolerance
    D. galactose tolerance

153. The following results were obtained from an anemic person: Serum Iron - 30 ug/dl (Reference range - 70 - 150 ug/dl) UIBC - 420 ug/dl and TIBC - 450 ug/dl. Which of the following disorders would be most likely to produce these results?

    A. thalassemia major
    B. hemosiderosis
    C. iron deficiency
    D. nephrosis

154. Which of the following enzymes has the greatest stability at room temperature?

    A. amylase   C. isocitrate dehydrogenase
    B. alpha-HBDH   D. acid phosphatase

155. During the performance of serum glucose levels utilizing the glucose oxidase method, which of the following enzymes is NOT used?

    A. glucose oxidase   C. hexokinase
    B. peroxidase   D. glucomutarotase

156. Which of the following methods of glucose determination is the lease sensitive?

    A. hexokinase   C. ortho-toluidine
    B. glucose oxidase   D. glucose dehydrogenase

157. Which of the following methods of glucose determination is utilized by the Beckman glucose analyzer?

    A. hexokinase   C. ortho-toluidine
    D. glucose oxidase   D. glucose dehydrogenase

158. According to the National Diabetes Data Group, what is the recommended dose of glucose to be used as a glucose challenge for a glucose tolerance test?

    A. 25 gm   C. 75 gm
    B. 50 gm   D. 100 gm

159. According to the recommendations of the National Diabetes Data Group, which of the following is the recommended dose of glucose to be used as a challenge for the determination of gestational diabetes?

    A. 25 gm   C. 75 gm
    B. 50 gm   D. 100 gm

160. In Waldenstrom's macroglobulinemia, which of the following types of immunoglobulin predominates?

    A. IgA   C. IgG
    B. IgE   D. IgM

161. Which of the following complement complexes is known as the recognition unit?

    A. C1   C. C5678
    B. C4b2a   D. none of the above

162. The Fab fragment of an immunoglobulin contains which of the following?

    A. the variable portion of the light chain only
    B. the entire light chain and the variable portion of the heavy chain only
    C. the entire light chain and the variable and 1st constant domain of the heavy chain
    D. the entire heavy chain only

163. The overall structure of immunoglobulin molecules is held together by:

    A. peptide bonds   C. disulfide bonds
    B. hydrogen bonds   D. all of the above

164. Which of the following, concerning Bence-Jones protein, is NOT true?

    A. synthesized independently of myeloma proteins
    B. nearly always identical to the heavy chains of the patients disease
    C. precipitates on heating to 45 to 60°C
    D. can be measured by the Ouchterlony double diffusion technique

165. The genetic ability to produce specific IgE when naturally exposed to certain materials which are harmless to the rest of the population, is referred to as:

    A. cell mediated immunity   C. atopy
    B. anaphylaxis   D. urticaria

166. Which of the following is not considered to be a phagocytic cell?

    A. T-lymphocyte   C. monocyte
    B. polymorphonuclear leukocyte   D. tissue macrophage

167. Which of the following chemical grades is used for the analysis of trace metals?

    A. Analytical Reagent Grade (AR)   C. Technical grade
    B. Chemically Pure Grade (CP)   D. Practical grade

168. In the life cycle of the malarial parasites, which of the following stages of development is the one transmitted from the mosquito to the human host?

    A. sporozoite   C. ookinete
    B. merozoite   D. schizont

169. Which of the following is the largest of the nematodes that parasitize humans?

    A. Ancylostoma duodenale   C. Ascaris lumbricoides
    B. Necator americanus   D. Enterobius vermicularis

170. Which of the following tapeworms requires two intermediate hosts?

    A. Echinococcus granulosus   C. Taenia saginata
    B. Taenia solium   D. Diphyllobothrium latum

171. Which of the following organisms is capable of development to the adult stage in humans?

    A. Toxocara canis   C. Onchocerca volvulus
    B. Ancylostoma braziliensis   D. Dirofilaria immitis

172. Which of the following hormones is NOT secreted by the anterior pituitary gland?

    A. Thyroid stimulating hormone (TSH)
    B. Adrenocorticotrophic hormone (ASTH)
    C. Antidiuretic hormone (ADH)
    D. Growth hormone (GH)

173.   Which of the following disease states will exhibit a decrease in the ketogenic steroids?

    A.   Addison's disease   C.   adrenal hyperplasia
    B.   Cushing's syndrome   D.   precocious puberty

Questions 174-185

Directions.   For each of the numbered items select the appropriate lettered response. Do not use the same letter more than once.

174.   capsule
175.   DNA replication
176.   FAD
177.   electron transport systems

    A.   mesosome
    B.   2 ATP's
    C.   erythromycins
    D.   Quellung reaction
    E.   cytochrome C

178.   rouleaux formation
179.   agglutination
180.   neutropenia
181.   Downey cells

    A.   agranulocytosis
    B.   red cells in stacks of coins
    C.   clumps of RBC's
    D.   atypical lymphocytes

182.   acute myelogenous leukemia
183.   Ig A multiple myeloma
184.   chronic myelogenous leukemia
185.   Hodgkin's disease

    A.   flame cells
    B.   Philadelphia chromosome
    C.   Reed-Sternberg cells
    D.   Auer rods

Questions 186-194

Directions.   Select the one BEST answer for each of the following statements. Circle the appropriate response on the answer sheet.

186.   Using the criteria established by the National Diabetes Data Group, which of the following is TRUE?

    A.   an individual of 60 years of age is said to be diabetic if he/she has a fasting glucose of 135 mg/dl and a two hour post prandial glucose of 210 mg/dl
    B.   a child (under 16 years of age) is said to be a diabetic if he/she has a fasting glucose of 135 mg/dl and a two hour post prandial of 210 mg/dl
    C.   an individual of 60 years of age is said to be diabetic if he/she has a fasting glucose of 145 mg/dl and a two hour post prandial of 195 mg/dl
    D.   a child (under 16 years of age) is said to be diabetic if he/she has a fasting glucose of 145 mg/dl and a two hour post prandial glucose of 210 mg/dl

187.   In the determination of diabetes insipidous, which of the following tests will provide the most useful data?

    A.   C-peptide assay   C.   insulin tolerance assay
    B.   vasopressin assay   D.   hemoglobin A_1C assay

188.   Glycosylated hemoglobin assays are most useful for which of the following?

    A.   reactive hypoglycemia
    B.   daily monitoring of diabetes mellitus
    C.   daily monitoring of diabetes insipidous
    D.   long term monitoring of diabetes mellitus

189. Glycosylated hemoglobin determination utilizes which of the following?

    A. serum and red blood cells   C. serum but not red blood cells
    B. red blood cells alone   D. plasma

190. Sodium nitroprusside is utilized in the urease method of Blood Urea Nitrogen
      assay to do which of the following?

    A. intensify the yellow color produced by the diazine derivative
    B. catalyze the acid hydrolysis of the diacetyl monoxime
    C. to hydrolize urea to the ammonium ion and carbonate
    D. to catalize the formation of a blue indophenol

191. Because of the high levels of uric acid that may be erroneously produced by the
      increase of urea nitrogen in patients with high levels of ascorbic acid, which
      of the following should be undertaken?

    A. if the phosphotungstate method was utilized, repeat the test using the uricase-
        neocuprine method
    B. if the urease-neocuprine method was utilized, repeat the test using the
        phosphotungstate method
    C. neutralize the ascorbic acid and repeat the phosphotungstate procedure
    D. neutralize the ascorbic acid and repeat the uricase-neocuprine procedure

192. During a routine chemical examination of a patient admitted for dehydration, a
      patient was found to have an elevated total protein and an elevated albumin level.
      Which of the following is true?

    A. the A/G ratio remains unchanged
    B. the A/G ratio decreases
    C. the A/G ratio increases
    D. the A/G ratio decreases, but returns to normal after rehydration

193. Which of the following may have an effect on a person's ability to metabolize
      glucose properly?

    A. age   C. both A and B
    B. sex   D. neither A nor B

194. According to the O'Sullivan and Mahan criteria for the diagnosis of gestational
      diabetes, which of the following doses of glucose should be used as a challenge?

    A. 50 gm   C. 100 gm
    B. 75 gm   D. 200 gm

Questions 195-200

Directions. Select and circle the one BEST answer for each of the following statements utilizing the information presented in either the following graph, tracing,
table or laboratory data.

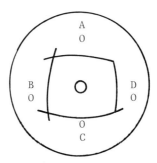

The central reservoir contains antibodies to two dissimilar antigens. One or both antigens are present in each surrounding well.

195.   Wells containing identical antigens are:

A.   A and B   D.   D and A
B.   B and C   E.   B and D
C.   C and D

196.   Wells containing totally dissimilar antigens are:

A.   A and B   C.   D and A
B.   C and D   D.   A and C

197.   Antigens in wells B and D would react like:

A.   A and B   D.   D and A
B.   B and C   E.   C and A
C.   C and D

198.   More than one antigen is contained in:

A.   A   D.   D
B.   B   E.   B and C
C.   C

199.   In order to make the best decision, a laboratory manager should:

A.   consult only with laboratory supervisors
B.   consult only with the bench technologists
C.   consult only with the pathologists
D.   be certain he/she has all the facts

200.   The person responsible for purchasing laboratory reagents:

A.   need not know anything about the laboratory
B.   should know about the laboratory and testing
C.   should try to save money
D.   should buy substitute reagents

Steps To Take After You Finish
The Diagnostic Test

STEP ONE   Work the diagnostic questions as a pretest; do this before you study medical technology topics and skills in this book. TIME yourself according to the suggested four hour limit. If you do not finish in the allotted time, draw a line below the last question you completed. Score your answers using only the Answer Key. Make a conscious effort not to remember correct answers from the key in order to avoid affecting your post test scores.

STEP TWO   Now that you have taken the Diagnostic Test (under actual examination conditions, we hope), count the number of correct answers that you scored on the test. For each incorrect answer, deduct $\frac{1}{4}$ of a correct answer. This will yield your "raw score." What is your percentile ranking (refer to the table)? If your approximate percentile ranking is above 90, you can be reasonably certain that you meet the minimum pass level for most of the medical technology registry or certification examinations. Before the Diagnostic Test was approved for this publication, it was tried out by a generous sampling of students who were about to take the actual test. The results of this sampling provide the basis for this Percentile Ranking Table. Although the Table is not official, it will give you a reasonably good idea of how you would stand with others taking the same test.

STEP THREE   You are urged to use the results of the Diagnostic Test in a scientifically diagnostic manner. Pinpoint the areas in which you show your greatest weakness. Do not be discouraged if you have done poorly on the Diagnostic Test. Now, get to work immediately to eliminate your weaknesses by using the coded answer key and doing the practice questions in the designated areas. Continue your study until you are ready to work the Diagnostic Test again.

STEP FOUR   When you have strengthened the weak areas indicated by the Diagnostic Test take the Test again. Use the post-test answer form and maintain the same time schedule. So that you may simulate a first administration to the best extent possible, do not refer to the pre-test answer sheet or key.

STEP FIVE   Score your answers for the post-test, using the key and compare your scores from the first testing with the second testing. If you have learned from the study experience between the two testings, this should be reflected in considerably higher scores for the second test. You may also want to compare your performance on each question for both times you worked it to see if you were consistent in performance. Question-by-question study and review of the explanatory answers can help you become more familiar with the questions, with how various question types work, and with the kinds of mistakes you tend to make on each type.

Percentile Ranking Tables

(Unofficial)

Approximate Percentile Ranking	Score* On Test	Approximate Percentile Ranking	Score* On Test	Approximate Percentile Ranking	Score On Test	Approximate Percentile Ranking	Score* On Test
99	197–200	79	139–140	59	111–112	39	71–72
98	193–196	78	137–138	58	109–110	38	69–70
97	189–192	77	135–136	57	107–108	37	67–68
96	185–188	76	133–134	56	105–106	36	65–66
95	181–184	75	131–132	55	103–104	35	63–64
94	177–180	74	129–130	54	101–102	34	61–62
93	173–176	73	127–128	53	99–100	33	59–60
92	169–172	72	125–126	52	97–98	32	57–58
91	165–168	71	124	51	95–96	31	55–56
90	161–164	70	123	50	93–94	30	53–54
89	159–160	69	122	49	91–92	29	51–52
88	157–158	68	121	48	89–90	28	49–50
87	155–156	67	120	47	87–88	27	47–48
86	153–154	66	119	46	85–86	26	45–46
85	151–152	65	118	45	83–84	25	43–44
84	149–150	64	117	44	81–82	24	41–42
83	147–148	63	116	43	79–80	23	39–40
82	145–146	62	115	42	77–78	22	37–38
81	143–144	61	114	41	75–76	21	35–36
80	141–142	60	113	40	73–74	0–20	0–34

*After ¼ of a correct answer has been deducted for each incorrect answer.

Diagnostic Test Answer Key

In order to help pinpoint your weaknesses, the specific area of each question is indicated in parentheses after the answers. Refer to textbooks, other study material and the explanatory answers wherever you are incorrect.

SUBJECT AREA CODES

(1) Procedures in Microbiology
(2) Bacteriology
(3) Mycology
(4) Parasitology
(5) Virology
(6) Immunology/Serology
(7) Immunohematology
(8) Hematology
(9) Nuclear Medicine

(10) Clinical Chemistry
(11) Toxicology
(12) Endocrinology
(13) Urinalysis
(14) Body Fluid Analysis
(15) Cytogenetics/Cytology
(16) Quality Control/Laboratory Safety
(17) Laboratory Management

ANSWER KEY

1.	A	(6)	21.	C	(7)	41.	C	(4)
2.	C	(6)	22.	B	(7)	42.	D	(4)
3.	E	(16)	23.	A	(2)	43.	E	(15)
4.	B	(8)	24.	D	(2)	44.	B	(12)
5.	D	(8)	25.	B	(2)	45.	C	(9)
6.	C	(8)	26.	C	(2)	46.	A	(9)
7.	A	(8)	27.	A	(2)	47.	C	(11)
8.	C	(11)	28.	C	(2)	48.	E	(11)
9.	A	(11)	29.	C	(10)	49.	D	(8)
10.	B	(11)	30.	B	(10)	50.	D	(8)
11.	D	(11)	31.	D	(10)	51.	D	(4)
12.	B	(2)	32.	D	(10)	52.	B	(4)
13.	D	(2)	33.	D	(10)	53.	B	(13)
14.	E	(2)	34.	C	(10)	54.	E	(13)
15.	C	(2)	35.	A	(10)	55.	D	(3)
16.	C	(13)	36.	B	(14)	56.	A	(3)
17.	B	(13)	37.	D	(14)	57.	A	(3)
18.	A	(13)	38.	D	(5)	58.	B	(3)
19.	A	(7)	39.	D	(5)	59.	A	(3)
20.	C	(7)	40.	A	(4)	60.	B	(6)

61.	B	(6)	108.	D	(6)	155.	C	(10)
62.	C	(6)	109.	B	(6)	156.	C	(10)
63.	B	(6)	110.	C	(6)	157.	B	(10)
64.	C	(6)	111.	C	(6)	158.	C	(10)
65.	D	(8)	112.	D	(6)	159.	D	(10)
66.	D	(8)	113.	B	(10)	160.	D	(6)
67.	C	(8)	114.	B	(10)	161.	A	(6)
68.	A	(8)	115.	B	(10)	162.	C	(6)
69.	C	(8)	116.	A	(10)	163.	D	(6)
70.	B	(4)	117.	A	(10)	164.	B	(6)
71.	D	(4)	118.	B	(10)	165.	C	(6)
72.	B	(4)	119.	B	(10)	166.	A	(6)
73.	D	(7)	120.	C	(10)	167.	A	(16)
74.	D	(7)	121.	C	(10)	168.	A	(4)
75.	A	(7)	122.	C	(10)	169.	C	(4)
76.	B	(7)	123.	B	(7)	170.	D	(4)
77.	A	(7)	124.	D	(7)	171.	C	(4)
78.	C	(1)	125.	D	(7)	172.	C	(12)
79.	D	(1)	126.	B	(7)	173.	A	(12)
80.	B	(1)	127.	B	(7)	174.	D	(2)
81.	C	(1)	128.	A	(7)	175.	A	(2)
82.	C	(14)	129.	C	(15)	176.	B	(2)
83.	B	(14)	130.	A	(15)	177.	E	(2)
84.	D	(10)	131.	B	(14)	178.	B	(0)
85.	A	(10)	132.	A	(5)	179.	C	(8)
86.	D	(10)	133.	D	(5)	180.	A	(8)
87.	A	(10)	134.	C	(5)	181.	D	(8)
88.	C	(10)	135.	A	(12)	182.	D	(8)
89.	B	(10)	136.	A	(12)	183.	A	(8)
90.	C	(2)	137.	C	(4)	184.	B	(8)
91.	C	(2)	138.	C	(4)	185.	C	(8)
92.	B	(2)	139.	D	(4)	186.	D	(10)
93.	C	(2)	140.	D	(9)	187.	B	(10)
94.	A	(2)	141.	C	(9)	188.	D	(10)
95.	E	(2)	142.	C	(8)	189.	B	(10)
96.	D	(2)	143.	E	(8)	190.	D	(10)
97.	B	(8)	144.	C	(8)	191.	A	(10)
98.	D	(8)	145.	A	(8)	192.	A	(10)
99.	C	(8)	146.	D	(8)	193.	A	(10)
100.	A	(8)	147.	A	(8)	194.	C	(10)
101.	E	(8)	148.	C	(13)	195.	D	(6)
102.	A	(11)	149.	B	(13)	196.	A	(6)
103.	A	(9)	150.	C	(13)	197.	A	(6)
104.	B	(9)	151.	C	(10)	198.	C	(6)
105.	C	(13)	152.	B	(10)	199.	D	(17)
106.	E	(13)	153.	C	(10)	200.	B	(17)
107.	D	(6)	154.	A	(10)			

Explanatory Answers

1. (A) Immunoglobulins are classified by the type of heavy chain present in their structure. IgA has alpha chains, IgD has delta chains, IgE has epsilon chains, IgG has gamma chains and IgM has mu chains.

2. (C) The major histocompatibility complex is a locus on the somatic chromosome number 6.

3. (E) The goals of quality control programs are to assure the precision and accuracy of test results, to check the technical performance of laboratory personnel, to check the performance of laboratory equipment, and to check the performance of reagents.

4. (B) Periodic acid-schiff (PAS) reaction detects the presence of intracellular glycogen.

5. (D) Sudan Black B stains various lipids, such as sterols, phospholipids, and neutral fats.

6. (C) New methylene blue is a supravital stain, meaning it stains cells while they are still living, this is the only method that can be used to stain the RNA remnants found in red cells known as reticulocytes. Brilliant cresyl blue may be used for staining reticulocytes also.

7. (A) Prussian blue stain is used to detect iron in body tissues. Iron will stain positively with Prussian blue.

8. (C) The generic name for LSD is lysergic acid diethylamine.

9. (A) The generic name for PCP is phencyclidine.

10. (B) The generic name for mellaril is thioridizine.

11. (D) The generic name for elavil is amitriptyline.

12. (B) All active transport mechanisms require ATP and thus are energy requiring.

13. (D) GDP is the electron acceptor in substrate level phophorylation, so called because the ATP is produced at the level of the Krebs cycle and not in the ETS.

14. (E) Chloramphenicol is notorious for causing aplastic anemia. For this reason, patients receiving chloramphenicol therapy must have their blood closely monitored.

15. (C) Each passage of NADH through the respiratory chain generates three molecules of ATP.

16. (C) Bence-Jones protein is associated with multiple myeloma. Approximately 50 to 80% of patients having multiple myeloma have a Bence-Jones protein in their urine.

43

17. (B) The Tamm-Horsfall mucoprotein is associated with urinary casts. Tamm-horsfall mucoprotein makes up the matrix of urinary casts.

18. (A) Amylase, a pancreatic enzyme, is normally found in the urine. Since the molecular weight of amylase is similar to that of albumin, it is normally excreted by the kidney in small amounts. Amylase is the only enzyme that is <u>normally</u> found in urine.

19. (A) Anti-Fy^a, anti-E, and anti-Kell are all IgG antibodies.

20. (C) Anti-M is an IgM antibody.

21. (C) Penney Sutter and Matthew are antigens in the Kell blood group.

22. (B) Cartwright is a blood group with three known phenotypes Y+(a+b-), Y+(a+b+), Y+(a-b+).

23. (A) Listeria monocytogenes can cause a fatal meningitis, has a characteristic type of motility due to the presence of bipolar flagella. Exposure to cold enhances the growth of Listeria.

24. (D) Listeria is a gram positive rod not a coccus.

25. (B) The members of the genus Bacillus are aerobic, spore forming bacilli. Woolsorter's disease is another name for anthrax. The causative agent of anthrax belongs to the genus Bacillus.

26. (C) Members of the genus Bacillus are gram positive, therefore, gram negative is not applicable.

27. (A) The rickettsia are intracellular, are spread by insects, and one species causes scrub fever or tsutsugamushi.

28. (C) Chlamydia are responsible for psittacosis or parrot fever and is unrelated to rickettsia.

29. (C) The therapeutic range of salicylate for arthritic patients is 15 - 30 mg/dl. Levels below 15 - 30 mg/dl are not in the therapeutic range, and levels of 40 - 60 mg/dl are considered to be toxic.

30. (B) Salicylates are converted to salicylic acid and the trinder reaction is based on the formation of violet colored complexes formed between the phenol group of the salicylic acid and the ferric ions in the reagent. The mercuric salt is utilized to precipiate the proteins present.

31. (D) Theophylline is the drug used for the therapeutic management of asthma. Phenytoin, primidone and phenobarbital are used for the therapeutic management of seizures.

32. (D) Hepatotoxicity, due to over-dosage of acetaminophen is related to all three of the criteria listed, the dose of the drug ingested, the plasma half-life, and the plasma concentration.

33. (D) The measurement of serum phenytoin is used to assess the adequate control of epileptic patients receiving anti-epiletic therapy. Theophylline is assayed to determine therapeutic management of asthmatic patients, while salicylate and acetaminophen levels are used to assess either arthritic therapy or overdosage.

34. (C) The plasma half-life of phenytoin is approximately 24 hours with a range of 18 - 30 hours.

35. (A) The rate of gastrointestinal absorption of lead is greater in children than in adults.

36. (B) Fructose determinations of seminal fluid are utilized to assess germinal cell activity. Germinal cell activity is associated with androgenic hormones. There is an inverse relationship between fructose

levels and spermatazoa counts. The
higher the fructose level, the lower
the spermatazoa count.

37. (D) The total protein concentration
is higher in exudative effusions than
in transudative effusions.

38. (D) Although adults in the general
population are not usually infected
with hepatitis B, certain persons,
by profession or drug habit, could
be considered risks due to exposure.
Medical technologists and blood banking specialists, working with contaminated blood, are considered risks.
Other hospital staff members, not
exposed to the contaminated blood,
have minimal or no risk at all of
contracting the disease.

39. (D) The highest HBV concentration
would be found in the blood (and
serous fluids) of carriers or individuals suffering with an acute HBV
infection.

40. (A) Piroplasmosis is another name
for babesiosis.

41. (C) In the life cycle of Paragonimus
westermani, the first intermediate
host (a species of snail) produces
cercariae which infect the fresh
water crab.

42. (D) In the life cycle of Paragonimus
westermani, the cercariae that invade
the fresh water crab develop into
metacercariae. When humans ingest
improperly cooked fresh water crabs
which contain metacercariae, the
human then acquires the infection.

43. (E) Nondisjunction occurs when
chromosomes fail to separate properly
during meiosis. Consequently some
cells receive two chromosomes-21 and
Down's syndrome results.

44. (B) The Porter-Silber method produces a yellow pigment when corticosteroids react with phenylhydrazine.

45. (C) Labeled iodine will appear in
stomach acid, saliva and urine;
hydroxyapatite is a calcium phosphate complex and does not bind
iodine.

46. (A) ^{131}I-albumin is used to assay
plasma volume because it is measurable in small quantities, leaves
the blood slowly, and the patient
need not fast at all; beta rays are
not penetrable enough to be used
for scanning.

47. (C) After breath samples, the order
of preference is: capillary samples,
venous samples and arterial samples.
Urine samples are not considered to
be suitable for assay due to the
effects of pooling of the urine.

48. (E) While toxicity due to overdose
is the formost consideration in
cases of abuse of drugs, it must be
of ultimate concern that the patient
may have an allergy to the specific
drug which may lead to anaphylactic
reaction, urticaria and other mani-
festations of allergic reactions.
Anaphylaxis is by far the most
serious and the only life-threatening one listed.

49. (D) The reticulocyte count is
increased because the bone marrow,
if it is functioning properly, is
trying to compensate for the drop
in hgb value. As the red cells are
hemolyzed, the hgb value is
decreased, the hgb that is being
liberated is bound by the haptoglobin
molecule, this increase in binding
accounts for the drop in the detected
level. Bilirubin is a degradation
product of hemoglobin and is
increased because of the breakdown
of the liberated hgb.

50. (D) All of these tests will show
characteristic changes in DIC. The
platelet count will be decreased
because the platelets are being
utilized in clot formation as are
the clotting factors which will
affect both the PT and APTT. There

is also fibrinolysis occurring in the microcirculation which contributes the circulating fibrin degradation products.

51. (D) All of the organisms listed involve the liver during some stage of development in humans. Fasciola hepatica and Opistorchis sinensis are liver flukes. Plasmodium vivax undergoes an exoerythrocytic stage of development in the liver. Echinococcus granulosus frequently causes the formation of hydatid cysts in the liver.

52. (B) Both Taenia saginata and Toxoplasma gondii may be acquired through the ingestion of improperly cooked beef.

53. (B) The Clinitest method of glucose determination is a modification of the Benedict's test and measures the presence of reducing substances. Fructose and ascorbic acid are both reducing substances and therefore would give a positive reaction with this method. Sucrose is not a reducing sugar and therefore would not react with the method. Strong oxidants likewise would not react with the reagent.

54. (E) Oliguria is a term used to describe decreased urinary output. Normal urinary output is 1200 to 1500 mgl, therefore, a 24 hour volume of 600 ml would be considered to be oliguria.

55. (D) Actinomyces isaelii, the causative agent of actinomycosis is not, in fact, a fungus, it is one of several organisms included in the higher bacteria and does not reproduce by the formation of either asexual or sexual sporulation.

56. (A) Candida albicans produces blastospores and chlamydospores, both of which are asexual types of spores.

57. (A) Cladosporium carrionii forms branching chains of conidia, which are asexual spores.

58. (B) Absidia species are members of the class zygomycetes which reproduce through the formation of zygospores which are a type of sexual sporulation.

59. (A) Sporothrix schenkii is a dimorphic fungus which in its yeast phase produces blastospores and in its mold phase produces conidia, both of which are asexual types of spores.

60. (B) The direct antiglobulin test (direct Coomb's test) is utilized for the detection of cell bound IgG molecules.

61. (D) Lymphotoxin is heat labile and is inactivated at 56°C. All of the other choices are stable at 56°C.

62. (C) C5a, a complement fraction, is considered to be the major chemotactic factor. While other substances such as microbial products, polymorphonuclear products and lymphokines also assist in chemotaxis, they are considered to be minor factors.

63. (B) In the typical case of atopic sensitization, the cytotropic IgE is bound to mast cells, which are sometimes referred to as tissue basophils.

64. (C) Heparin, which is released along with histamine, histadine, bradykinnin and other kinnins and slow reacting substance anaphylactic, works as an anticoagulant while the others work as agents to increase vascular permeability, slow contraction of smooth muscle, cause prolonged contraction of smooth muscle and vasodilate.

65. (D) HbS moves faster than HbC but slower than HbA.

66. (D) Schumm's test is used to detect methemalbumin.

67. (C) Only the statement regarding the reading of the hematocrit tubes by omitting the buffy coat is accurate.

68. (A) The smaller the gauge the larger the berul.

69. (C) Erythropoietin is produced in man primarily in the kidney.

70. (B) Schistosoma mansoni is classified as a trematode or fluke. All of the other choices are cestodes.

71. (D) Of the choices offered, Balantidium coli is most likely to be the largest. While trophozoites of Entamoeba histolytica may be as large as 60 microns, trophozoites of Balantidium coli may be as large as 100 microns or more.

72. (B) Pediculus humanus, the human body louse, is an important vector for endemic typhus.

73. (D) Components prepared in an open system have an outdate of 24 hours.

74. (D) Because the person inherits Le and Se, he/she will be a secretor and have Le^a in his/her saliva. Because they are a bombay (hh), he/she will not have the ABO antigens in his/her saliva. Also, because he/she does not inherit H, he/she cannot convert Le^a to Le^b, therefore there will only be Le^a in the saliva.

75. (A) An antibody which reacts at the immediate spin saline phase and not at 37°C will be an IgM antibody. Anti-M is the only IgM antibody listed here.

76. (B) In autoimmune hemolytic anemia the direct antiglobulin test would be positive. This distinguishes this type of anemia from all other types. The Donath-Lansteiner test is used in the diagnosis of paroxysmal cold hemoglobinuria (PCH). The Kleihauer-Betke test is used to enumerate the number of fetal red blood cells present in the maternal circulation after delivery.

77. (A) A delayed transfusion reaction should be suspected and the direct antiglobulin test should be performed and careful observation for a microscopic mixed field reaction. The direct antiglobin test will rapidly become negative as the sensitized transfused red blood cells are cleared by the RE system.

78. (C) Large numbers of epithelial cells, along with varied types of bacteria in a gram stain of "sputum", are consistent with normal oral constituents and are therefore not indicative of what may be or may not be present in the sputum. To culture such specimens is a waste of time and money.

79. (D) Transtracheal aspiration is the best way to collect sputum which is full of contaminating oral flora. In routine practice, however, this is not practical for obvious reasons. Most of the time, satisfactory specimens can be collected if the patient is carefully instructed to produce sputum from deep within the lungs. Bronchoscopic specimens, if carefully collected, are also satisfactory. Rinsing the mouth with antiseptic is not recommended. In decreasing order of suitability the choices are: D,B,C.

80. (B) Urines, which cannot be transported or cultured within a reasonable amount of time, should be refrigerated to prevent alteration of the colony count. Choice A might lead to increased numbers of bacteria, choice C would kill any bacteria. Choice D, although reasonable, is not necessary if there is a refrigerator nearby in which to place the urine.

81. (C) Suprapubic aspiration of urine is an invasive procedure and, for this reason, these specimens assume the same degree of importance as spinal fluids and transtracheal aspirations. Furthermore, any organism isolated from a suprapubic tap is significant, regardless of quantity. In this particular situation, although the accuracy of the colony count would be suspect, the significance of any growth and subsequent course of treatment would remain unchanged. It should be noted, however, on the preliminary and final reports that the colony count is questionable.

82. (C) Actinomycosis produces a purulent exudative effusion into the pleural space.

83. (B) The cerebrospinal fluid glucose concentration is a reflection of the serum glucose concentration, normally being approximately 40 to 60% of the serum glucose levels. In hyperglycemia the serum glucose level would be elevated therefore the cerebrospinal fluid glucose would also be elevated.

84. (D) The conversion of glucose values from mg/dl to SI units is a straightforward calculation as follows:

$$70 \text{ mg/dl} \times \frac{10 \text{ dl}}{1 \text{ liter}} \times \frac{1g}{1000 \text{ mg}} \times \frac{1 \text{ mol}}{180 \text{ g}}$$

$$= 70 \times \frac{1}{100} \times \frac{1}{180} \quad \text{mol/liter}$$

$$= 0.00388 \text{ mol/liter} = 3.88 \text{ mmol/liter}$$

85. (A) In uncompensated metabolic alkalosis, the pH will be increased with no change in the pCO_2. Whereas in a fully compensated metabolic alkalosis, the pH will be normal with an increased pCO_2.

86. (D) None of the responses are correct. In a fully compensated metabolic acidosis, the pH will be normal and there will be a decreased pCO_2.

87. (A) The enzyme aldolase is used to determine muscle disorders and is not affected by liver dysfunction.

88. (C) Pseudocholinesterase is the enzyme measured to determine toxic exposure to organophosphate insecticides.

89. (B) In accordance with the recomendations of the National Diabetes Data Group (NDDG), if an individual has a fasting blood glucose of less than 140 mg/dl, even with an elevated 2 hour post-prandial, the diagnosis of diabetes mellitus cannot be made and therefore, this patient is presumed to have impaired glucose metabolism until otherwise determined through a glucose tolerance test.

90. (C) The so-called "safety pin" appearance on gram stain is characteristic of Yersinia pestis.

91. (C) K. pneumoniae, a normal inhabitant of the human gut, is a non-motile gram negative rod responsible for some acute pneumonias. It utilizes the butylene glycol pathway for the metabolism of glucose and, therefore, is methyl red negative.

92. (B) Beta lactamose production (the basis for resistance to penicillin) is mediated by bacterial plasmids.

93. (C) Teichoic acids comprise the antigenic portions of gram positive organisms.

94. (A) Erythromycin antibiotics exert their effort on the ribosomes of bacteria thereby inhibiting protein synthesis.

95. (E) Oxygen is the terminal electron acceptor in the respiratory chain of bacteria that possess an electron transport system.

96. (D) Pyruvate is the end product of fermentation. It in turn may be converted to acids or alcohols or it

can proceed through the citric acid cycle, of those bacteria having the citric acid cycle.

97. (B) Leukemic reticuloendothliosis, also known as hairy cell leukemia was first described in 1958, it occurs primarily in middle-aged men and is characterized by splenomegaly, pancytopenia and characteristic cells found in the blood, marrow, and spleen.

98. (D) Erytholeukemia, erythremic myelosis, also known as DiGuglielom's syndrome occurs in acute or sometimes chronic form. It is characterized by a white count that can be slightly decreased or moderately elevated, myeloblasts and immature granulocytes, and immature red cells in the peripheral blood.

99. (C) Myelofibrosis, aleukemic myelosis, agnogenic myeloid metaplais are all synonyms for a myeloproliferative disease characterized by an abnormal proliferation of erythroid, myeloid and other hematopoietic precursors, there is also some fibrosis of the bone marrow present and the spleen and liver show some myeloid metaplasia.

100. (A) Alder-Reilly anomaly is inherited as a receissive trait, and is a disease of mucopolysaccaride metabolism. Morphologically it is characterized by larger than normal azurophilic granules, which may be easily confused with granulations due to toxic states.

101. (E) Thalassemia major, Cooley's anemia, homozygous B-thalassemia are all synonyms for a disorder in which there is no normal HgbA formed. The only hemoglobin present is HgbF with variable amounts of HbgA2. Clinically there is severe anemia and other severe complications.

102. (A) The serum creatinine levels should be determined at least every other day to insure adequate kidney function. Additionally, the serum levels of gentamycin both peak and trough levels should be assayed at least twice a week during therapy.

103. (A) Using isotopes with short half-lives decreases the radiation exposure of the patient and decreases interference with subsequent tests. Biological clearance rate is dependent upon the nature of the compound and not the radioactivity; effective half-life is decreased by isotopes with short half-lives.

104. (B) Scintigraphy is used in the detection of tumors and ectopic tissue; hypothyroidism and hyperthyroidism are best detected by measuring serum thyroxine and TSH levels.

105. (C) The dipstick methods for the determination of blood in the urine will react with red blood cells, hemoglobin and myoglobin. Bilirubin will not react with the reagent.

106. (E) Polyuria is a term used to describe increased urinary output. Normal urinary output is 1200 to 1500 ml, therefore, a 24 hour volume of 2500 ml would be considered to be polyuria.

107. (D) Some patients with the cytotropic IgE antibody to Hymenoptra venom have been found to carry the antibody for up to 20 years.

108. (D) All of the drugs listed are capable of causing an autoimmune hemolytic anemia. Penicillin may cause a hemolytic reaction by either of two methods: 1, by acting as a hapten and functioning as an exogenous antigen, and 2, by effecting an innocent bystander mechanism through the transfer of complement. Quinidine may bring about a hemolytic reaction through an innocent bystander-exogenous antigen mechanism. Aldomet (methyldopa) acts differently, in that it acts as an endogenous antigen by creating a surface change in the red cell membrane rendering it recognizable as "non-self" to the immune system.

109. (B) All of the choices listed are considered to be lymphokines. Interferon is a lymphokine that is responsible for the mediation of antiviral activities. MIF (migration inhibitory factor) prevents the migration of phagocytic cells away from the cite of inflammation, MAF (macrophage activating factor) enhances the phagocytic activity of the phagocytic cells in the area of the inflammation and chemotactic factor chemically draws phagocytic cells to the area of inflammation.

110. (C) While IgA does occur in different polymeric forms, has two subclasses and is the principle antibody found in excretions, it does not bind complement.

111. (C) IgE is the immunoglobulin most frequently associated with allergic reactions. IgE is the cytotropic antibody that attaches to the mast cells after a primary challenge with an allergin.

112. (D) While foreigness to the host, complexity of structure and size are requisits for immunogenicity, many immunogens do not contain DNA or RNA.

113. (B) The alpha cells of the pancreas are responsible for the production of glucagon. Ironically, the beta cells of the same organ are responsible for its antagonist, insulin.

114. (B) A serum sample that has an increased amount of triglycerides or chylomicrons may appear to have a creamy layer on top of a turbid layer.

115. (B) In humans, amylase splits starch molecules at their alpha-1,4-glycosidic bonds of the starch chains producing glucose molecules, maltose molecules, and dextrins.

116. (A) During electrophoresis of human proteins, the major groups of proteins migrate, from fastest to slowest, in the following manner: albumin, alpha-globulins, beta-globulins, and gamma-globulins.

117. (A) In an acute myocardial infarction, the LD isoenzyme LD 1 will exceed the concentration of LD 2. Normally, the inverse is true.

118. (B) Hemolysis will have an affect (that of elevating) the total LD value, while it does not affect the CK, CK-MB or LD1/Total LD ratio.

119. (B) If the patient has had an acute myocardial infarction, the total CK is most likely to be elevated, since this enzyme rises the fastest following the damage that results from acute myocardial infarction. The other enzymes listed may ultimately be elevated, but are usually within normal limits on admission.

120. (C) A normal free thyroxin index (FTI) is usually associated with euthyroidism, whereas an elevated FTI is associated with hyperthyroidism, and a decreased FTI is associated with hypothyroidism.

121. (C) The diagnosis of reactive hypoglycemia requires plasma glucose nadirs to be below 50 mg/dl with a corresponding decrease in plasma cortisol levels within 30 to 60 minutes following the nadir of glucose concentration.

122. (C) Decreased levels of serum magnesium are associated with acute pancreatitis, malnutrition, malabsorption and alcoholism, while increased levels are associated with uremia, vitamin-D-intoxication, and treatment of dwarfism with human growth hormone.

123. (B) Fetal hemoglobin (hemoglobin F) is resistant to acid elution, whereas adult hemoglobin (hemoglobin A) is not. When fetal RBC's are exposed to an acid environment, the hemoglobin F will <u>not</u> "leak" out of the red blood cells.

124. (D) The previously identified Fy^a antibody cannot be ignored because if the recipient were reexposed to the Fy^a antigen this could stimulate a rapid secondary antibody-antigen response with resultant decreased survival of the transfused RBC. The units should be screened for the Fy^a antigen and only Fy^a negative units should be transfused.

125. (D) The baby is Rh positive and the maternal anti-D has crossed the placenta and bound to the D antigen sites causing the positive direct Coombs. Because of the high antibody titer, all of the available D antigen binding sites have been utilized, therefore, there is none left for the anti-D antisera. To determine the baby's correct type, a partial heat elution should be performed to remove some of the maternal anti-D. These cells should be used to retype the baby.

126. (B) Galactose is added to the precursor chain to produce B substance. N-acetyl-galactosamine is added to the precusor chain to produce A substance.

127. (B) Dolichos biflorus (A, lectin) will react with only A, antigens. This is useful in identifying subgroups of A which will react with anti-A antisera, but not with A, lectin.

128. (A) Anti-hr' is anti-$\overline{C}$. Units which will be compatible must be $\overline{C}$ negative. A conversion for Weiner to Fisher-Race reveals that the only compatible units would be R^1R^1.

$$R^1R^1 = DC\overline{e}/DC\overline{e}$$
$$R^1R^2 = DC\overline{e}/Dc\overline{E}$$
$$R^1r + DC\overline{e}/dc\overline{e}$$
Rh negative is usually $d\overline{c}\overline{e}/d\overline{c}\overline{e}$

129. (C) Since the disease is rare, the father is most likely heterozygous for Huntington's chorea (Hh). All of the father's children would then have a 50% chance of inheriting the dominant allele.

130. (A) Depending upon which cells are examined, one or two Barr bodies could be found. Some of this person's cells are XX and have one Barr body, but other cells are XXXY and have two Barr bodies.

131. (B) Amniotic fluid creatinine levels of 1.0 or less are indicative of fetal prematurity. Fetal immaturity, therefore, would suggest fetal lung immaturity.

132. (A) Studies have indicated that Reye syndrome seems associated with salicylate usage for the treatment of chickenpox or childhood influenza-like infections. Reye syndrome can be serious and even life threatening. Survivors have been reported to suffer permanent brain damage.

133. (D) An individual is considered immune to rubeola if he/she has either laboratory proof of immunity, diagnosis by a physician, or evidence of vaccination with live rubeola vaccine.

134. (C) The togaviruses are arthropod-borne viruses and are the etiologic agents of yellow fever, dengue fever and eastern and western equine encephalitis.

135. (A) The normal range for plasma levels of growth hormone in males is 0-8 ng/ml, while in females it is 0-30 ng/ml.

136. (A) The normal levels of VMA for infants is less than 83 ug/kg/day. Therefore, the value of 75 ug/kg/day would not be considered abnormal.

137. (E) Only Taenia solium infection would not be acquired by someone on a strict vegetarian diet since humans acquire this infection through the ingestion of improperly cooked pork. Fasciola hepatica and Fasciolopsis buski are acquired through the ingestion of fresh water

vegetation containing the encysted metacercariae. Schistosoma mansoni is not related to dietary habits and the infection is acquired through exposure of the skin to contaminated water.

138. (C) Echinococcus infection is acquired from dogs, while toxoplasmosis may be acquired from the family cat, and Toxocara infections may be acquired from both cats and dogs. Schistosoma infections are acquired by exposing the skin to contaminated water.

139. (D) All of the organisms listed may be acquired through the ingestion of improperly cooked meats.

140. (D) The harmful effects of radiation depend upon the energy, penetrability, ability to ionize and concentration, which in turn depends upon half-life.

141. (C) ^{99m}Tc has a half-life of 6 hours, emits a o.14 Mev gamma, and is easily separated from its parent compound, molybdenum. It does not emit beta particles.

142. (C) It is thought that polycythemia vera is caused by the proliferation of an abnormal stem cell, causing the increase in the associated cell lines, i.e., erythrocytes, platelets, and leukocytes. The increase in leukocytes alkaline phophatase is due to an increase in enzyme activity in the cells.

143. (E) Macroploycytes are most commonly associated with folate and B12 deficiencies. They are giant neutrophils (diameter greater than 16 um.) and they posses 6-14 nuclear lobes. The manner in which these cells are formed is unknown, it has been suggested that one cell division may be skipped during maturation resulting in the hypersegmentation.

144. (C) Patients with certain viral infections, patients that have taken particular drugs, and post-transfusion patients may develop a thrombocytopenia due to antibody formation against the platelets.

145. (A) Neutropenia is an abnormal decrease in the circulating neutrophils. The mechanism of drug induced neutropenia is not known with certainty. Some drugs may suppress granulopoiesis, while other may cause destruction of the cells within the bone marrow, via the immune system. Hyperspleism can result in neutropenia due to increased destruction or sequestration of the cells within the spleen.

146. (D) Thrombocytosis (increase in platelet count) may occur with inflammatory disorders, i.e., rheumatoid arthritis, also in carcinomas. It may also occur as a result of iron deficiency anemia and following splenectomy (no splenic pooling of platelets).

147. (A) Schistocytes and spherocytes will be present on a smear if the patient really has DIC. The red cells are being broken and fragmented while circulating through the fibrin meshwork (clots) that are formed throughout the circulating system in DIC.

148. (C) Tolbutamide, penicillin, Gantrisin, other antibiotics, and para-aminosalicylic acid are all known to cause false positive reactions with the sulfosalicylic acid method of protein determination.

149. (B) Radiographic iodine preparations will cause elevations of the specific gravity when performed with the urinometer or the refractometer. The osmolality is not affected by radiographic dyes. The dipstick method for specific gravity is not affected by these dyes because they are not ionic and therefore do not react with the reagent.

150. (C)   The formation of urinary casts is dependent on meeting three criteria, 1: an acid pH; 2: a high solute concentration; and, 3: the presence of Tamm-horsfall mucoprotein. An alkaline pH will prohibit the formation of casts.

151. (C)   The metallochromic dye, calgamite, is used in the colorimetric determination of serum magnesium. Under alkaline conditions, the calgamite forms pink colored calgamite-magnesium complexes.

152. (B)   The D-xylose tolerance test is used to diagnose malabsorption states, while the tolbutamide tolerance test may be useful in the diagnosis of patients suspected of having adenomas of the pancreatic cells, the fructose tolerance test is used primarily for the detection of heriditary enzyme deficiences, and the galactose tolerance test is used for the detection of heriditary enzyme deficiencies.

153. (C)   The results presented in this question are consistent with those found in iron deficiency anemia. In thalassemia major and hemosiderosis, there would be a marked elevated serum iron with low Total Iron Binding capacity. In nephrosis, there would be a low serum iron with a low UIBC and TIBC.

154. (A)   At room temperature, serum amylase is stable for one month while a Alpha-HBDH is unstable at room temperature. Isocitrate dehydrogenase is stable for 5 hours. Acid phosphatase is stable for 4 hours.

155. (C)   Hexokinase is the enzyme that is NOT used in the glucose oxidase method. All of the other enzymes listed play an important role in the determination of serum glucose concentrations utilizing the glucose oxidase procedure.

156. (C)   The ortho-toluidine method is the least sensitive and least specific of the methods listed. The ortho-toluidine method is based on the principle that aromatic amines, in hot acid solutions, produce colored derivatives. While this procedure was once adequate, the other methods listed are enzymatic procedures which are far more specific and ultimately more sensitive.

157. (B)   The Beckman glucose analyzer utilizes the glucose oxidase method with an electrode that measures the rate of glucose utilization.

158. (C)   The recommended dose for a glucose challenge for the glucose tolerance test as recommended by the NDDG is 75 gms. This is a comprise between the European challenge of 50 gms and the former U.S. challenge of 100 gms.

159. (D)   The dose recommended for the diagnosis of gestational diabetes is 100 gms. This 100 gms is consistent with the recommendations of O'Sullivan and Mahan with respect to the diagnostic criteria for the determination of gestational diabetes.

160. (D)   Waldenstrom's macroglobulinemia is characterized by the production of IgM.

161. (A)   Cl, which is a polymer made up of three subunits Clq, Clr and Cls, is referred to as the recognition unit in the complement cascade.

162. (C)   When immunoglobulins are cleaved with enzymes for study purposes, cleavage of the Fab fragment leaves the entire light chain and the variable and 1st constant domain of the immunoglobulin intact.

163. (D)   The overall structure of the immunoglobulin molecule is maintained by all three of the options listed. Peptide bonds, disulfide bonds, hydrogen bonds and van der Walls forces are all utilized to maintain the primary, secondary, tertiary and quartrinary structure of these proteins.

164. (B)   While Bence-Jones proteins are synthesized independently of the myeloma protein, precipitate at 45 to 60°C and can be measured by the Ouchterlony double diffusion technique, they are nearly always identical to the light chains of the patients disease, NOT the heavy chains.

165. (C)   Atopy is classically defined as the genetic ability to produce specific IgE when naturally exposed to certain materials which are harmless to the rest of the population.

166. (A)   Lymphocytes in general, whether T-lymphocytes or B-lymphocytes, are not phagocytic cells. All of the other choices listed are phagocytic cells.

167. (A)   Analytical reagent grade chemicals are recommended for trace metal analysis because of high level of purity.

168. (A)   When an infected mosquito bites a human, sporozoites travel from the salivary glands of the mosquito into the humans blood. These are rapidly cleared from the blood by the reticuloedothelial cells of the liver where they begin the exoerythrocytic stage of development in humans.

169. (C)   Ascaris lumbricoides is the largest of the nematodes listed, averaging about 25 to 35 cm in length while the other choices rarely exceed 13 mm in length.

170. (D)   Diphyllobothrium latum, the fish tapeworm, requires two intermediate hosts, the first of which is a minute crustacean known as Cyclops, the second being the fresh water fish which ingests the larva bearing Cyclops.

171. (C)   Onchocerca volvulus is the only one of the choices which is capable of developing to adulthood in the human. The other choices are all animal parasites. While these animal parasites may infect humans, the infection is usually accidental and development to the adult stage is not possible since the human is not the definitive host.

172. (C)   Antidiuretic hormone (ADH) is secreted by the posterior pituitary gland. Thyroid stimulating hormone, growth hormone, and adrenocorticotrophic hormone are all secreted by the anterior pituitary gland.

173. (A)   There is a decrease in the excretion of ketogenic steroids in Addison's disease. All of the other conditions listed will characteristically show increases in the ketogenic steroids.

174. (D)   The Quellung reaction forms the basis for identifying encapsulated organisms through the use of antibodies specific to capsular antigens. It has often been used to identify Streptococcus pneumonia, but can be used to identify any organism with a capsule. All that is needed is the specific antibody to that organism's capsule.

175. (A)   The mesosome (a sort of invagination of the cell membrane of bacteria) is thought to be the site of DNA replication in bacteria.

176. (B)   Each passage of FAD through the respiratory chain (ETS) generates two molecules of ATP.

177. (E)   Cytochrome C is the final cytochrome in the ETS before final electron passage to oxygen.

178. (B)   Rouleaux formation is the arrangement of red cells in rolls or stacks.

179. (C)   Agglutination is the aggragation or clumping of red cells.

180. (A)   Neutropenia and agranulocytosis mean the same, a reduction in neutrophilic leukocytes.

181. (D)   Downey cells are an early method of classifying a typical lymphocytes

found in infectious mononucleosis.

182. (D) Auer rods are azurophilic cytoplasmic inclusions which are rod-
shaped. They are found in myeloblast-
sin acute myelogenous leukemia.

183. (A) Plasma cells that can be morphologically identified as "flame" cells
seem to be found most often in IgA
multiple myeloma.

184. (B) Approximately 90% of all patients
with CML have an abnormal chromosome,
the Philadelphia chromosome (Phl), due
to a translocation.

185. (C) Hodgkin's disease is a lymphopro-
liferative disorder that is thought to
represent a proliferation of malignant
cells, called Reed-Sternberg cells.

186. (D) According to the NDDG and subsequent journal articles, the diagnosis
of diabetes mellitus in children and
elderly people can only be made if
the fasting glucose and the two hour
post prandial meet the specific
criteria of: a fasting glucose over
140 mg/dl and a two hour post prandial glucose of 200 or more. The
other examples presented would be
temporarily diagnosed as impaired
glucose metabolism.

187. (B) The diagnosis of diabetes
insipidous would depend, in part,
on the vasopressin assay to determine the kidney's response to
either endogenous or exogenous
vasopressin.

188. (D) The Glycosylated hemoglobin
determination is most useful in the
long term monitoring of diabetic
control. The glycosylation of a
normal hemoglobin fraction is a non-
reversible process which is useful
in establishing the degree of control
over a period of 80 to 120 days.

189. (B) Glycosylated hemoglobin utilizes
the red cells only. Red blood cells
are lysed and the resulting hemoly-
sate is electrophoresed to determine

the percentage of glycosylated
hemoglobin.

190. (D) The sodium nitroprusside is
utilized in the urease method of
BUN determination. It is a catalyst
in the reaction enhancing the formation of the blue indophenol.

191. (A) When utilizing the phosphotungstate method, false high levels of
uric acid may be observed because
of drug interference. To confirm
false high uric acid concentrations,
the uricase method may be used in
addition to the phosphotungstate
method.

192. (A) Since in cases of dehydration,
and other causes of hemoconcentra-
tion, the total protein, and consequently both the serum albumin and
serum globulins rise in the same
proportion, there is no change in
the A/G ratio.

193. (A) An individual's age has a
direct relationship with his/her
ability to metabolize glucose. This
makes the glucose tolerance test
difficult, at best, to interpret.
Sex, on the other hand, has little
to do with an individuals ability
to metabolize glucose, with the
rare exception of the pregnant
woman.

194. (C) The screening test described
by O'Sullivan and Mahan, as well as
the glucose tolerance testing procedure recommended by them, is
based on an oral challenge of 100 gm
of glucose. This differs from the
criteria established by the NDDG
for other glucose tolerance testing
where the recommended glucose
challenge is 75 gm.

195. (D) The fused precipitation band
between A and D is characteristic
of reactions of identity.

196. (A) When antigens are totally
dissimilar, precipitation bands are
independent of one another and
therefore cross.

197. (A) Since A is identical to D, B would react with D exactly as it does with A.

198. (C) The antigen in C is partially identical to both B and D. B and D are not identical. Therefore, C must contain more than one antigen.

199. (D) In order to make the best decision or to resolve a problem, a laboratory manager should try to obtain all the facts in the situation.

200. (B) Laboratory quality begins with reagent quality. The purchasing agent should know how the laboratory functions and should avoid substitute reagents unless these have been proven to be as good and as reliable as those reagents recommended by the vendor.

CHAPTER 3

Procedures in Microbiology

Directions. Select the one BEST answer for each of the following statements. Circle
the appropriate response on the answer sheet.

1. Loeffler's medium is used as a primary isolation medium for:

    A. Streptococcus pyogenes   D. Haemophilus pertussis
    B. Klebsiella pneumoniae   E. Corynebacterium diphtheriae
    C. Mycobacterium tuberculosis

2. The agar content in a blood agar plate may be increased to 5% to inhibit:

    A. the growth of gram positive bacteria
    B. the growth of gram negative bacteria
    C. hemolysis
    D. swarming
    E. pigmentation

3. The first laboratory result which suggests the diagnosis of a rickettsial disease
   is the:

    A. yolk sac culture   D. API test
    B. Dick test   E. Schick test
    C. Weil-Felix reaction

4. The BEST single test for differentiating the pathogenic from non-pathogenic
   staphylococci is:

    A. mannitol fermentation
    B. coagulase slide or tube test
    C. salt tolerance
    D. pigmentation
    E. hemolysis on blood agar

5. Ebullition of gas after hydrogen peroxide has been poured over clones either in an
   agar slant or in a plate indicates a positive:

    A. catalase test   D. indole test
    B. citrate test   E. coagulase test
    C. esculin test

6. Filter paper disks saturated with either antibiotics, chemicals or ointments may be employed to test their inhibitory action upon various microorganisms. The diameter of the zone of inhibition around the disks determines:

   A. the antimicrobial power and diffusibility of the test chemical
   B. the test chemical's ability to denature proteins
   C. the test chemical's ability to inhibit cell wall synthesis
   D. the test chemical's ability to inhibit enzyme action
   E. none of the above

7. Although fungi may be examined macroscopically, both fungi and yeasts may be stained satisfactorily using:

   A. Castaneda
   B. Giemsa
   C. Safranin
   D. methylene blue
   E. lactophenol cotton blue

8. Sabouraud dextrose agar should be used to promote the growth of:

   A. rickettsias
   B. viruses
   C. fungi
   D. bacteria
   E. PPLO's

9. Although rickettsias are gram negative, the gram stain results are frequently unsatisfactory. Better staining results could be obtained using:

   A. an acid fast stain
   B. the Dorner method
   C. the Ziehl-Neelsen method
   D. Giemsa stain
   E. methylene blue

10. The Albert stain is a meta-chromatic granule stain recommended for staining:

    A. Haemophilus influenza
    B. Mycobacterium tuberculosis
    C. Mycobacterium leprae
    D. Corynebacterium diphtheriae
    E. Proteus vulgaris

11. Three common enrichment broths used to enhance the growth of the enterobacteriaceae are:

    A. GN, selenite, and tetrathionate
    B. thioglycollate, trypticase soy, and GN
    C. nutrient, brain heart infusion, and Todd-Hewitt
    D. GN, Loeffler's medium, and tryptophane
    E. GN, tetrathionate, and lactophenol cotton blue medium

12. Autoclave sterilization of laboratory media usually requires the following pressure, temperature and time relationships:

    A. 15 lbs. pressure, 100°C for 15 minutes
    B. 20 lbs. pressure, 110°C for 10 minutes
    C. 15 lbs. pressure, 121°C for 15 minutes
    D. 15 lbs. pressure, 105°C for 15 minutes
    E. 15 lbs. pressure, 115°C for 15 minutes

Questions 13-16

Directions. One, some, or all of the responses for each of the following statements
may be correct. Indicate your response as follows:

A. if items 1 and 3 are correct
B. if items 2 and 4 are correct
C. if three of the items are correct
D. if all of the items are correct
E. if only one of the items is correct

13. The following commercially developed procedures rapidly identify members of the
enterobacteriaceae:

1. API system
2. Enterotube system
3. Pathotec system
4. R/B system
5. MiniTek system

14. The oxidase test may be helpful in identifying:

1. Staphylococci
2. Neisseria
3. Klebsiella
4. Pseudomonas
5. Treponema

15. Bismuth sulfite agar is recommended for the isolation of:

1. Salmonella typhi only
2. Salmonella typhi and other salmonellae
3. Salmonellae and Shigellae
4. Shigella dysenteriae only
5. Shigella dysenteriae and other shigellae

16. Urease test broth may be used to detect urease producing bacteria. Proteus
strains are well known urease producers. However, members of the following genera
may also produce urease:

1. Brucella
2. Mycobacterium
3. Bacillus
4. Salmonella
5. Klebsiella

Questions 17-21

Directions. The following statements contain numbered blanks. For each numbered blank
there is a corresponding set of lettered responses. Select the BEST answer from each
lettered set.

The agent of Legionnaire's disease not only causes a serious respiratory disease but
it is also extremely difficult to isolate. To date, most isolations have been by
__17__. However, __18__ supplemented with other materials serves as a satisfactory
growth medium.

17. A. egg yolk sac
B. horse inoculation
C. Middlebrook 7H10 Agar
D. Castaneda media
E. rhesus monkey inoculation

18. A. blood agar
    B. chocolate blood agar
    C. Mueller-Hinton agar

    D. Middlebrook agar
    E. McBride medium

Hajna medium is a clinical preservative recommended for the transportation, preservation and isolation of members of the __19__ groups. This medium is also recommended for the transportation and preservation of sputa containing members of the __20__ and __21__ .

19. A. Staphylococci and Streptococci
    B. Mycobacterium and Klebsiella
    C. Salmonella and Shigella
    D. Neisseria and Treponema
    E. Corynebacterium and Listeria

20. A. Streptococci
    B. Staphylococci
    C. Bacilli

    D. Haemophilus
    E. Klebsiella

21. A. Mycobacterium
    B. Streptococci
    C. Staphylococci

    D. All of the above
    E. None of the above

Questions 22-30

Directions. Select the one BEST answer for each of the following statements. Circle the appropriate response on the answer sheet.

22. Antigens of meningococci and pneumococci may be rapidly detected in spinal fluid by:

    A. counterimmunoelectrophoresis
    B. Thayer-Martin test
    C. chromatography
    D. spectroscopy
    E. Schlichter test

23. The biochemical basis for differentiating the Salmonellae and Shigellae bacteria from the coliform bacteria is that the coliform bacteria ferment:

    A. glucose
    B. galactose
    C. lactose

    D. sucrose
    E. maltose

24. Aspergillosis is a necrotizing disease of the lungs caused by the fungus Aspergillus. Diagnosis of this disease depends upon the detection of the fungus in the lung tissue and identification of its cultural characteristics. Pus containing the fungus may be observed microscopically in wet mounts having:

    A. 10% potassium hydroxide
    B. 10% sodium chloride
    C. 10% sodium hydroxide

    D. 10% potassium chloride
    E. 10% copper sulfate

25. Rabies occurs in many warm blooded animals. Rabies is usually transmitted to humans via the bite of an infected animal. Clinical diagnosis of rabies in infected animals, such as dogs, is dependent upon the isolation of:

    A. Nissl bodies   D. Herpes virus
    B. Negri bodies   E. a rickettsia
    C. metachromatic granules

26. Reactions on TSI agar: Acid butt
                             Alkaline slant
                             Gas in butt
                             H_2S produced

    These reactions could be produced by:

    A. Salmonella   D. Citrobacter
    B. Proteus   E. All of the above
    C. Edwardsiella

27. Sheep blood is recommended for the isolation of the beta-hemolytic streptococci because sheep blood inhibits the growth of a normal throat commensal which is also beta hemolytic. This throat commensal is:

    A. Staphylococcus aureus
    B. Haemophilus hemolyticus
    C. Corynebacterium diphtheriae
    D. Lactobacillus catenaforme
    E. Bordetella pertussis

28. The Ziehl-Neelsen carbolfuchsin stain is recommended to stain:

    A. Corynebacterium diphtheriae
    B. Mycobacterium tuberculosis
    C. Diplococcus pneumoniae
    D. Klebsiella pneumoniae
    E. Pseudomonas aeruginosa

29. Lactose negative bacteria, such as Salmonella and Shigella, produce small colorless clones on the following agars:

    A. EMB   D. All of the above
    B. XLD   E. None of the above
    C. SS

30. In the Weil-Felix test, the OX19 strain of Proteus is agglutinated by serum of patients suffering with:

    A. typhoid fever   D. scarlet fever
    B. paratyphoid fever   E. rheumatic fever
    C. typhus fever

Questions 31-36

Directions. The column on the left contains 3 scientifically related categories while the column on the right contains 4 items which may illustrate scientific phenomena or processes. Three of the items in the column on the right relate to only one of the categories in the column on the left. FIRST, indicate the category in which the 3 processes or phenomena belong. SECOND, indicate the one process or phenomenon which is not related to that category.

Category

Phenomenon

31. A. Staphylococcus aureus
     B. Streptococcus pyogenes
     C. Escherichia coli

32. A. coagulase positive
     B. salt tolerant
     C. mannitol fermentation
     D. lactose fermentation

33. A. Proteus vulgaris
     B. Escherichia coli
     C. Salmonella typhi

34. A. metallic sheen in EMB
     B. lactose fermentation
     C. "swarmer"
     D. catalase positive

35. A. Clostridia
     B. Staphylococci
     C. Salmonella

36. A. Thioglycollate broth
     B. Brewer jar
     C. Gas pack
     D. Mueller-Hinton broth

Questions 37-54

Directions. Select the one BEST answer for each of the following statements. Circle the appropriate response on the answer sheet.

37. The normal amount of blood in blood agar plates is:

     A. 1.5%
     B. 10%
     C. 5%
     D. 15%
     E. 2%

38. Collection and transportation of specimens is important in anaerobic bacteriology. The best way to collect anaerobic bacteria is by:

     A. swabs
     B. aspiration
     C. tubing
     D. vials

39. Laboratory diagnosis of infectious mononucleosis is dependent upon the detection of heterophile agglutinins in the serum of patients with the disease. To facilitate the diagnosis of infectious mononucleosis, the following technique is used:

     A. slide tests using horse red blood cells
     B. gel electrophoresis
     C. absorption techniques
     D. Weil-Felix reaction
     E. yolk sac culture

40. When plating beta hemolytic streptococci, the blood agar plates should be in-cubated in an environment with a reduced oxygen tension because:

    A. streptolysin O will be inactivated
    B. streptolysin S will be inactivated
    C. both streptolysins S and O will be inactivated
    D. the X factor will be inactivated
    E. the V factor will be inactivated

41. On blood agar, differential disks may be used to differentiate the group A beta hemolytic streptococci from other groups of the beta hemolytic streptococci. This differential disk would contain:

    A. ampicillin   D. penicillin
    B. bacitracin   E. streptomycin
    C. chloramphenicol

42. The best procedure to differentiate Listeria monocytogenes from Corynebacterium species is:

    A. Giemsa stain   D. motility
    B. Gram stain   E. acid fast stain
    C. oxidase test

43. The gram stain of a sputum specimen reveals gram positive cocci in chains and in pairs. Numerous small alpha hemolytic clones are observed on a sheep blood agar plate. Which of the following tests would assist in determining whether the bacteria are alpha streptococci or pneumococci?

    A. bacitracin sensitivity   D. optochin susceptibility
    B. catalase   E. none of the above
    C. esculin hydrolysis

44. Antimicrobial susceptibility tests of fungi have not been developed to the degree that they have for bacteria. To date, most tests and antimicrobial therapy of mycotic infections is limited to:

    A. amphotericin B   D. polymyxin E
    B. penicillin G   E. vancomycin
    C. polymyxin B

45. The agar most frequently used for sensitivity testing is:

    A. Lowenstein-Jensen   D. Mueller-Hinton
    B. Todd-Hewitt   E. Middlebrook 7H10
    C. Fletcher's semisolid medium

46. For serological identification of the streptococci, the streptococci are grown in:

    A. Thayer-Martin broth   D. Mueller-Hinton broth
    B. Hajna broth   E. Cary and Blair medium
    C. modified Todd-Hewitt broth

47. Fletcher's medium supplemented with 8-10% rabbit serum enhances the growth of:

    A. Clostridia   D. Corynebacteria
    B. Leptospira   E. Mycobacteria
    C. Streptococci

48. An acceptable method of determining the pH of solid media is to check the pH:

    A. on the solid agar in a tube or plate
    B. from an aliquot sample before autoclaving
    C. from an aliquot sample after autoclaving
    D. one day after preparing the media
    E. one week after preparing the media

49. The Dorner method is used to stain:

    A. flagella   D. spores
    B. capsules   E. cell membranes
    C. cell walls

50. Blood was drawn from a patient and a blood count was made. A marked increase in monocytes was observed. From another blood sample drawn from the same patient, the bacteriologist isolated a non-sporeforming, non-encapsulated, gram positive rod which produced small translucent beta hemolytic clones on blood agar and was catalase positive, methyl red positive, indole and hydrogen sulfide negative. The cause of the high monocyte count is most probably:

    A. infectious mononucleosis   D. Listeria murrayi
    B. Listeria grayi   E. All of the above
    C. Listeria monocytogenes

51. Spinal fluids, which cannot be cultured immediately, should not be stored at refrigerator temperature because:

    A. refrigeration favors the growth of psychrophilic organisms
    B. Hemophilus and Neisseria species are adversely affected by cold temperatures
    C. the sensitivity patterns of most microorganisms are permanently changed after exposure to the cold
    D. all of the above

52. Stool specimens left at room temperature for an extended period of time would be unsuitable for the isolation of:

    A. Escherichia coli   C. group D streptococcus
    B. Salmonella species D. Shigella species

53. Of the following methods of collection the least acceptable for the collection of specimens for anaerobic culture is:

    A. gassed out tubes   C. sterile syringe and needle
    B. routine sterile swabs   D. commercial anaerobic transport systems

54. Material received from a vaginal washing upon gram-stain showed the presence of gram positive cocci in small chains. After incubation, there was growth on the blood agar plate but not on EMB. Colonies on the blood agar plate exhibited beta hemolysis and were positive in the CAMP test. These organisms might also be expected to:

    A. be resistant to penicillin
    B. be sensitive to low dose bacitracin
    C. hydrolyze sodium hippurate
    D. grow in 6.5% NaCl

Explanatory Answers

1. (E) Loeffler's medium may be used for primary isolation of Corynebacterium diphtheriae

2. (D) Swarming is generally inhibited by increasing the agar content of the medium to five percent. This is particularly beneficial when plating Proteus species.

3. (C) The Weil-Felix test using Proteus antigens is frequently used in laboratories to diagnose rickettsial diseases. The complement fixation test may also be used for the same diagnostic purpose.

4. (B) Pathogenic staphylococci strains are coagulase positive. Either the coagulase tube or slide test demonstrates "free" coagulase and is therefore the best single test for differentiating the pathogenic and non-pathogenic staphylococci.

5. (A) Gas production by clones covered by hydrogen peroxide indicates a positive catalase test.

6. (A) The diffusibility and antimicrobial power of either an antibiotic, ointment or chemical affects the diameter of the zones of inhibition on agar plates.

7. (E) Lactophenol cotton blue may serve as a stain for fungi and yeast.

8. (C) Sabouraud dextrose agar is a medium of choice for enhancing the growth of fungi.

9. (D) The Giemsa stain or Castaneda methods are highly effective for staining rickettsiae.

10. (D) The Albert stain is a differential stain recommended for staining Corynebacterium diphtheriae.

11. (A) Because of the varied flora in feces, GN, selenite and tetrathionate broths are media of choice used to enhance the growth of the enterobacteriaceae.

12. (C) Generally, autoclave sterilization requires 15 lbs. of steam pressure to attain 121°C. This pressure and temperature are generally maintained for 15 minutes. However, the sterilization time may be extended if large volumes of materials are being sterilized.

13. (D) Each of the designated procedures is a commercial preparation used to identify enterobacteriaceae.

14. (B) Neisseria and Pseudomonas strains produce indophenol oxidase and therefore give a positive oxidase test.

15. (E) Bismuth sulfite agar is recommended for the identification of S. typhi and other salmonellae.

16. (C) Urease activity is observed by

members of the genera Brucella, Mycobacterium and Bacillus. Some Sarcina strains may also exhibit urease activity. However, Proteus is the only member of the enterobacteriaceae to demonstrate urease production.

17. (A) Legionnaire's disease is believed to be caused by a unique short, gram negative bacillus. To date, most isolations have been either by egg yolk sac or guinea pig inoculation.

18. (C) Mueller-Hinton agar, supplemented with L-cysteine hydrochloride and ferric pyrophosphate, serves as an isolation medium.

19. (C) Hajna is a clinical preservative recommended for the transportation and isolation of the Salmonella-Shigella group and other gram negative bacteria.

20. (E) Hajna is a medium which is recommended as a preservative of Klebsiella in sputum samples.

21. (A) Mycobacterium tuberculosis is preserved in sputa specimens during transportation. Hajna is not recommended for either gram positive or spore forming microorganisms.

22. (A) Counterimmunoelectrophoresis (CIE) has provided rapid and specific diagnosis of pneumococci and meningococci antigens in spinal fluid.

23. (C) The coliform bacteria are lactose fermenters while the Salmonellae and Shigellae are not.

24. (A) Cultural characteristics of Aspergillus are easily observed in a wet mount containing 10% potassium hydroxide.

25. (B) Confirmation of rabies in animals is dependent upon the presence of Negri bodies in the brain tissues of infected animals.

26. (E) Members of the genera Salmonella, Proteus, Citrobacter and Edwardsiella could produce acid butts, alkaline slants, gas and H_2S in TSI.

27. (B) Haemophilus hemolyticus is normally found in the upper respiratory tract. Since this bacterium is beta hemolytic, it may be thought to be clones of beta streptococci. However, a gram stain will differentiate the gram positive Streptococci from the gram negative Haemophilus.

28. (B) Mycobacteria do not readily stain by the gram method. However, good results are obtained with the Ziehl-Neelsen carbofuchsin method.

29. (D) Lactose negative Salmonella and Shigella produce colorless clones on all the media listed.

30. (C) OX19 strains of Proteus should be used for the serological diagnosis of typhus fever.

31. (A) Staphylococcus aureus is coagulase positive, salt tolerant and ferments mannitol.

32. (D) Lactose fermentation is the process unrelated to the category.

33. (B) E. coli organisms do produce a metallic sheen on EMB due to lactose fermentation and E. coli is catalase positive.

34. (C) E. coli organisms are not swarmers.

35. (A) Clostridia are anaerobic and grow best in Thioglycollate broth under the anaerobic conditions of a Brewer jar with a gas pack.

36. (D) Mueller-Hinton broth is used primarily for susceptibility testing and is unrelated to this question.

37. (C) Normally, blood agar plates contain 5% blood. This is sufficient to provide luxuriant bacterial growth.

38. (B) Aspiration with a syringe is the best means of collecting anaerobic bacteria. Closing off the end of the needle with a hard stopper basically creates an anaerobic environment. Swabbing should be discouraged. When swabs must be used, the sterilized swabs should be placed in tubes containing oxygen free gas. A gassing cannula would have to be used to inhibit the entrance of air.

39. (A) In recent years slide tests using horse red cells have been devised in order to more easily and quickly diagnose infectious mononucleosis. Horse red blood cells are recommended over sheep red blood cells, since the test using horse red blood cells is more sensitive and just as reliable.

40. (A) Streptolysin O is oxygen labile and will be inactivated unless the blood agar plates are incubated in a reduced oxygen environment.

41. (B) The Group A beta hemolytic streptococci grown on blood agar plates may be inhibited by differential disks containing 0.04 units of bacitracin. The other groups of beta hemolytic streptococci will not be inhibited by bacitracin.

42. (D) Listeria monocytogenes is motile while Corynebacterium species are not.

43. (D) The optochin test is presently the most common test used to differentiate the Streptococcus pneumoniae from other alpha hemolytic streptococci. The pneumococci are optochin susceptible.

44. (A) Amphotericin B is an antibiotic which has been used for fungal susceptibility tests.

45. (D) The Mueller-Hinton agar is used for the determination of antibiotic susceptibility by the disk and agar-dilution method.

46. (C) Todd-Hewitt broth, modified, is the medium used to grow streptococci for serological identification.

47. (B) Fletcher's medium promotes the growth of Leptospira organisms.

48. (C) Aliquot samples of autoclaved media can be used to determine the pH.

49. (D) The Dorner method is employed to stain spores.

50. (C) Listeria monocytogenes does cause a sharp increase in monocytes. It may be involved in bacteremia and therefore be isolated from blood and produce all the biochemical results listed.

51. (B) The most common causes of bacterial meningitis (hemophilus and neisseria) are killed by cold temperatures. Although A is true, it is not a prime consideration when spinal fluids cannot be attended to immediately. Answer C has no basis in fact.

52. (D) Shigella species rapidly die (due to pH changes) if stool specimens are left at room temperature for extended periods (Lennett & Spaulding).

53. (B) Oxygen is very toxic to most anaerobes and for this reason most anaerobes will die if specimens are collected on a swab. All the other methods listed are acceptable for the collection of anaerobic speciments (Konnerman).

54. (C) CAMP positive beta hemolytic streptococci belong to Lancefield group B. Group B streptococci also hydrolyze sodium hippurate.

Bibliography and Recommended Readings

Braude, Abraham I. Microbiology. 1982. W. B. Saunders Company. Philadelphia.

Finegold, Sydney M. and William J. Martin. Diagnostic Microbiology. Sixth Edition.
    1982. The C. V. Mosby Company. St. Louis.

Koneman, Elmer and Stephen Allen, V. R. Dowell, Jr. and Herbert Sommers. Color Atlas
    and Textbook of Microbiology. Second Edition. 1983. J. B. Lippincott Company.
    Philadelphia.

Volk, Wesley A. Essentials of Medical Microbiology. Second Edition. 1982. J. B.
    Lippincott Company. Philadelphia.

CHAPTER 4

Bacteriology

Directions. The column on the left contains 3 scientifically related categories while the column on the right contains 4 items which may illustrate scientific phenomena or processes. Three of the items in the column on the right relate to only one of the categories in the column on the left. FIRST, indicate the category in which the 3 processes or phenomena belong. SECOND, indicate the one process or phenomenon which is not related to that category.

	Category		Phenomenon
1.	A. Treponema B. Neisseria C. Herpes	2.	A. syphilis B. lactose fermentation C. darkfield illumination D. TPI
3.	A. Staphylococcus citreus B. Staphylococcus aureus C. Salmonella typhi	4.	A. coagulase positive B. gram negative C. mannitol fermentation D. hemolytic
5.	A. bacillus B. coccus C. spirochete	6.	A. syphilis B. yaws C. pinta D. shingles
7.	A. diphtheria B. plague C. tuberculosis	8.	A. pseudomembrane B. acid fast C. Loeffler's medium D. Corynebacterium
9.	A. Shigella dysenteriae B. Salmonella typhi C. Vibrio comma	10.	A. El Tor biotype B. 6.8 pH C. 9.6 pH D. "rice stools"
11.	A. Streptococcus B. Staphylococcus C. Proteus	12.	A. Dick test B. Schick test C. erythrogenic toxin D. scarlet fever

Category   Phenomenon

13. A. Streptococcus pyogenes   14. A. beta hemolytic
    B. Streptococcus faecalis   B. mouse virulence test
    C. Streptococcus pneumoniae   C. Neufeld reaction
                                           D. inulin fermentation

15. A. Yersinea   16. A. rat flea
    B. Brucella   B. pneumonic plague
    C. Borrelia   C. waterborne
                                           D. bubonic plague

17. A. Brucella   18. A. X factor
    B. Haemophilus   B. V factor
    C. Yersinia   C. gram positive
                                           D. "satellite" phenomenon

19. A. Corynebacterium   20. A. acid fast
    B. Mycobacterium   B. photochromogens
    C. Clostridium   C. scotochromogens
                                           D. catalase negative

Questions 21-45

Directions. Select the one BEST answer for each of the following statements. Circle
the appropriate response on the answer sheet.

21. Statistics indicate that approximately 15-20% of the population are healthy
    carriers of Neisseria meningococci. What type of specimen would be collected to
    detect these carriers?

    A. cerebrospinal fluid   D. sputum
    B. external nares   E. throat
    C. feces

22. Clostridium perfringens is the causative agent of:

    A. food poisoning   D. shock
    B. gas gangrene   E. trauma
    C. tetanus

23. Which of the following bacteria is non-motile, does not produce H_2S, does not
    utilize citrate as a sole carbon source, ferments mannitol, and produces indole?

    A. Shigella   D. Escherichia
    B. Proteus   E. Edwardsiella
    C. Salmonella

24. The causative agent of Hansen's disease is:

    A. Mycobacterium leprae   D. Brucella suis
    B. Mycobacterium tuberculosis   E. Borrelia buccalis
    C. Vibrio comma

25. An agent responsible for pneumonia which is gram negative, encapsulated and ferments lactose is:

    A. Streptococcus pneumoniae　　D. Staphylococcus
    B. Haemophilus influenzae　　　 E. Streptococcus pyogenes
    C. Klebsiella pneumoniae

26. Serodiagnostic tests have facilitated and accelerated laboratory diagnosis of disease. The antistreptolysin O (ASO) test is frequently used to identify:

    A. Staphylococcus aureus　　　 D. Staphylococcus epidermidis
    B. Streptococcus faecalis　　　 E. Streptococcus pyogenes
    C. Streptococcus pneumoniae

27. Which of the following usually demonstrates the greatest resistance to chemical disinfectants and heat?

    A. Mycobacteria　　　　　　　 D. Corynebacteria
    B. Spirochetes　　　　　　　　 E. Yersinia
    C. Rickettsiae

28. Bacille Calmette Guerin (BCG) is a:

    A. pleomorphic bacterium
    B. spore forming bacterium
    C. normal inhabitant of the digestive tract
    D. mutant form of Bordetella pertussis
    E. vaccine against tuberculosis

29. Clostridium tetanus is the causative agent of tetanus. The symptoms of tetanus are caused by:

    A. endotoxin　　　　　　　　　 D. exotoxin
    B. spore　　　　　　　　　　　 E. endotoxin and exotoxin
    C. capsule

30. A patient has a rash over most of the body. Tests were performed and a positive Schultz-Charlton "blanching reaction" was observed. The patient has:

    A. measles　　　　　　　　　　 D. rheumatic fever
    B. chicken pox　　　　　　　　　E. "shingles"
    C. scarlet fever

31. Salmonella enteritidis and Staphylococcus aureus both may cause:

    A. dysentry　　　　　　　　　　D. respiratory disorders
    B. pneumonia　　　　　　　　　 E. urinary infections
    C. food poisoning

32. When a positive urease test is observed, the test organisms converted urea to:

    A. tryptophan　　　　　　　　　D. nitrates
    B. ammonia　　　　　　　　　　 E. urea
    C. indole

33. A cholera victim is brought into a clinic. The first thing to do for this patient is:

    A. an antigen-antibody titer
    B. a Kirby-Bauer susceptibility test
    C. administer antibiotics
    D. reconstitute the fluid loss
    E. isolate the causative agent

34. The Proteus strain generally sensitive to penicillin is:

    A. Proteus vulgaris   D. Proteus rettgeri
    B. Proteus mirabilis   E. None of the above
    C. Proteus morganii

35. Which Proteus strain does not produce indole?

    A. Proteus vulgaris   D. Proteus rettgeri
    B. Proteus mirabilis   E. Proteus inconstans
    C. Proteus morganii

36. The "rice water stool" is characteristic of patients with:

    A. Salmonella typhi   D. Salmonella paratyphi
    B. Shigella dysenteriae   E. All of the above
    C. Vibrio cholerae

37. The causative agent of boils, carbuncles, styes and impetigo is:

    A. Staphylococcus epidermidis   D. Streptococcus viridans
    B. Staphylococcus aureus   E. Erysipelothrix rhusiopathiae
    C. Streptococcus pyogenes

38. Hyaluronidase is a virulence factor which:

    A. destroys leucocytes
    B. dissolves the substance which cements cells together
    C. inhibits phagocytosis
    D. induces hemolysis
    E. causes vascular clots

39. Streptokinase is an antigenic exotoxin produced by Streptococcus pyogenes which:

    A. dissolves clots and may cause intravascular bleeding
    B. breaks down hyaluronic acid
    C. causes intravascular clotting
    D. breaks down streptolysin O
    E. causes beta hemolysis

40. A person recovered from cholera. The immunity occurring after an attack of cholera is:

    A. permanent
    B. not permanent but having at least a 5 year duration
    C. slight and short lived
    D. at least 3 years in duration
    E. at least 2 years in duration

41. Clostridium botulinum is the cause of botulism. It is not the bacterium itself which causes the disease but rather its:

    A. spore   D. flagella
    B. capsule   E. cell wall
    C. exotoxin

42. A young child has numerous skin ulcers in the head region. Material was collected from the bluish purulent lesion and brought to the laboratory for analysis. A gram negative, motile, non sporeforming, oxidase positive, disinfectant resistant bacillus was believed to be the causative agent. This agent is most likely:

    A. Proteus vulgaris   D. Proteus mirabilis
    B. Pseudomonas aeruginosa   E. Pseudomonas fluorescens
    C. Pseudomonas mallei

43. A patient had a soft chancre of the genitalia. A gram stained smear demonstrated small gram negative rods arranged in tangled chains. Based on this limited information you could conclude that the cause of the chancroid could be:

    A. Treponema pallidum   D. Haemophilus haemolyticus
    B. Haemophilus ducreyi   E. Herpesvirus 2
    C. Neisseria gonorrhea

44. The cell wall of certain bacterial species may be removed by treating these bacterial cells with:

    A. a 10% sodium chloride solution   D. DNase
    B. EDTA   E. lysozyme
    C. a 30% sodium chloride solution

45. Halophilic bacteria are:

    A. "heat-loving" bacteria
    B. "cold-loving" bacteria
    C. bacteria which grow best at moderate temperatures
    D. "salt-loving" bacteria
    E. spore-bearing bacteria

Questions 46-55

Directions. One, some, or all of the responses for each of the following statements may be correct. Indicate your response as follows:

A. if items 1 and 3 are correct
B. if items 2 and 4 are correct
C. if three of the items are correct
D. if all of the items are correct
E. if only one of the items is correct

46. Staphylococcus epidermidis is:

1. catalase negative
2. coagulase negative
3. mannitol positive

4. salt tolerant
5. motile

47. Salmonella typhi is:

1. a gram negative rod
2. usually motile by peritrichous flagellation
3. H_2S positive
4. indole negative
5. a facultative anaerobe

48. Shigella dysenteriae is:

1. a strict aerobe
2. non-motile
3. indole positive

4. H_2S positive
5. catalase positive

49. Proteus vulgaris is:

1. a "swarmer"
2. strict aerobe
3. indole positive

4. lactose fermenter
5. H_2S negative

50. Endotoxin shock is caused by the release of endotoxin by gram negative bacteria. This is a dynamic syndrome which is usually associated with hospitalized patients. Cancer, hepatic cirrhosis, diabetes mellitus, and urinary, intestinal, biliary tract or gynecologic surgery seem to predispose the patients to this syndrome. The organism most frequently involved in endotoxin shock is:

1. Clostridium botulinum
2. Escherichia coli
3. Proteus species

4. Pseudomonas aeruginosa
5. Clostridium perfringens

51. Bacterial phagocytosis by either neutrophils, monocytes or reticuloendothelial cells is enhanced by the presence of opsonins on the surface of bacteria. Opsonins are:

1. foreign antigens
2. RNA particles
3. antibodies

4. neutralizing agents
5. enzymes

52. Streptococcus (Diplococcus) pneumoniae are:

    1. lancet shaped
    2. gram positive
    3. encapsulated
    4. spore forming
    5. motile

53. According to the Lancefield classification, group A streptococci account for more than 90% of the human streptococci infections. Group B streptococci cause:

    1. scarlet fever
    2. endocarditis
    3. mastitis in cows
    4. genital infections in dogs
    5. respiratory infections

54. Gas gangrene is caused by Clostridia. The strains of Clostridia implicated in gas gangrene are:

    1. Clostridium perfringens
    2. Clostridium septicum
    3. Clostridium tetani
    4. Clostridium botulinum
    5. Clostridium novyi

55. The development of gummas throughout various organs of the body is associated with:

    1. gonorrhea
    2. meningitis
    3. syphilis
    4. streptococcus infections
    5. pneumonia

Questions 56-62

Directions. Select and circle the one BEST answer for each of the following statements utilizing the information presented in either the following graph, tracing,
table or laboratory data.

Although typhoid fever is considered primarily an intestinal infection, the typhoid
bacilli do invade the body and may be recovered from either the feces, blood or urine.

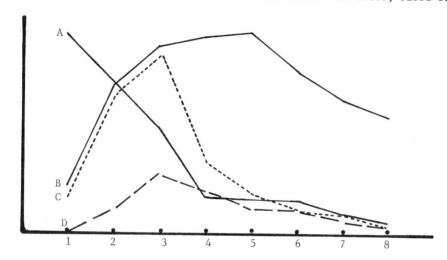

Time of Infection in Weeks

56. Profile A illustrates:

    A. a predominance of typhoid bacilli in the blood
    B. a predominance of typhoid bacilli in the urine
    C. a predominance of typhoid bacilli in the feces
    D. antibody formation

57. Profile B illustrates:

    A. a predominance of typhoid bacilli in the blood
    B. a predominance of typhoid bacilli in the urine
    C. a predominance of typhoid bacilli in the feces
    D. antibody formation·

58. Profile C illustrates:

    A. a predominance of typhoid bacilli in the blood
    B. a predominance of typhoid bacilli in the urine
    C. a predominance of typhoid bacilli in the feces
    D. antibody formation

60. Profile D illustrates:

    A. a predominance of typhoid bacilli in the blood
    B. a predominance of typhoid bacilli in the urine
    C. a predominance of typhoid bacilli in the feces
    D. antibody formation

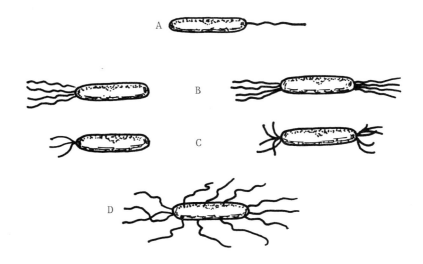

Motility was generally accepted as presumptive evidence that bacteria were flagellated. Today electron microscopy demonstrates different flagellar arrangements and types. This information may be of taxonomic and diagnostic value. If type A flagellation is referred to as monotrichous then:

60. Type B flagellation is referred to as:

    A. peritrichous   C. lophotrichous
    B. multitrichous   D. paratrichous

61. Type C flagellation is referred to as:

    A. peritrichous   C. lophotrichous
    B. multitrichous   D. paratrichous

62. Type D flagellation is referred to as:

    A. peritrichous   C. lophotrichous
    B. multitrichous   D. paratrichous

Questions 63-100

Directions. Select the one BEST answer for each of the following statements. Circle the appropriate response on the answer sheet.

63. A gram negative, non-encapsulated, non-sporeforming rod which produces a green metallic sheen on EMB and is colorless on SS and believed to be the agent responsible for Winkler's disease of the newborn is:

    A. Escherichia coli   D. Enterobacter aerogenes
    B. Escherichia freundi   E. Escherichia intermedia
    C. Enterobacter cloaca

64. Pseudomonas aeruginosa belongs to the order:

    A. Eubacteriales
    B. Pseudomonodales
    C. Actinomycetales
    D. Myxobacterales
    E. Chlamydobacterales

65. Streptococcus pyogenes, Staphylococcus aureus and Proteus vulgaris belong to the order:

    A. Pseudomonodales
    B. Chlamydobacteriales
    C. Eubacteriales
    D. Actinomycetales
    E. Myxobacterales

66. The Salmonella most frequently involved in Salmonella food poisoning is:

    A. Salmonella typhi
    B. Salmonella typhimurium
    C. Salmonella paratyphi
    D. Salmonella gallinarum
    E. Salmonella schottmuelleri

67. Motility is a factor which aids in the identification of the Salmonellae. Which of the following is non-motile?

    A. Salmonella typhi
    B. Salmonella typhimurium
    C. Salmonella enteritidis
    D. Salmonella gallinarum
    E. Salmonella paratyphi

68. If an endotoxic bacterium is a non-encapsulated, flagellated pathogen, it would contain:

    A. only the H antigen
    B. both the H and O antigens
    C. H, O and K antigens
    D. only the K antigen
    E. only the O antigen

69. Capsules are associated with:

    A. resistance to heat
    B. resistance to cold
    C. resistance to salt
    D. virulence
    E. hemolysis

70. Most Clostridia species are:

    A. microaerophilic
    B. obligate aerobes
    C. facultative anaerobes
    D. facultative aerobes
    E. obligate anaerobes

71. Diagnosis of a certain infectious agent was difficult. Cultures from a foul smelling purulent lesion in the nasopharynx produced the following results:

    1. gram negative pleomorphic rods
    2. strictly anaerobic
    3. non-sporeforming
    4. the patient demonstrated the classic symptoms of septicemia but growth was not observed in blood cultures after 48-72 hours of incubation
    5. excessive gas production by the organisms

    Although the diagnosis is not conclusive, which of the following could this agent be?

    A. Clostridium perfringens   D. Haemophilus ducreyi
    B. Bacteroides funduliformis   E. Neisseria gonococci
    C. Clostridium novyi

72. Gonorrhea is one of the most frequently reported communicable diseases. However, not all gonorrhea is contracted by the venereal route. The newborn may be threatened with blindness if untreated. This condition is referred to as:

    A. keratosis   D. bacteremia
    B. gonococcemia   E. septicemia
    C. ophthalmia

73. The etiologic agent responsible for either bubonic, pneumonic or septicemic plague is:

    A. Yersinia pseudotuberculosis   D. Yersinia pestis
    B. Yersinia enterocolitica   E. Pasteurella septica
    C. Pasteurella haemolytica

74. The main vector for the transmission of the plague is the:

    A. mosquito   D. guinea pig
    B. rat flea   E. dog flea
    C. fly

75. Members of this genus are gram negative, motile and rod shaped. A few of the species are chromogenic and produce a red, non-water soluble pigment. Recently some of the members of the genus have been implicated in septicemia, pulmonary and urinary tract infections. One member of this genus could be:

    A. Pseudomonas fluorescens   D. Serratia marcescens
    B. Pseudomonas aeruginosa   E. Staphylococcus citreus
    C. Sarcina lutea

76. The Kauffmann-White antigenic scheme provides a long list of serotypes which aid the serologic identification of:

    A. Shigellae   D. Streptococci
    B. Salmonellae   E. Escherichiae
    C. Staphylococci

77. The O antigens, or somatic antigens in bacteria are heat stable and are located in the:

    A. capsule   D. cell wall
    B. spore   E. nucleoid
    C. cell membrane

78. Haemophilus influenzae and Haemophilus parainfluenzae require a phosphopyridine nucleotide factor to enhance their growth. Staphylococcus aureus strains produce this factor. A spot inoculation of S. aureus on plates previously seeded with Haemophilus enhances the growth of the Haemophilus clones. This relationship is referred to as:

    A. amensalism   D. satellitism
    B. parasitism   E. all of the above
    C. mutualism

79. Streptomycin destroys susceptible bacteria by inhibiting protein synthesis. The site of streptomycin action in the susceptible bacteria is believed to be the:

    A. cell wall   D. nucleoid
    B. ribosomes   E. flagella
    C. cell membrane

80. Penicillin interferes with cell wall synthesis in sensitive bacteria. Generally penicillin is most effective against gram positive bacteria, however this antibiotic has been highly effective against the gram negative:

    A. Escherichia coli   D. Pseudomonas aeruginosa
    B. Salmonella typhi   E. Salmonella enteritidis
    C. Neisseria gonorrhea

81. In a growing culture, which of the cells would be most resistant to disinfectants?

    A. young actively growing cells
    B. cells at the stationary growth phase
    C. all of the cells would be equally susceptible
    D. all of the cells would be equally resistant
    E. older cells

82. Which of the following would be employed to maintain bacteria at a constant population and constant multiplication rate?

    A. lyophilization   D. mineral salt solution
    B. chemostat   E. serial dilution
    C. coulter counter

83. Bacterial conjugation has been studied in several E. coli strains. In bacterial conjugation, each donor bacterium transfers "sex factors" to the recipient bacterium. This "sex factor" is made up of:

    A. DNA only   C. DNA and RNA
    B. RNA only   D. none of the above

84. Most disease causing bacteria and most non-pathogenic bacteria utilize organic carbon as their nutrient source. Based on their organic carbon requirement, these bacteria are referred to as:

    A. autotrophic
    B. chemosynthetic
    C. heterotrophic
    D. pathogenic
    E. chemolithotropic

85. These nonsporeforming, pleomorphic, anaerobic rods are the most numerous bacteria in the human intestine. As many as 10^9 of this bacterium have been found in a gram of feces. Some species are pathogenic and may be implicated in peritonitis, urogenital tract lesions, nasopharynx lesions and rectal abscesses. This bacterium belongs to the genus:

    A. Clostridium
    B. Bacteroides
    C. Salmonella
    D. Proteus
    E. Escherichia

86. The sulfonamides are effective against pathogenic bacteria. Sulfonamide action:

    A. inhibits cell wall synthesis
    B. involves competitive action with folic acid
    C. involves competitive action with para-aminobenzoic acid
    D. involves non-competitive action with para-aminobenzoic acid
    E. inhibits cell wall peptidoglycan synthesis

87. The following antibiotics inhibit bacterial cell wall synthesis:

    A. penicillins
    B. cephalosporins
    C. bacitracin
    D. vancomycin
    E. all of the above

88. Bacitracin is an antibiotic produced by the spore forming bacillus:

    A. Bacillus subtilis
    B. Bacillus cereus
    C. Bacillus lichenformis.
    D. Bacillus megaterium
    E. Bacillus anthracis

89. Bacteria have been implicated in dental caries. Several bacteria are involved but one organism secretes an extracellular dextransucrase which forms a glucan. This glucan adheres to the surface of the tooth and brings bacteria into close contact with tooth enamel. The bacterium in question is:

    A. Streptococcus lactis
    B. Streptococcus mutans
    C. Streptococcus pyogenes
    D. Streptococcus epidermidis
    E. none of the above

90. Staphylococci secrete the enzyme staphylokinase which causes:

    A. clot formation
    B. lysis of clots
    C. destruction of hyaluronic acid
    D. leukocyte destruction
    E. destruction of phagocytes

91. Nonfermentative, gram negative bacilli were isolated from the sputum of patients with cystic fibrosis. These produced blue-green mucoid colonies with a grapelike odor and a zone of hemolysis. This nonfermentative, gram negative bacillus may be suspected to be a member of the genus:

    A. Comamonas
    B. Flavobacterium
    C. Serratia
    D. Pseudomonas
    E. Alcaligenes

92. An enteric gram negative bacillus which is best cultured by isolating in an alkaline peptone water having a pH ranging from about pH 9.0 - 9.6 is:

    A. Shigella dysenteriae
    B. Salmonella typhi
    C. Proteus vulgaris
    D. Vibrio cholerae
    E. Shigella sonnei

93. A halophilic bacterium responsible for gastroenteritis due to the consumption of contaminated <u>seafood</u>:

    A. Staphylococcus epidermidis
    B. Salmonella enteritidis
    C. Salmonella typhimurium
    D. Staphylococcus aureus
    E. Vibrio parahaemolyticus

94. The brucellae are obligate parasites and the causative agents of undulant fever. Isolation and identification of the brucellae are essential for clinical diagnosis. The body material which most frequently provides positive cultural results is:

    A. feces
    B. urine
    C. cerebrospinal fluid
    D. blood
    E. sputum

95. Proteus mirabilis is generally:

    A. monotrichous
    B. multitrichous
    C. lophotrichous
    D. peritrichous
    E. atrichous

96. Friedlander's bacillus is the same as:

    A. Bacillus anthracis
    B. Streptococcus pneumoniae
    C. Klebsiella pneumoniae
    D. Yersinia pestis
    E. Clostridium botulinum

97. Which characteristic is most useful in differentiating between Citrobacter and Salmonella?

    A. lysine decarboxylase
    B. H$_2$S production in TSI slants
    C. indole production
    D. urease production
    E. both B and C of the above

98. A sputum specimen is sent to the laboratory. A gram stain demonstrates many gram positive cocci in chains and in pairs. Numerous small alpha hemolytic clones are observed on the primary sheep blood agar plate. The technician cannot decide whether these are clones of alpha streptococci or pneumococci. Which of the following tests would provide identification?

A. esculin hydrolysis   C. catalase results
B. optochin susceptibility   D. bacitracin susceptibility

99. The reason that a person can have a "strep" throat and not get scarlet fever is:

A. the person is resistant to Streptococcus pyogenes
B. the person is immune to the erythrogenic toxin but not Streptococcus pyogenes
C. the person is immune to the erythrogenic toxin and resistant to Streptococcus pyogenes
D. the person is not susceptible to the Schultz-Charlton reaction

100. Most of the beta hemolytic streptococci responsible for infections in humans belong to Lancefield's group:

A. A   D. D
B. B   E. all of the above
C. C

Questions 101-121

Directions. For each of the numbered items select the appropriate lettered response. Do not use the same letter more than once.

101. scarlet fever   A. Group A streptococci
102. whooping cough   B. Staphylococcus aureus
103. plague   C. Yersinia pestis
                            D. Haemophilus influenzae
                            E. Bordetella pertussis

104. "pink eye"   A. Haemophilus ducreyi
105. chancroid   B. Haemophilus influenzae
106. "pseudomembrane"   C. Treponema pallidum
                            D. Corynebacterium diphtheriae
                            E. Haemophilus aegyptius

107. enteric fever   A. Shigella
108. dysentery   B. Staphylococci
109. rheumatic fever   C. Salmonella
                            D. Vibrio
                            E. Streptococci

110. pinta   A. Treponema vincentii
111. yaws   B. Treponema pallidum
112. trench mouth   C. Treponema carateum
                            D. Borrelia recurrentis
                            E. Treponema pertenue

113. anthrax
114. gas gangrene
115. stillbirths or abortions

A. Listeria
B. Treponema
C. Clostridium
D. Salmonella
E. Bacillus

116. leprosy
117. relapsing fever
118. Vincent's angina

A. Mycobacterium
B. Corynebacterium
C. Bacteroides
D. Yersinia
E. Borrelia

119. puerperal sepsis
120. food poisoning
121. tuberculosis

A. Klebsiella
B. Staphylococci
C. Streptococci
D. E. coli
E. Mycobacterium

Questions 122-137

Directions. Select the one BEST answer for each of the following statements. Circle the appropriate response on the answer sheet.

122. Bacteria in the genus Enterobacter can be differentiated from those in the genus Klebsiella by:

A. gram stain
B. motility

C. lactose fermentation
D. rod shape

123. Citrobacter is a genus of the Enterobacteriaceae which were formerly classified as the:

A. Aerobacter group
B. Providence group
C. Pasteurella group

D. Bethesda-Ballerup group
E. none of the above

124. Members of the genus Proteus are generally noted for their:

A. rapid lactose fermentation
B. rapid growth rate
C. pathogenicity
D. resistance to antibiotics
E. rapid motility which is characterized by "swarming" on agar plates

125. Streptodornase is the general name given to streptococcal enzymes which degrade:

A. intercellular cement
B. DNA
C. RNA

D. coenzymes
E. fibrin

126. The CDC has recommended that standard disk diffusion methods and quantitative dilution test methods be changed for Neisseria gonorrhoeae and Haemophilus species because these are:

    A. fastidious
    B. non-fastidious
    C. obligate aerobes
    D. microaerophilic

127. Bacteria which form colorless colonies on EMB, MacDonkey, XLD, and SS agars do so because they are:

    A. lactose negative
    B. lactose positive
    C. sucrose negative
    D. galactose negative

128. TSI agar contains:

    A. lactose
    B. sucrose
    C. glucose
    D. all of the above

129. The dye in TSI indicative of carbohydrate fermentation is:

    A. methyl red
    B. safranin
    C. phenol red
    D. methylene blue

130. Acid-fast bacilli produce the enzyme:

    A. coagulase
    B. oxidase
    C. dihydrolase
    D. catalase

131. A gram negative rod has produced an alkaline slant and an acid butt on TSI. Which of the following fermented?

    A. lactose
    B. sucrose
    C. glucose
    D. glucose and sucrose
    E. maltose

132. Neisseria gonococci and Neisseria meningococci have the ability to oxidize:

    A. urea
    B. para-amino-benzoic acid
    C. benzidine dihydrochloride
    D. tetramethyl-p-phenylenediamene dihydrochloride

133. Certain bacteria produce the enzyme tryptophanase which breaks down the amino acid tryptophan. With Kovac's reagent this would produce:

    A. a positive oxidase test
    B. a positive urease test
    C. a positive esculin test
    D. a positive citrate test
    E. a positive indole test

134. Bordet-Gengou cough plates are used to isolate:

    A. Bordetella pertussis
    B. Mycobacterium tuberculosis
    C. Streptococcus pneumoniae
    D. Klebsiella pneumoniae

135. The TPI, VDRL, Kahn, and Eagle tests are used to provide presumptive identification of:

    A. N. gonorrhoeae   C. H. Ducreyi
    B. T. pallidum   D. H. influenza

136. Cultures of bacteria and fungi may be preserved for a year or more when:

    A. the slant is covered with ethanol
    B. the slant is covered with acetone
    C. the slant is covered with mineral oil
    D. the slant is covered with buffered saline

137. Albert's stain is used to identify the causative agent of:

    A. scarlet fever   C. rheumatic fever
    B. diphtheria   D. pneumonia

Questions 138-140

Directions. The following statements contain numbered blanks. For each numbered blank there is a corresponding set of lettered responses. Select the BEST answer for each lettered set.

Most 138 and some staphylococci grow in the presence of 100 ug/ml potassium tellurite and reduce the tellurite to tellurium. The tellurium is the absorb in the cells. The colonies of bacteria which grow on tellurite agar appear 139 to 140 in color.

138.		139.		140.	
A.	Streptococci	A.	greenish	A.	brown
B.	Mycobacteria	B.	bluish	B.	black
C.	Corynebacteria	C.	grayish	C.	purple
D.	Salmonella	D.	pinkish	D.	red
E.	Shigella	E.	transparent	E.	white

Questions 141-145

Directions. For each of the numbered items, select the appropriate lettered response. Do not use the same letter more than once.

141. S. aureus   A. oxygen labile
142. streptolysin S   B. protein synthesis
143. streptolysin O   C. thymidine synthesis
144. chloramphenicol   D. coagulase
145. sulfonamide   E. oxygen stable

Questions 146-150

Directions. For each of the numbered items, select the appropriate lettered response. Do not use the same letter more than once.

146. gonococci   A. syphilis
147. chancre   B. fertility factor
148. F$^+$ cell   C. PMN leukocytes
149. Pseudomonas aeruginosa D. pyocyanin
150. Enterobacteriaceae   E. endotoxin

Questions 151-169

Directions. Select the BEST answer for each of the following statements. Circle the appropriate response on the answer sheet.

151. Pure cultures of S. pneumoniae can be identified by:

A. gram stain only
B. gram stain and hemolysis on blood agar
C. "omni-serum" and capsular swelling
D. gram stain and no hemolysis on blood agar

152. Bacteria, which produce catalase, utilize which of the following as final electron acceptor during electron transport?

A. NAD   D. carbon dioxide
B. FAD   E. oxygen
C. alcohol

153. Ethylhydrocupreine is non-bacteriostatic for most alpha hemolytic streptococci. However, an exception to this case is:

A. S. pneumoniae   C. S. sanguis
B. S. mitis   D. S. mutans

154. The Kinyoun stain can be used to examine:

A. all bacteria   C. acid-fast bacteria
B. aerobic bacteria only D. anaerobic bacteria only

155. Clinically, plasminogen levels are decreased due to patients receiving therapeutic treatment with:

A. streptolysin   C. hormones
B. streptokinase   D. antibiotics

156. Neisseria species are aerobic and demonstrate high activity levels of:

A. oxidase   C. deoxyribonuclease
B. tryptophanase   D. trypticase

Questions 157-160

Directions. For each of the numbered items select the appropriate numbered response. Do not use the same letter more than once.

157. Schick test   A. tuberculosis
158. Dick test   B. scarlet fever
159. Kahn test   C. tularemia
160. Vollmer test   D. diphtheria
                           E. syphilis

Questions 161-169

Directions. Select the one BEST answer for each of the following statements. Circle
the appropriate response on the answer sheet.

161. Sheep blood inhibits the growth of:

    A. H. ducreyi   D. S. mitis
    B. S. aureus   E. none of the above
    C. H. influenzae

162. The ONPG (ortho-nitrophenyl-Beta-D-galactopyranoside) test should be used to
      determine:

    A. oxidase
    B. bile solubility
    C. catalase
    D. late lactose fermenters from non lactose fermenters

163. In 1928, Todd discovered that certain streptococci hemolyzed red blood cells.
      Streptolysin S and O were later found to be the hemolysins responsible.
      However, streptolysin O is oxygen labile and its hemolytic action may be
      inhibited by:

    A. proteins   D. cholesterol
    B. 5% agar   E. starch
    C. carbohydrates

164. Which of the following should be maintained as a stock culture to check for
      encapsulated unknowns?

    A. E. coli   D. all of the above
    B. S. pyogenes   E. B and C only
    C. K. pneumoniae

165. Rapid freeze-drying of bacteria is called:

    A. precipitation   D. sterilization
    B. agglutination   E. lyophilization
    C. coagulation

166. Certain members of the genera Bacillus and Clostridium are similar in that
      both are:

    A. gram negative   D. fastidious
    B. encapsulated   E. anaerobic
    C. spore formers

167. An acid-fast bacillus is isolated which produces an orange pigment when grown
      either in the presence of light or in darkness. This bacillus could be
      referred to as:

    A. photochromogen   D. scotochromogen
    B. M. tuberculosis   E. microaerophilic
    C. BCG

168. Drying kills many bacteria. Some, however, will live in dried material for months. Which of the following has been found to live in dried sputum for weeks and even months?

    A. N. gonococci
    B. M. tuberculosis
    C. S. pyogenes
    D. N. meningococci
    E. S. aureus

169. Flavescens, sicca, subflava belong to the genus:

    A. Neisseria
    B. Haemophilus
    C. Pseudomonas
    D. Streptococcus

Questions 170-174

Directions. For each of the numbered items, select the appropriate lettered response. Do not use the same letter more than once.

170. gram negative rod which is longer and narrower than Enterobacteriaceae; oxidizes glucose; cytochrome oxidase produced; acctamide utilized; pigment produced

171. gram positive, lancet shaped cocci in pairs; alpha hemolytic; most strains encapsulated; bile soluble; optochin sensitive

    A. S. agalactiae

    B. Haemophilus species

    C. Ps. aeruginosa

172. gram positive coccus; beta hemolytic but some strains non-hemolytic; narrow zones of hemolysis; positive CAMP test

    D. S. pneumoniae

    E. Campylobacter jejuni

173. pleomorphic cells with bipolar staining; hemolysis variable; needs X and V factors for growth

174. comma or corkscrew shaped gram negative bacillus; cytochrome oxidase produced; naladixic sensitive

Questions 175-179

Directions. One, some or all of the responses for each of the following statements may be correct. Indicate your response as follows:

A. if items 1 and 3 are correct
B. if items 2 and 4 are correct
C. if 3 of the items are correct
D. if all of the items are correct
E. if only one of the items is correct

175. Systems used to rapidly identify the Enterobacteriaceae are:

   1. Abbott MS-2   3. R/B tube system
   2. API 20E   4. N/F system

176. The "Omni-serum" is used to determine the presence of:

   1. spores   4. F^+ factor
   2. capsules   5. fimbrae
   3. cell walls

177. The following species belong to the genus Enterobacter:

   1. aerogenes   4. sonnei
   2. cloacae   5. alvei
   3. agglomerans

178. The following may be implicated in acute bronchitis:

   1. S. pneumoniae   4. H. influenzae
   2. S. pyogenes   5. B. pertussis
   3. S. aureus

179. Pleuropulmonary anaerobic bacterial infections:

   1. never occur
   2. are non-existent
   3. rarely occur
   4. occur frequently enough that a laboratory should be prepared to handle
      these specimens

Questions 180-184

Directions. Select the BEST answer for each of the following statements. Circle the
appropriate response on the answer sheet.

180. Bacteria that grow at temperatures ranging from $10^{\circ}C$ - $20^{\circ}C$ are, by definition,
    classified as:

   A. psychrophilic   C. mesophilic
   B. thermophilic   D. "cold loving" bacteria

181. K antigens seem to interfere with:

   A. antibody production   D. spore formation
   B. phagocytosis   E. F factor
   C. electron transport

182. E. coli K 1 strains are etiologic agents of:

   A. neonatal meningitis   C. "swimmer's ear" infection
   B. diarrhea of the newborn   D. pink eye

183. The natural habitat for Clostridium botulinum is:

    A. canned foods   D. water
    B. pickled fish   E. pork
    C. soil

184. Strains, of which of the following, are serotyped by the Kauffman-White scheme?

    A. Salmonella   D. Staphylococcus
    B. Shigella   E. Streptococcus
    C. Enterobacter

Questions 185-189

Directions. For each of the numbered items, select the appropriate lettered response. Do not use the same letter more than once.

185. Gram positive "drumstick-like" bacillus; strict anaerobe; alpha to beta hemolysis on horse blood agar; grows as a rhizoidal film with a filamentous edge of growth

186. large gram positive thick rod; oval spores which may be centrally or subterminally located; colonies are translucent with a granular surface; colonies are irregular or circular; hemolysis on blood agar

    A. Clostridium sporogenes

    B. Clostridium novyi

187. gram positive rod; not a strict anaerobe but can be microaerophilic; has large distended, oval subterminal spore; colonies are circular and grayish white, narrow zone of hemolysis on horse blood agar

    C. Clostridium tetanus

    D. Clostridium histolyticum

    E. Clostridium botulinum

188. gram positive rod, strict anaerobic; large subterminal spores; irregular or circular semitranslucent colonies; lobulated edges may be seen on the colonies

189. strongly gram positive rod; spores are oval and subterminal; umbonate colonies; colonies are opaque with a grayish white center; colonies may be flat, irregular or circular with rhizoidal edges; no hemolysis

Explanatory Answers

1. (A) Treponema pallidum is the causative agent of syphilis. Dark-field illumination and the treponema pallidum immobilization test (TPI) aid in the identification of T. pallidum.

2. (B) Lactose fermentation is not a biochemical testing result relevant for the identification of Treponema pallidum.

3. (B) Staphylococcus aureus is co-agulase positive, hemolytic on blood agar and ferments mannitol.

4. (B) The related category is not gram negative but rather gram positive.

5. (C) A spirochete causes syphilis, yaws and pinta.

6. (D) Shingles is caused by a virus and is therefore unrelated to the category in question.

7. (A) The causative agent of diphtheria is a member of the genus Corynebacterium. It grows best on Loeffler's medium and it does characteristically produce a pseudo-membrane in the throat.

8. (B) The agent responsible for diphtheria is not acid fast.

9. (C) Vibrio comma is the causative agent of Asiatic cholera which is characterized by the "rice stools," grows best at an alkaline pH (9.6)

and has an El Tor biotype.

10. (B) Vibrio comma organisms do not grow well at a neutral or slightly acidic (6.8) pH. An alkaline environment enhances their growth.

11. (A) A streptococcal infection causes scarlet fever. The erythro-genic toxin is responsible for the scarlatinal rash. The role of the erythrogenic toxin in scarlet fever was established by George and Gladys Dick and is referred to as the Dick test.

12. (B) The Schick test is used to measure a person's susceptibility or immunity to diphtheria.

13. (C) Streptococcus penumoniae or-ganisms ferment inulin and their capsular type may be identified by the Neufeld (quellung) reaction. The white mouse is extremely suscep-tible to these pneumococci and therefore the mouse virulence test may be useful to identify strepto-coccus pneumoniae in mixed cultures.

14. (A) Streptococcus pneumoniae strains are not beta hemolytic.

15. (A) Yersinia pestis is the causa-tive agent of the bubonic, pneumonic and septicemic plague. The rat flea is the main vector for trans-mission of the plague to humans.

16. (C) The plague is not a waterborne infection.

17. (B) Certain members of the genus Haemophilus require the X and V factors for growth and demonstrate "satellitism" when grown on blood agar with strains of Staphylococci, Pneumococci or Neisseriae.

18. (C) Haemophilus species are NOT gram positive but are small gram negative rods.

19. (B) The Mycobacteria are acid fast bacilli which are capable of producing pigmentation either after exposure to light (photochromogens) or remaining in the dark (scotochromogens).

20. (D) The Mycobacteria are catalase positive.

21. (E) A swabbing of the throat would be necessary to determine carriers of N. meningococci.

22. (B) Clostridium perfringens is one of the clostridia responsible for gas gangrene.

23. (D) Members of the genus Escherichia are generally non-motile, fail to produce H_2S, produce indole, do not utilize citrate and ferment mannitol.

24. (A) Hansen's disease is the name frequently used to designate leprosy. Mycobacterium leprae is the causative agent of Hansen's disease.

25. (C) Klebsiella pneumoniae are short, gram negative, encapsulated bacilli which ferment lactose.

26. (E) The ASO test has been advocated to aid in the identification of Streptococcus pyogenes infections.

27. (A) Some of the non-spore forming mycobacteria are more resistant to certain disinfectants and heating than are some of the spore forming pathogens. Mycobacterium tuberculosis is particularly resistant

in dried sputum.

28. (E) BCG is a vaccine of live tubercle bacilli used to immunize against tuberculosis. This immunization process was introduced by Calmette and Guerin in 1925. The virulence of the tubercle bacilli is reduced because the organisms are grown on a medium containing bile. The use of BCG as an immunizing agent is still controversial.

29. (D) The tetanus exotoxin is one of the most potent toxins known. The exotoxin acts upon body nerves and muscles to cause the characteristic tetanus symptoms.

30. (C) The erythrogenic toxin causes the scarlet fever rash. When scarlet fever antitoxin is injected into the skin of a person with scarlet fever, the rash fades or "blanches." This reaction is referred to as the Schultz-Charlton reaction.

31. (C) Salmonella enteritidis and Staphylococcus aureus may cause food poisoning.

32. (B) Urease producing organisms convert urea to ammonia.

33. (D) Due to the excessive fluid loss caused by cholera, it is imperative to replace the fluid loss.

34. (B) Only Proteus mirabilis strains are usually sensitive to penicillin.

35. (B) Proteus mirabilis does not produce indole. All other Proteus strains do.

36. (C) Profuse diarrhea caused by Vibrio cholerae results in the characteristic "rice water stool."

37. (B) Staphylococcus aureus strains may cause boils, carbuncles, styes and impetigo.

38. (B) Hyaluronidase dissolves hyaluronic acid which acts as an

intercellular cement to hold cells together. The breakdown of the intercellular cement permits bacterial penetration into tissues.

39. (A) Streptokinase lyses fibrin and therefore may induce intravascular bleeding.

40. (C) An attack of cholera provides no great protection against a second attack. The immunity occurring after an attack is very brief and the risk of reinfection is only slightly less than that of the initial infection.

41. (C) The Clostridium botulinum exotoxin is believed to be the most deadly. The exotoxin, not the bacterium, causes the disease.

42. (B) Pseudonomas aeruginosa is a human pathogen, which may be a primary invader but more commonly is a secondary invader which may be involved in abscesses, wound infections, skin infections or bronchopneumonia. Pigments, pyocyanin and fluorescein give Ps. aeruginosa its characteristic bluish color on agar or in a pus filled lesion.

43. (B) Haemophilus ducreyi is a gram negative rod which causes chancroid.

44. (E) Lysozyme digests some of the polysaccharides in the cell wall of certain bacteria and inhibits proper cell wall synthesis. The resulting protoplasts are vulnerable to environmental conditions and could lyse if not properly treated.

45. (D) Halophilic bacteria grow best in high salt concentrations and are therefore usually referred to as being "salt-loving" or salt tolerant bacteria.

46. (B) Staphylococcus epidermidis is coagulase negative and salt tolerant. However, contrary to the statement, Staphylococcus epider-

midis is catalase positive, mannitol negative and non-motile.

47. (D) All of the items are correct. Salmonella typhi is a gram negative, facultative anaerobe which is indole negative, H_2S positive and usually motile due to peritrichous flagellation.

48. (B) Shigella dysenteriae is non-motile and H_2S positive. Furthermore, this bacterium is a facultative anaerobe, catalase negative and indole negative.

49. (A) Proteus is not only a swarming bacterium which is indole positive but is also a facultative anaerobe, non-lactose fermenter and H_2S producer.

50. (C) Three of the items are correct. Escherichia coli, Proteus species, and Pseudomonas aeruginosa are frequently involved in endotoxin shock. The Clostridia release exotoxins.

51. (E) Only one of the items is correct. Opsonins are antibodies which cover the surface of bacteria to facilitate phagocytosis.

52. (C) Streptococcus pneumoniae are lancet shaped, gram positive, encapsulated diplococci. However, they are non-spore formers and are non-motile.

53. (E) The group B streptococci are responsible for mastitis in cows.

54. (C) Clostridium perfringens is the most important species associated with gas gangrene, but Clostridium septicum and Clostridium novyi are also involved in gas gangrene.

55. (E) Gummas develop during the tertiary stage of syphilis. The gummas affect any tissue but especially bone, the central nervous system and the cardiovascular system.

56. (A) Profile A illustrates a predominance of tubercle bacilli in the blood.

57. (D) Profile B demonstrates antibody formation against the tubercle bacilli.

58. (C) Profile C illustrates the predominance of tubercle bacilli in feces.

59. (B) Profile D shows the presence of tubercle bacilli in urine.

60. (B) Type B flagellation is multitrichous. Multitrichous flagellation typically consists of more than one flagellum at or near both ends of the bacterium. Furthermore, each flagellum bears more than two curves.

61. (C) Type C flagellation is lophotrichous. This type of flagellation is made up of more than one flagellum at one or both ends of the bacterium and each flagellum has only one or two curves.

62. (A) Type D flagellation is peritrichous. Peritrichous flagellation is characterized by flagella extending from all sides of the cell even perhaps including the ends of the bacterial cell.

63. (A) Escherichia coli is believed responsible for infant diarrhea and it does produce a green metallic sheen on EMB and translucent clones on SS agar.

64. (B) Pseudomonas aeruginosa belongs to the order Pseudomonodales.

65. (C) Streptococcus pyogenes, Staphylococcus aureus and Proteus vulgaris each belong to the order Eubacteriales.

66. (B) Salmonella typhimurium is the most frequent cause of Salmonella food poisoning. Salmonella **enteritidis** has also been implicated with food poisoning.

67. (D) Salmonella gallinarum is a gram negative rod which is usually non-motile.

68. (B) A pathogen which is non-encapsulated will not contain the capsular K antigen, but will contain the somatic O antigen since the bacterium is disease producing, and the flagellar H antigen since it is flagellated.

69. (D) Capsules contribute to the virulence of certain species of bacteria. Many capsules are anti-phagocytic and inhibit or resist ingestion by phagocytes.

70. (E) Most Clostridia species are anaerobic. A few are aerotolerant, but these are the exceptions.

71. (B) The diagnosis of bacteroides infections is sometimes difficult. Strict anaerobic conditions are essential for culture and sufficient growth may not be evidenced for several weeks. Bacteroides funduliformis is the bacteroides species most frequently implicated in disease.

72. (C) If the mother is infected with N. gonorrheae, the newborn may contact gonorrheal ophthalmia which could, if not treated, lead to blindness.

73. (D) Yersinia pestis is the causative agent of the bubonic, pneumonic and septicemic plague. This disease has a high mortality rate in humans.

74. (B) The rat flea is the main vector for the transmission of the plague. Human beings are the accidental hosts of the rat flea.

75. (D) Once thought to be non-pathogenic, Serratia marcescens has recently been implicated in urinary and pulmonary infections as well as septicemia. S. marcescens is a gram negative, motile rod which produces a red non-water soluble pigment at ambient temperature.

76. (B) The Kauffmann-White antigenic scheme facilitates the serologic identification of Salmonella.

77. (D) The heat stable O, or somatic antigen, is located mainly in the bacterial cell wall.

78. (D) Satellitism is a form of commensalism whereby the S. aureus clones produce a factor required for the luxuriant growth of the Haemophilus strains.

79. (B) The main site of action of streptomycin seems to be the ribosomes so that there is an error in the genetic code. Other cellular damage occurs as a result.

80. (C) Although resistant strains have become widespread in recent years, penicillin has been highly effective against Neisseria gonorrhea.

81. (E) Young actively growing cells are most susceptible to disinfectants while older or more mature cells are more resistant.

82. (B) A continuous flow apparatus referred to as a chemostat maintains a constant population and constant multiplication rate. The chemostat is commonly used in bacterial physiology and bacterial genetic studies.

83. (A) The donor cell or male cell, transfers genetic material referred to as "sex factors" to the recipient, or female bacterium. These "sex factors" are made up of DNA.

84. (C) Bacteria which utilize organic carbon for their nutrient requirements are classified as heterotrophic bacteria.

85. (B) Members of the genus Bacteroides are the predominant organisms in the normal human intestinal tract.

86. (C) Sulfonamide action is described as competitive. For bacteria to survive they must synthesize folic acid which is a B vitamin necessary for bacterial growth. Para-aminobenzoic acid (PABA) makes up part of the folic acid molecule. The sulfonamides are structurally similar to PABA and the enzyme which usually incorporates PABA into folic acid mistakenly attaches to PABA and consequently cannot synthesize folic acid.

87. (E) The penicillins, cephalosporins, bacitracin and vancomycin each inhibit cell wall synthesis.

88. (C) Bacillus lichenformis produces bacitracin. Bacitracin is primarily bactericidal against gram positive bacteria but may be effective against gonococci and meningococci.

89. (B) Streptococcus mutans secretes an extracellular dextransucrase which forms a glucan. As the streptococci in the glucan plaques ferment, lactic acid forms and tooth decalcification and decay result.

90. (B) Staphylokinase is an enzyme secreted by staphylococci which lyses clots and may cause intravascular bleeding.

91. (D) Pseudomonas strains are frequently isolated from the sputum of patients with cystic fibrosis. These organisms do produce zones of hemolysis, grapelike odors and blue-green mucoid clones.

92. (D) Vibrio cholerae grow best in an alkaline medium. The alkalinity of the medium also suppresses the growth of other intestinal bacteria.

93. (E) Vibrio parahaemolyticus can cause food poisoning due to the consumption of contaminated seafood. V. parahaemolyticus is halophilic for it grows in a medium containing 7% to 8% NaCl. Although Staphylococcus aureus also causes gastroenteritis and although it too is

halophilic, it is not commonly associated with food poisoning due to the consumption of contaminated seafoods.

94. (D) Blood is the body fluid which most frequently provides positive isolation of the brucellae.

95. (D) Proteus mirabilis is a swarmer and demonstrates peritrichous flagellation.

96. (C) Klebsiella pneumoniae is often referred to as Friedlander's bacillus.

97. (A) Lysine decarboxylase activity facilitates differentiation between Salmonella and Citrobacter. Salmonella demonstrates lysine decarboxylase activity.

98. (B) The optochin test is widely used to differentiate pneumococci from other alpha hemolytic streptococci. Optochin inhibits the growth of pneumococci.

99. (B) A person may be susceptible to Streptococcus pyogenes but resistant or immune to the erythrogenic toxin elicited by that bacterium.

100. (A) The great majority of the beta hemolytic streptococci which infect humans belong to Lancefield's group A.

101. (A) Group A streptococci which produce the erythrogenic toxin cause scarlet fever. The erythrogenic toxin produces the characteristic scarlet fever rash.

102. (E) Whooping cough is an acute infection of the respiratory tract caused by Bordetella pertussis.

103. (C) Yersinia pestis is the etiologic agent of the plague.

104. (E) Haemophilus aegyptius is the bacterium responsible for a common conjunctivitis generally referred to as "pink eye." The infection may be diagnosed as mild or severe and smears or cultures grown on chocolate blood agar will identify the causative agent.

105. (A) Haemophilus ducreyi is the etiologic agent of the venereal disease referred to as chancroid.

106. (D) Corynebacterium diphtheriae strains cause diphtheria which is an acute respiratory infection. Dead tissue cells, red blood cells, host leukocytes and bacteria mass together to form a pseudomembrane in the host's throat.

107. (C) Salmonella typhi causes typhoid fever. Typhoid fever is commonly referred to as enteric fever.

108. (A) Shigella dysenteriae is the etiologic agent of dysentery.

109. (E) Beta hemolytic streptococci may cause rheumatic fever.

110. (C) Treponema carateum is the etiologic agent of pinta, a disease which occurs primarily in Central and South America.

111. (E) Treponema pertenue is the causative agent of yaws, a disease which appears restricted to the tropics. Yaws spreads from person to person either by direct contact with open ulcers or by vectors, such as flies.

112. (A) Treponema vincentii along with Bacteroides melaninogenicus seems implicated in trench mouth--also referred to as Vincent's angina.

113. (E) Anthrax is mainly a disease of cattle, goats and sheep. Humans contract Bacillus anthracis through the skin by contact with the hides of infected animals or by inhaling the spores from contaminated hides.

114. (C) Clostridium perfringens is the agent most frequently responsible for gas gangrene. However, Clostridium novyi, Clostridium septicum and Clostridium histolyticum may also be part of the "gas gangrene group" of bacteria.

115. (A) Listeria infections during pregnancy may result in an abortion or stillbirth.

116. (A) Mycobacterium leprae is the etiologic agent of leprosy.

117. (E) Borrelia species may cause relapsing fever in humans. The body louse and ticks may serve as vectors. Humans contract the infection from the bite of the infected body louse or tick.

118. (C) Bacteroides melaninogenicus and Treponema vincentii have both been implicated with Vincent's angina, also called trench mouth.

119. (C) Beta hemolytic streptococci are responsible for puerperal sepsis, a postpartum infection of the uterus.

120. (B) Many coagulase positive staphylococci produce enterotoxin, which when ingested may cause food poisoning.

121. (E) Mycobacterium tuberculosis is the causative agent of tuberculosis.

122. (B) The bacteria in the genus Enterobacter are motile while the Klebsiellae are not.

123. (D) Members of the genus Citrobacter were formerly known as the Bethesda-Ballerup bacteria.

124. (E) Bacteria in the genus Proteus demonstrate swarming on agar plates due to their rapid motility.

125. (B) Streptodornase enzymes degrade DNA and contribute to the spread of streptococcal infections.

126. (A) Modification of the disk and dilution test methods have been recommended, by the Center for Disease Control, for susceptibility testing of N. gonorrhoeae and Haemophilus species because these bacteria have fastidious nutritional requirements. N. gonorrhoeae should be subcultured on chocolate agar and in a carbon dioxide environment; chocolatized Mueller-Hinton agar is recommended for Haemophilus species.

127. (A) Bacteria which are colorless on EMB, MacConkey, XLD, and SS agars are lactose negative.

128. (D) TSI agar contains lactose, sucrose and glucose.

129. (C) Phenol red is the dye used to designate carbohydrate fermentation in TSI.

130. (D) Acid fast bacilli produce catalase. Catalase may be detected by the breakdown of hydrogen peroxide and subsequent formation of gas bubbles on plates of acid-fast bacteria.

131. (C) An alkaline slant and an acid butt on TSI indicate glucose fermentation.

132. (D) N. gonococci and N. meningococci produce indophenol oxidase and thus oxidize tetramethyl-p-phenylene-diamine dihydroxychloride to yield a positive oxidase test.

133. (E) Kovac's reagent is used to test for indole.

134. (A) Bordetella pertussis is the causative agent of whooping cough. B. pertussis is difficult to grow outside of the body. Pearl-like clones form after 3-4 days of incubation on Bordet-Gengou agar.

135. (B) The TPI (Treponema pallidum immobilization), Kahn, Eagle, and Kline diagnostic tests are used to identify T. pallidum.

136. (C) Bacteria and fungi slants may be preserved for a year or more if the slant is covered with mineral oil.

137. (B) Albert's stain is used to identify Corynebacterium diphtheriae, the causative agent of diphtheria.

138. (C) Most Corynebacteria grow in 100 ug/ml potassium tellurite.

139. (C) The Corynebacteria convert the potassium tellurite to tellurium. Grayish clones can be observed on tellurite agar. The clones may darken as indicated in the next answer.

140. (B) The grayish Corynebacteria clones, on tellurite agar, can range in color from grayish to jet black.

141. (D) Most S. aureus strains are coagulase positive.

142. (E) Streptolysin S is a non-antigenic peptide which is oxygen stable. It is produced by actively growing and resting streptococcal cells. Many A, C and G streptococci produce this hemolysin.

143. (A) Streptolysin O is a protein antigen which is oxygen labile. Most members of group A, C, and G streptococci produce this hemolysin.

144. (B) Chloramphenicol inhibits peptide bond formation so that protein synthesis ceases. This antibiotic binds to the larger moiety of the ribosome.

145. (B) The sulfulonamides are collectively referred to as transcription inhibitors because they inhibit the synthesis of thymidine and the purines. The sulfonamides are structural analogs of PABA and compete with the PABA to interfere in the formation of folic acid, a coenzyme necessary to synthesize thymidine and purines.

146. (C) Gonococci have been found on and within PMN leukocytes shortly after phagocytosis.

147. (A) The chancre is the primary lesion of syphilis.

148. (B) The F^+ cell is a bacterial cell which contains the fertility factor as an extrachromosomal component. The F^+ cell has the ability to donate the factor to the F^- bacterial cell.

149. (D) Pyocyanin is the water and chloroform soluble pigment formed by most Pseudomonas aeruginosa. Pyocyanin usually produces a green or bluish-green color around the clones.

150. (E) All Enterobacteriaceae form endotoxin.

151. (C) Pure cultures of S. pneumoniae can be identified by capsular swelling. "Omni-serum" has been used by some laboratories as a rapid testing procedure to identify the capsular polysaccharides. "Omni-serum" contains capsular antibodies.

152. (E) During electron transport, oxygen is the final electron acceptor for catalase forming bacteria.

153. (A) Ethylhydrocupreine, more commonly known as optochin, inhibits S. pneumoniae. Optochin inhibition by optochin helps in the differentiation of S. pneumoniae from other alpha-hemolytic streptococci.

154. (C) The Kinyoun test is used to examine acid-fast bacteria. Some use this procedure as a modification of the Ziehl-Neelsen technique.

155. (B) Plasminogen is a beta globulin in the euglobulin fraction of plasma. Decreased levels of plasminogen have been reported due to therapeutic treatment with streptokinase.

156. (A) Neisseria species are oxidase producers.

157. (D) The Schick test is a skin test used to determine immunity to diphtheria toxin.

158. (B) The Dick test is a skin test for immunity to scarlet fever toxin.

159. (E) The Kahn test is a flocculation test for reagin, produced during syphilis infection.

160. (A) The Vollmer test is a skin test for tuberculin immunity.

161. (C) Sheep blood inhibits the growth of Haemophilus influenzae; rabbit or horse blood enhances the growth of this bacterium.

162. (D) The ONPG test is used to differentiate late lactose fermenting bacteria from non-lactose fermenters.

163. (D) Streptolysin O is oxygen labile and its action may be inhibited by cholesterol.

164. (C) K. pneumoniae cultures should be maintained to check for suspected encapsulated bacteria.

165. (E) Lyophilization is the process whereby bacteria, or other substances, are rapidly frozen at low temperatures and vacuum dried.

166. (C) Certain members of the genus Bacillus and Clostridium are similar in that they are spore formers.

167. (D) An acid-fast bacillus which, produces an orange pigment when grown in the presence of light or in darkness, is called a scotochromogen.

168. (B) Air drying kills many bacteria, however, M. tuberculosis retains its viability in dry sputum for months.

169. (A) Neisseria is the genus. The bacteria are N. flavescens, N. subflava and N. sicca.

170. (C) Pseudomonas aeruginosa is the gram negative rod that is longer and narrower than the Enterobacteriaceae; oxidizes glucose; produces cytochrome oxidase; utilizes acetamide and produces the pigment pyocyanin.

171. (D) S. pneumoniae is a gram positive lancet shaped coccus found in pairs; is alpha hemoloytic, encapsulated, bile soluble and inhibited by optochin.

172. (A) S. agalactiae is the bacterium described.

173. (B) Species of Haemophilus are pleomorphic in shape and demonstrate bipolar staining. These may or may not hemolyze blood and need X and V growth factors.

174. (E) Campylobacter jejuni is a comma or corkscrew shaped gram negative bacillus that produces cytochrome oxidase and is naladixic sensitive.

175. (C) Three of the systems: Abbott MS-2, API 20E, and R/B are used to identify the Enterobacteriaceae.

176. (E) "Omni-serum" is a reagent which contains antibodies to capsular polysaccharides.

177. (C) Aerogenes, cloacae and agglomerans are the species belonging to the genus Enterobacter. (Laboratory Medicine, vol. 14, no. 6, June, 1983, using API and MS-2 identification)

178. (D) S. pneumoniae, S. pyogenes, S. aureus, H. influenzae, and B. pertussis are pathogens which may cause acute bronchitis.

179. (E) Because there are large numbers of anaerobes in the oropharynx, pleuropulmonary anaerobic infections are not uncommon. Laboratories should be prepared to culture these anaerobes as routine laboratory practices.

180. (C) Bacteria that grow at 10°C - 20°C are called mesophiles.

181. (B) K antigens are polysaccharides that promote pathogenicity by interfering with phagocytosis.

182. (A) E. coli K 1 strains are responsible for a high number of neonatal meningitis cases.

183. (C) The natural habitat of C. botulinum is the soil but these do grow in contaminated foods, under appropriate conditions.

184. (A) Salmonella species are serotyped using the Kauffman-White scheme.

185. (C) The characteristics listed identify Clostridium tetanus.

186. (E) Clostridium botulinum is the bacterium described.

187. (D) Clostridium histolyticum is the bacterium described.

188. (B) The traits listed describe Clostridium novyi.

189. (A) The characteristics presented relate to Clostridium sporogenes.

Bibliography and Recommended Readings

Berquist, Lois. M. Microbiology for the Hospital Environment. 1981. Harper and Row Publishers. New Yor.

Braude, Abraham I. Microbiology. 1982. W. B. Saunders Company. Philadelphia.

Finegold, Sydney M. and William J. Martin. Diagnostic Microbiology. Sixth Edition. 1982. The C. V. Mosby Company. St. Louis.

Freeman, Bob A. Burrow's Textbook of Microbiology. Twenty-First Edition. 1979. W. B. Saunders Company. Philadelphia.

Fuerst, Robert. Microbiology in Health and Disease. Fifteenth Edition. 1983. W. B. Saunders Company. Philadelphia.

Koneman, Elmer, et.al. Color Atlas and Textbook of Microbiology. Second Edition. 1983. J. B. Lippincott Company. Philadelphia.

Raphael, Stanley S. Lynch's Medical Laboratory Technology. Fourth Edition. 1983. W. B. Saunders Company. Philadelphia.

Volk, Wesley A. Essentials of Medical Microbiology. Second Edition. 1982. J. B. Lippincott Company. Philadelphia.

JOURNALS

Laboratory Medicine. January, 1983, Volume 14, Number 1; February, 1983, Volume 14, Number 2; June, 1983, Volume 14, Number 6; July, 1983, Volume 14, Number 7.

CHAPTER 5

Mycology

Directions. Select the one BEST answer for each of the following statements. Circle the appropriate response on the answer sheet.

1. None of the pathogenic fungi are:

   A. aerobic
   B. anaerobic
   C. spore formers
   D. yeast like
   E. heterotrophic

2. The majority of the pathogenic fungi are in the class:

   A. Phycomycetes
   B. Ascomycetes
   C. Basidiomycetes
   D. Deuteromycetes

3. Cryptococcosis is caused by Cryptococcus neoformans and is primarily a disease of the:

   A. urinary system
   B. skin
   C. reproductive system
   D. pulmonary system
   E. circulatory system

4. Cryptococcus neoformans in specimens is best observed by:

   A. acid fast preparation
   B. Giemsa stain
   C. a negative contrast stain
   D. gram stain
   E. lactophenol blue

5. Yeasts may be observed in unstained pus, sputum or exudates using:

   A. methylene blue
   B. lactophenol blue
   C. methanimine silver
   D. safranin red
   E. India ink

6. In the past, central nervous system cryptococcosis was highly fatal. Which of the following has reduced the mortality rate to less than ten percent?

   A. penicillin G
   B. amphotericin B
   C. polymyxin B
   D. ampicillin
   E. streptomycin

7. Of all the pathogenic systemic fungi, which of the following is perhaps the most nutritionally fastidious?

   A. Cryptococcus neoformans
   B. Histoplasma capsulatum
   C. Blastomyces dermatiditis
   D. Paracoccidiodes brasiliensis
   E. Coccidiodes immitis

8. Chancriform lesions of the skin may be characteristically caused by:

   A. Sporothrix schenckii
   B. Candida granuloma
   C. Paracoccidiodes brasiliensis
   D. Allescheria boydii
   E. Candida albicans

9. Griseofulvin is an antibiotic produced by Penicillium griseofulvum and is an active fungistatic agent against:

   A. the systemic fungi
   B. the mycetomas
   C. histoplasmosis
   D. the dermatophytes
   E. cryptococcosis

10. Capsule formation is uncharacteristic of most fungi or yeasts, however it is prominent in:

    A. Penicillium griseofulvum
    B. Cryptococcus neoformans
    C. Trichophyton rubrum
    D. Tinea capitis
    E. Candida albicans

11. Histoplasmosis is a disease of the pulmonary system of fungal origin acquired by inhaling:

    A. mycelia of a fungus
    B. infected animal hair
    C. spores produced by a free living fungus
    D. Cryptococcus spores
    E. Trichophyton spores

12. Data demonstrate that fungal infections are controlled by cellular immune mechanisms. However, which of the following also has been implicated in preventing the spread of many fungal infections?

    A. basophils
    B. eosinophils
    C. monocytes
    D. neutrophils
    E. lymphocytes

13. On Sabouraud Dextrose agar, Sporothrix schenckii forms brownish wrinkled mold colonies. However, on blood agar plates incubated at 37°C the same fungus appears as:

    A. greenish mold colonies
    B. white rough colonies
    C. pink smooth colonies
    D. brownish smooth colonies
    E. creamy yeast colonies

14. The etiologic agent of ringworm is:

    A. Microsporum canis   D. Epidermophyton floccosum
    B. Trichophyton tonsurans   E. Microsporum audouinii
    C. Trichophyton schoenleinii

15. Athlete's foot is most often caused by either Trichophyton mentagrophytes or Epidermophyton floccosum. This superficial mycosis is also commonly referred to as:

    A. Tinea capitis   D. Tinea versicolor
    B. Tinea cruris   E. Tinea pedis
    C. Tinea unguium

16. Maduromycosis is a chronic and commonly deforming disease frequently caused by Allescheria boydii. Diagnosis may be made on the basis of clinical observation and by identifying the causative agent in KOH mounts of pus from lesions. If Allescheria boydii is the infecting agent the pus will contain:

    A. brown granules   D. no granules
    B. yellowish to white granules E. red to brown granules
    C. black granules

17. Chromblastomycosis is worldwide in distribution. Typical itchy cauliflower-like ulcerations occur on the arms or legs of workers exposed to contaminated soil or splinters. Pus smears show black yeast-like cells that occur in tetrads. This dark pigment is also observed in the mycelial colonies grown on Sabouraud dextrose agar. The causative agent is most likely a member of the genus:

    A. Cladosporium   D. Microsporum
    B. Phialophora   E. Allescheria
    C. Candida

18. Fungi can be distinguished from all bacteria except the mycoplasmas in that the plasma membrane of fungi contain:

    A. sterols   D. mannan
    B. dipicolinic acid   E. cellulose
    C. chitin

19. A swab containing pus was inoculated onto Sabouraud dextrose agar plates. After incubation at 37°C for 3 or 4 days, smooth, cream-colored pasty colonies were observed. Microscopic examination revealed oval budding cells and some pseudo-mycelia. Chlamydospore production was later observed on Czapek Dox agar. The infectious agent is most likely a:

    A. Cryptococcus   D. Nocardia
    B. Candida   E. Microsporum
    C. Saccharomyces

20. Candida albicans occurs primarily as an ovoid to spherical budding yeast. Although C. albicans is a dimorphic fungus which has the ability to form true mycelia, it frequently forms pseudomycelia. Consequently, C. albicans has been said to exist in two forms. These are forms:

    A. M and P
    B. M and Y
    C. C and M
    D. C and P
    E. none of the above

21. Fungi may be nutritionally classified as:

    A. autotrophic
    B. chemolithotrophic
    C. photoautotrophic
    D. heterotrophic
    E. photolithotrophic

22. Systemic mycoses may involve any body tissue or organ. When the disease has spread the mycosis is referred to as:

    A. exogenous
    B. extracellular
    C. disseminated
    D. metastasized
    E. endogenous

23. Mycology includes both:

    A. bacteria and fungi
    B. fungi and algae
    C. fungi and yeasts
    D. fungi and viruses

24. A fungus which is believed to multiply in the various cells of the reticulo-endothelial system is involved primarily in a pulmonary infection which resembles tuberculosis. This is a dimorphic fungus which on Sabouraud agar produces conidia bearing hyphae and appears yeast-like on blood agar. Which of the following could this dimorphic fungus be?

    A. Histoplasma capsulatum
    B. Trichophyton mentagrophytes
    C. Aspergillus fumigatus
    D. Microsporum canis
    E. Candida albicans

25. Mothers with vaginal candidiasis can transmit the infection to the newborn. The infectious agent most frequently involved in vaginal candidiasis is:

    A. Candida parapsilosis
    B. Candida tropicalis
    C. Candida pseudotropicalis
    D. Candida albicans
    E. Candida guilliermondi

26. A patient complained of drowsiness, headache, fever and unilateral paralysis. A series of tests revealed an abscess in the brain. X-rays also showed minor pulmonary lesions. Blood samples, plated out on Sabouraud Dextrose agar, demonstrated brown, branching, septate hyphae. The causative agent is most likely:

    A. Candida albicans
    B. Geotrichum candidum
    C. Aspergillus fumigatus
    D. Trichosporon beigelii
    E. Cladosporium bantianum

27. A yeast-like organism was isolated from a sputum specimen. On corn meal agar this yeast-like organism produced mycelia with thick-walled terminal chlamydospores. This organism would most likely be:

    A. Candida tropicalis
    B. Candida albicans
    C. Candida parapsilosis
    D. Candida guilliermondi
    E. all of the above

28. Taxonomically, the fungi are:

    A. procaryotic
    B. eucaryotic
    C. eubacteriales
    D. myxobacterales
    E. beggiatoales

29. Corn meal agar is frequently used to grow fungi to induce:

    A. septate formation
    B. spore formation
    C. mycelia production
    D. cell wall synthesis
    E. all of the above

30. Most Candida infections are associated with the mouth and gastrointestinal tract. However, when Candida invades the tissues, inflammation and the formation of a white pseudomembrane is observed. When this occurs on the lips or in the mouth, the condition is referred to as:

    A. swarming
    B. inflammatory reaction
    C. thrush
    D. foaming
    E. blastospores

31. Dark green fungal colonies were isolated from the sputum of an arrested tubucular patient who had an old unresolved cavity lesion. The fungus is most likely:

    A. Aspergillus fumigatus
    B. Aspergillus niger
    C. Penicillium notatum
    D. Rhizopus oryzae
    E. Mucor corymbifera

32. Thick walled yeast cells bearing single buds attached by a broad base are observed in an aspirated clinical specimen. The etiologic agent could possibly be:

    A. Candida albicans
    B. Cryptococcus neoformans
    C. Geotrichum candidum
    D. Candida parapsilosis
    E. Blastomyces dermatitidis

Questions 33–38

Directions. Identify the following asexual spores produced by medically important fungi.

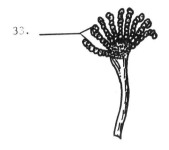

33.

A. spherule
B. arthrospore
C. conidia
D. blastospore
E. chlamydospore

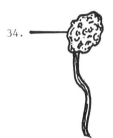

34.

A. spherule
B. arthrospore
C. conidia
D. blastospore
E. chlamydospore

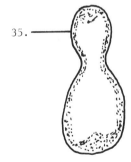

35.

A. conidia
B. arthrospore
C. chlamydospore
D. blastospore
E. spherule

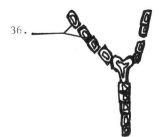

36.

A. conidia
B. arthrospore
C. chlamydospore
D. blastospore
E. spherule

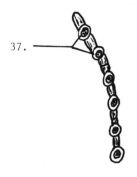

37.

A. conidia
B. arthrospore
C. chlamydospore
D. blastospore
E. spherule

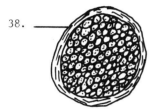

38.

A. conidia
B. arthrospore
C. chlamydospore
D. blastospore
E. spherule

Questions 39-41

Directions. Identify the following fungal components:

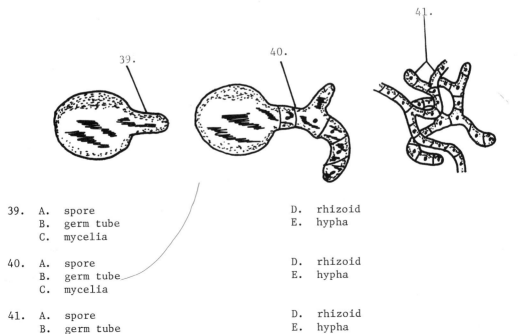

39. A. spore   D. rhizoid
     B. germ tube   E. hypha
     C. mycelia

40. A. spore   D. rhizoid
     B. germ tube   E. hypha
     C. mycelia

41. A. spore   D. rhizoid
     B. germ tube   E. hypha
     C. mycelia

Questions 42-45

Directions. Identify the fungal components specified in the following illustration.

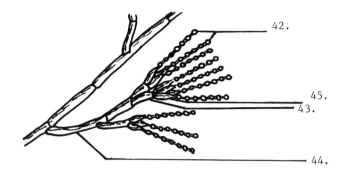

42. A. conidia
    B. conidiophore
    C. sporangium

    D. arthrospores
    E. chlamydospores

43. A. branches
    B. hyphae
    C. metulae

    D. vesicle
    E. sporangium

44. A. sporangium
    B. thallus
    C. conidia

    D. conidiophore
    E. hypha

45. A. hypha
    B. metula
    C. stalk

    D. stem
    E. sterigmata

Questions 46-60

Directions. Select the one BEST answer for each of the following statements. Circle the appropriate response on the answer sheet.

46. Microsporum canis, Microsporum fulvum, and Microsporum audouini each cause:

    A. dark blotches on the palms
    B. lesions in the lungs
    C. ringworm
    D. pneumonia
    E. abscesses in the kidneys

47. Histoplasma capsulatum, Blastomyces dermatitidis, Aspergillus fumigatus and Coccidiodes immitis are the etiologic agents of:

    A. superficial infections
    B. cutaneous infections

    C. systemic infections
    D. subcutaneous infections

48. The pathogenic actinomycetes are included in medical mycology, however, many workers consider the actinomycetes as transitional forms between:

   A. bacteria and algae
   B. blue green algae and bacteria
   C. fungi and yeasts
   D. fungi and algae
   E. bacteria and fungi

49. A disease common among gardeners and referred to as "rose fever" is caused by:

   A. Sporothrix schenckii
   B. Allescheria boydii
   C. Candida albicans
   D. Blastomyces dermatitidis
   E. Paracoccidioides brasiliensis

50. The yeast form of Histoplasma capsulatum is characteristically found in:

   A. kidney cells
   B. liver cells
   C. reticuloendothelial cells
   D. heart cells
   E. the gastrointestinal tract

51. A patient presents with a superficial skin lesion on the palm of his hands that resembles silver nitrate stains. Direct examination reveals dark colored septate hyphae and elongated budding cells. Direct culture on Sabouraud's agar at 30°C produces a young colony which is gray and which turns black within a few days. Which of the following organisms is most likely responsible for this lesion?

   A. Piedra hortae
   B. Cladosporium werneckii
   C. Cryptococcus neoformans
   D. Microsporum canis

52. Busse-Buschke's disease is caused by which of the following organisms?

   A. Cryptococcus neoformans
   B. Coccidioides immitis
   C. Histoplasma capsulatum
   D. Aspergillus fumigatus

53. Which of the following organisms is most frequently associated with the formation of "fungus balls" in bronchi?

   A. Cryptococcus neoformans
   B. Histoplasma capsulatum
   C. Aspergillus niger
   D. Paracoccidioidas brasiliensis

54. Darling's disease is caused by which of the following organisms?

   A. Cryptococcus neoformans
   B. Histoplasma casulatum
   C. Aspergillus niger
   D. Paracoccidioides brasiliensis

55. Gilchrist's disease is caused by which of the following organisms?

   A. Blastomyces dermatitidis
   B. Phialophora verrucosa
   C. Histoplasma capsulatum
   D. Sporothrix schenkii

56. Which of the following dermatophytes would not produce fluorescence when examined with ultraviolet light?

   A. Microsporum audouini
   B. Microsporum canis
   C. Microsporum gypseum
   D. Microsporum distortum

57. Which of the following types of spores is an asexual type of spore?

    A. zygospores   C. ascospores
    B. basidiospores   D. blastospores

58. Which of the following organisms is characterized by the formation of arthrospores?

    A. Cryptococcus neoformans   C. Candida albicans
    B. Geotrichum candidum   D. Aspergillus fumigatus

59. The production of germ tubes (pseudohyphae) is associated with screening for Candida albicans. Which of the following will also produce germ tubes?

    A. Candida stellatoidea   C. Candida parapsilosis
    B. Candida tropicalis   D. Candida krusei

60. Which of the following stains would be most useful in the identification of Histoplasma capsulatum?

    A. gram stain   C. acid-fast stain
    B. Wright's-Giemsa stain   D. methylene blue stain

Questions 61-65

Directions. One, some, or all of the responses for each of the following statements may be correct. Indicate your response as follows:

A. if items 1 and 3 are correct
B. if items 2 and 4 are correct
C. if three of the items are correct
D. if all of the items are correct
E. if only one of the items is correct

61. Which of the following organisms produce pulmonary disease?

    1. Aspergillus fumigatus   3. Cryptococcus neoformans
    2. Nocardia asteroides   4. Histoplasma capsulatum

62. Which of the following organisms are considered to be dimorphic?

    1. Cryptococcus neoformans   3. Candida albicans
    2. Histoplasma capsulatum   4. Blastomyces dermatitidis

63. Which of the following organisms produce an endothrix type of hair infection?

    1. Trichophyton rubrum   3. Trichophyton violaceum
    2. Trichophyton tonsurans   4. Trichophyton schoenleini

64. Which of the following organisms produce dark, olivaceous colonies on Sabouraud's agar?

    1. Phialophora verrucosa   3. Fonsecaea pedrosoi
    2. Trichophyton mentagraphytes 4. Microsporum canis

65. Which of the following media would not be suitable for Crytococcus neoformans?

    1. neopeptone-glucose with chloramphenicol
    2. neopeptone-glucose with cycloheximide
    3. brian-heart infusion agar
    4. blood agar

Questions 66-75

Directions. For each of the numbered words or phrases listed below, select the appropriate response as follows:

A. if the item is associated with A only
B. if the item is associated with B only
C. if the item is associated with both A and B
D. if the item is associated with neither A nor B

              A. skin infections
              B. pulmonary infections

66. Crytococcus neoformans
67. Phialophora verrucosa
68. Candida albicans
69. Sporothrix schenkii
70. Geotrichum candidum

              A. asexual spore production
              B. sexual spore production

71. Actinomyces israelii
72. Candida albicans
73. Cladosporium carrionii
74. Absidia corymbifera
75. Sporothrix schenkii

Explanatory Answers

1. (B) The pathogenic fungi are not anaerobic. All are aerobic and heterotrophic. Some fungi are spore formers, some are yeast-like and some are dimorphic.

2. (D) Most of the pathogenic fungi belong to the class Deuteromycetes.

3. (D) Cryptococcosis is a disease of the respiratory system contracted by the inhalation of the infectious agent. The infection may remain localized in the lungs or spread.

4. (C) The negative contrast stain provides good results in identifying Cryptococcus neoformans in laboratory specimens because of the presence of the wide capsule borne by most clinically significant isolates. The capsule appears as a clear area.

5. (E) India ink mixed with pus, sputum or exudate specimen will demonstrate the capsule around the thick-walled budding yeast cells.

6. (B) Amphotericin B is presently the only effective therapeutic agent for fungal infections and it is highly effective against CNS cryptococcosis.

7. (B) Histoplasma capsulatum is possibly the most fastidious systemic fungus. Although H. capsulatum will grow on Sabouraud Dextrose Agar (SDA), growth is enhanced on Brain-heart

infusion (BHI) blood agar or on a mixture of SDA and BHI.

8. (A) Sporothrix schenckii is a fungus which produces a lesion resembling the chancre of syphilis (the chancriform lesion).

9. (D) Griseofulvin is effective against the dermatophytes.

10. (B) Cryptococcus neoformans occurs in the form of a budding yeast with a polysaccharide capsule.

11. (C) Histoplasmosis is a disease of the pulmonary system contracted by inhaling spores produced by a free living fungus.

12. (D) Clinical and experimental data show that neutrophils play a role in protecting against the spread of fungal infections.

13. (E) On blood agar plates, the usually brownish wrinkled S. schenckii colonies appear as creamy yeast colonies.

14. (A) Ringworm, also referred to as tinea corporis, is most frequently caused either by Microsporum canis or Trichophyton mentagrophytes.

15. (E) The word "tinea" comes from a Latin root meaning "gnawing worm." This is misleading but the term has been employed to identify certain mycoses. Tinea is further classified

by its location on the body--tinea pedis referring to athlete's foot.

16. (B) If Allescheria boydii is the etiologic agent, KOH preparations show wide, swollen hyphae masses and the pus contains yellowish to white granules.

17. (B) Phialophora is one of the etiologic agents of chromoblasto-mycosis and is readily identified in pus by its black yeast-like cells. Cladosporium also causes chromoblastomycosis but it does not form a black pigment.

18. (A) The cytoplasmic membranes of fungi contain sterols. This distinguishes the fungi from all bacteria except the mycoplasmas.

19. (B) Chlamydospores are characteristic of the members of the genus Candida.

20. (B) Candida albicans may exist as either a budding yeast or it forms a pseudomycelium or a true mycelium. Consequently, either of the mycelial forms are referred to as mycelial (M) forms or as budding yeast as (Y) forms.

21. (D) Fungi are nutritionally classified as heterotrophic micro-organisms because they utilize organic carbons as an energy source, form CO_2 and require free oxygen for cell life and functions.

22. (C) The term dissemination is used to designate that a disease caused by a mycotic agent has spread from organ to organ.

23. (C) Mycology includes both the fungi and the yeasts.

24. (A) Histoplasma capsulatum replicates in the various cells of the reticuloendothelial system and does cause a pulmonary infection which may be chronic and resemble tuberculosis. H. capsulatum is also a dimorphic fungus.

25. (D) Several species of Candida have been implicated in disease. However, the most pathogenic and the most frequently involved in vaginal candidiasis is Candida albicans.

26. (E) Cladosporium bantianum is probably acquired by inhalation which leads to pulmonary lesions. The organisms are then carried to the brain via the bloodstream where they characteristically form abscesses. The presence of brown branching septate hyphae on Sabouraud Dextrose agar facilitates diagnosis.

27. (B) Chalmydospores distinguish Candida albicans from other Candida species.

28. (B) Fungi are taxonomically classified as eucaryotes.

29. (B) Many fungi can be identified by their spores. Corn meal is not an optimum growth medium, therefore spore production is enhanced when fungi are grown on this medium.

30. (C) When a white pseudomembrane forms on the lips or in the mouth due to a Candida infection, the condition is referred to as thrush.

31. (A) Aspergillus fumigatus is the predominant causative agent of aspergillosis and is primarily an infection of the respiratory tract. Dark green fungal colonies are observed on Sabouraud Dextrose agar.

32. (E) The thick walled yeast cells observed in the aspirated clinical specimen are possibly Blastomyces dermatitidis.

33. (C) The diagram illustrates conidia on a conidiophore.

34. (E) The structure illustrated is a chlamydospore.

35. (D) The structure illustrated is a blastospore. Blastospores arise from yeast and yeast-like cells.

36.   (B)   The asexual spore illustrated is an arthrospore.

37.   (C)   The fungal structure illustrated is a chlamydospore.

38.   (E)   A spherule is illustrated in the diagram.

39.   (B)   The fungal structure illustrated is the germ tube.

40.   (E)   The fungal component illustrated is a hypha.

41.   (C)   Mycelia are the fungal components illustrated.

42.   (A)   The fungal components illustrated are conidia.

43.   (C)   The metulae are just below the sterigmata and are illustrated in the diagram.

44.   (D)   The structure illustrated is collectively referred to as conidiophore.

45.   (E)   The structure illustrated is the sterigmata.

46.   (C)   Microsporum canis, Microsporum flavum and Microsporum audouini cause ringworm.

47.   (C)   Histoplasma capsulatum causes the disease, histoplasmosis. Blastomyces dermatitidis is the etiologic agent of blastomycosis. Aspergillus fumigatus causes aspergillosis and Coccidiodes immitis is an agent responsible for coccodioidomycosis. These are all systemic infections.

48.   (E)   The pathogenic actinomycetes are classified as belonging to the order Actinomycetales. However, many feel that they exhibit transitional characteristics between bacteria and fungi.

49.   (A)   Sporotrichosis, caused by Sporothrix schenckii, is common among gardeners since the disease is frequently associated with cuts from rose thorns contaminated with spores of S. schenckii.

50.   (C)   H. capsulatum yeast cells are characteristically found in reticuloendothelial cells and lymphocytes.

51.   (B)   Cladosporium werneckii is the causative agent of Tinea nigra. Tinea nigra is a superficial infection, usually on the palms of the hands, that is dark brown to black, resembling silver nitarte stains.

52.   (A)   Busse-Buschke's disease is a form of Cryptococcosis that involves bones and joints.

53.   (C)   Aspergillus niger is the causative agent of "fungus balls" which is a type of pulmonary aspergillosis.

54.   (B)   Darling's disease is another name for histoplasmosis. The name is a tribute to Dr. Samuel T. Darling who reported 3 fatal cases of the disease in 1905-1906.

55.   (A)   Gilchrist's disease is also known as blastomycosis and is caused by Blastomyces dermatitidis.

56.   (C)   Microsporum gypseum does not cause fluorescence of the involved hair, all of the other species of Microsporum listed as choices will produce fluorescence.

57.   (D)   Blastospores, which are produced in a budding fashion are asexual spores.

58.   (B)   Arthrospores, which are thick walled spores produced from fragmentation of hyphae, are characteristic of Geotrichum species.

59.   (A)   Candida albicans and Candida stellatoidea will both produce germ tubes while the other clinically important species of Candida will not.

60. (B) Wright's-Giemsa stain is most useful in the diagnosis and identification of Histoplasma capsulation. The Wright's-Giemsa stain will show a red stained, cup-shaped mass of protoplasm at the large end of an oval cell.

61. (D) All of the organisms listed as choices may produce a pulmonary infection.

62. (B) Both Histoplasma capsulation and Blastomyces dermatitidis are considered to be dimorphic fungi having both a yeast and a mold stage.

63. (C) Trichophyton violaceum, T. tonsurans, and T. schoenleini all produce and endothrix type of hair infection. Trichophyton rubrum produces an ectothrix type of infection.

64. (A) Phialophora verrucosa and Fonsecaea pedrosoi both produce dark colored colonies on Sabouraud's agar. Trichophyton mentagraphytes produces a white to pinkish colony and Microsporum canis produces a white colony with yellow to orange pigment on the reverse side of the colony.

65. (E) Neopeptone-glucose agar with cycloheximide inhibits growth of Cryptoccus.

66. (C) Although the most common site of infection with Cryptococcus neoformans is often thought to be the nervous system, cryptococcosis may be pulmonary, cutaneous, visceral, osseous or involve the central nervous system.

67. (A) Phialophora verrucosa is one of the causative agents of chromomycosis which is a chronic mycosis of skin and subcutaneous tissues.

68. (C) Candida albicans is associated with skin lesions, pulmonary infections, oral lesions, vulvovaginitis and septicemia.

69. (C) Sporotrichosis is generally considered to be a chronic, localized subcutaneous lymphatic mycosis, however, if dissemination of the mycosis occurs, the bones, joints, lungs, and central nervous system may become involved.

70. (B) Geotrichosis is a mycosis that is associated with the respiratory tract and the gastro-intestinal tract. No skin lesions are produced.

71. (D) Actinomyces israelii, the causative agent of actinomycosis is not, in fact, a fungus, it is one of several organisms included in the higher bacteria and does not reproduce by the formation of either asexual or sexual sporulation.

72. (A) Candida albicans produces blastospores and chlamydospores, both of which are asexual types of spores.

73. (A) Cladosporium carrionii branching chains of conidia, which are asexual spores.

74. (B) Absidia species are members of the class zygomycetes which reproduce through the formation of zygospores which are a type of sexual sporulation.

75. (A) Sporothrix schenkii is a dimorphic fungus which in its yeast phase produces blastospores and in its mold phase produces conidia, both of which are asexual types of spores.

Bibliography and
Recommended Readings

Al-Doory, Y. Laboratory Medical Mycology. 1980. Lea and Febiger. Philadelphia.

Boyd, R. F. and B. G. Hoerl. Basic Medical Microbiology. 1977. Little, Brown and Company. Boston.

Larone, D. H. Medically Important Fungi. 1976. Harper and Row Publishers. Hagerstown. Maryland.

McGinnis, M. R. Laboratory Handbook of Medical Mycology. 1980. Academic Press, Inc. New York.

Myrvik, Q. N., Pearsall, N. N. and R. S. Weiser. Fundamentals of Medical Bacteriology and Mycology. 1976. Lea and Febiger. Philadelphia.

CHAPTER 6

Parasitology

Directions. Select the one BEST answer for each of the following statements. Circle the appropriate response on the answer sheet.

1. An adult worm whose posterior is fatter than the anterior and whose egg is bile stained, oval, with bipolar plugs, describes the charactertistics of:

    A. whipworm
    B. pinworm
    C. hookworm
    D. large roundworm

2. The ova of Paragonimus westermani may be confused with those of:

    A. Schistosoma japonicum
    B. Diphyllobothrium latum
    C. Clonorchis sinesis
    D. Ancylostoma duodenale

3. Laboratory diagnosis of Naegleria is best demonstrated by:

    A. sputum
    B. feces
    C. blood
    D. spinal fluid (CSF)

4. A specimen has been standing in a laboratory overnight. Upon examination the next day you find many motile larvae which have a long buccal cavity. No ova are found. Identification of this organism is:

    A. Necator americanus, rhabditiform larvae
    B. Strongyloides stercoralis, rhabditiform larvae
    C. Strongyloides stercoralis, adult
    D. Necator americanus, filariform larvae

5. A condition by which man becomes infected with larvae of a species of Diphyllobothrium other than D. latum is known as:

    A. Sparaganosis
    B. Visceral larva migrans
    C. "ground itch"
    D. "miners itch"

6. A fecal specimen was received on a man who had returned from duty in Viet Nam. He is suspected of having Schistosomiasis. A direct mount and a zinc sulfate concentration procedure was done. However, no ova or parasites were found. Despite this the physician feels that the patient is infected with a Schistosoma species. How would you treat a second specimen which is sent to your laboratory?

    A. examine the smear more closely
    B. concentrate using formalin-ether technique
    C. recommend that the specimen be examined while warm
    D. process as usual using zinc sulfate but add a stained smear for examination

7. An 85 year old woman was admitted to the hospital with abdominal cramps and diarrhea of approximately one week's duration. She appeared cachectic and severely dehydrated and gave a history of eating poorly for several months prior to the onset of the above symptoms. The direct smear of a fecal specimen revealed an oval trophozoite measuring approximately 90 microns and containing a funnel shaped depression and a kidney shaped nucleus. Other inclusions were not visible. This organism was identified as:

    A. Entamoeba coli
    B. Giardia lamblia
    C. Balantidium coli
    D. Isospora belli

8. A slide stained with Wright's-Giemsa stain was received in the laboratory. The technologist saw the following:

    Size of cell: Normal
    Size of the parasite in the cell: Small, occupies less than 1/3 of the cell
    Number of parasites inside the RBC: 1 - 4
    Other characteristics: forms around the edge of the cell, some rings with two red dots

    This parasite is most likely:

    A. Plasmodium vivax
    B. Plasmodium malariae
    C. Plasmodium falciparum
    D. Babesia bigemina

9. A small child often plays in an unfenced yard containing a sandbox. The first attack of pneumonitis was treated as a bad cold. Slight diarrhea plus rectal itching suggested to the mother that the child might have pinworms. She was instructed to do three scotch tape preparations. All are negative upon examination. What would be the next step in diagnosis?

    A. examine three feces for Enterobius vermicularis
    B. recommend further scotch tape preparations since three are not conclusive
    C. recommend examination of three feces for Toxocara canis
    D. recommend examination of three feces for Ascaris lumbricoides

10. The golden-brown malarial pigment is a part of the identification of malarial species. The cells containing the most abundant amount of pigment are:

    A. gametocyte of Plasmodium falciparum
    B. gametocyte of Plasmodium malariae
    C. schizont of Plasmodium vivax
    D. schizont of Plasmodium malariae

11. Smears for the diagnosis of Plasmodium infections should be taken:

    A. after the fever breaks   C. after the chill period
    B. before the paroxysm   D. anytime during the attack

12. Eating "infected flour" may result in infection with:

    A. Taenia solium   C. Fasciolopsis buski
    B. Hymenolepsis diminuta   D. Taenia saginata

13. Paragonimus westermani is transmitted by:

    A. metacercaria on water plants
    B. metacercaria in fish
    C. metacercaria in crabs
    D. cercaria

Questions 14-20

Directions. One, some, or all of the responses for each of the following statements may be correct. Indicate your response as follows:

A. if items 1 and 3 are correct
B. if items 2 and 4 are correct
C. if three of the items are correct
D. if all of the items are correct
E. if only one of the items is correct

14. The adults of Ancylostoma duodenale may be distinguished from those of Necator americanus by the following:

    1. length of the buccal cavity
    2. presence or absence of teeth
    3. size of the worm
    4. characteristics of the caudal bursa

15. Parasites which are best concentrated by the zinc sulfate flotation technique include:

    1. Isospora belli   3. Trichuris trichiura
    2. Diphyllobothrium latum   4. Enterobius vermicularis

16. Morphologically a patient with Plasmodium vivax may demonstrate any or all of the following characteristics in his blood smear:

    1. enlarged red blood cells   3. amoeboid trophozoites
    2. Schüffner's granules   4. multiple infections

17. Adult worms of Ascaris lumbricoides may be found in:

    1. feces   3. sputum
    2. urine   4. blood

18. Parasites which may be transmitted by contaminated drinking water include:

    1. Entamoeba histolytica
    2. Ancylostoma duodenale

    3. Giardia lamblia
    4. Schistosoma mansoni

19. Organisms which may be transmitted by the bite of a mosquito include:

    1. Fasciola hepatica
    2. Plasmodium vivax

    3. Naegleria fowleri
    4. Wuchereria bancrofti

20. Autoinfection (self-infection) may be seen with patients who have "acquaintance" (i.e., infection) with:

    1. Enterobius vermicularis
    2. Taenia solium

    3. Strongyloides stercoralis
    4. Ancylostoma duodenale

Questions 21-24

Directions. For each of the numbered items select the appropriate lettered response. Do not use the same letter more than once.

Organism

21. Trypanosoma cruzi
22. Trypanosoma gambiense
23. Leishmania donovani
24. Loa loa

Vector

A. Phlebotomus
B. Reduviid bug
C. Anopheles mosquito
D. Tse-tse fly
E. Chrysops

25. Plasmodium vivax
26. Plasmodium ovale
27. Plasmodium malariae
28. Plasmodium falciparum

A. prefers young red blood cells
B. has fimbrinated edges of rbc's
C. has sausage shaped gametocyte
D. has band form trophozoites
E. prefers target cells

Questions 29-48

Directions. Select and circle the one BEST answer for each of the following statements utilizing the information presented in either the following graph, tracing,
table or laboratory data.

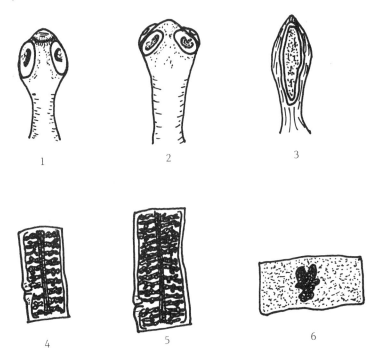

29. Which set of characteristics illustrated above are found in the cestode that
     may produce a vitamin B_{12} deficiency and anemia?

     A.   1 and 4   C.   2 and 6
     B.   1 and 5   D.   3 and 6

30. Which of the characteristics illustrated above belong to the organism that
     produces the disease known as Cysticercosis?

     A.   1 and 4   C.   1 and 5
     B.   2 and 5   D.   2 and 4

31. Which of the characteristics illustrated above belong to the organism that
     utilizes the pig as its intermediate host?

     A.   1 and 4   C.   1 and 5
     B.   2 and 5   D.   2 and 4

32. Which of the characteristics illustrated above belong to the organism which
     produces disease in man from the ingestion of improperly cooked beef?

     A.   1 and 4   C.   1 and 5
     B.   2 and 5   D.   2 and 4

Questions 33-39

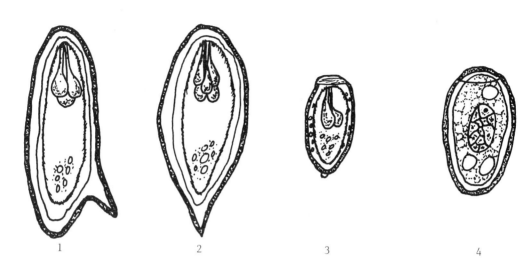

33. Which of the trematode ova illustrated above must be differentiated from the ova of a cestode that is quite similar in appearance?

    A. 1   C. 3
    B. 2   D. 4

34. Of the ova illustrated above, which one will characteristically be found in the urine of infected patients?

    A. 1   C. 3
    B. 2   D. 4

Match the ova illustrated above with their common names.

35. 1   A. the lung fluke
36. 2   B. oriental liver fluke
37. 3   C. urinary schistosomiasis
38. 4   D. Manson's bilharziasis
                                    E. the intestinal fluke

39. Which of the adult forms of the ova illustrated above would inhabit the blood stream?

    A. 1 and 2   C. 2 and 3
    B. 1 and 3   D. 3 and 4

Questions 40-43

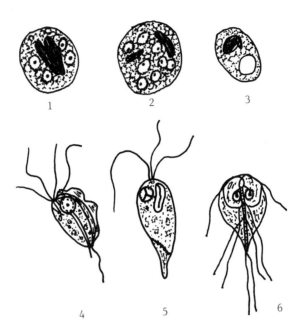

40. Which of the illustrations above belong to organisms that are pathogenic to man?

    A. 1, 2, and 6   C. 1, 3, and 4
    B. 1 and 6   D. 2, 3, and 5

41. Which of the non pathogens illustrated above is, if found in a stool specimen, evidence of <u>direct</u> fecal contamination?

    A. 2   C. 5
    B. 4   D. 6

42. The cyst illustrated as #3 above, when stained with Iodine, displays a characteristic large glycogen vacuole. Which of the following organisms does this cyst form belong to?

    A. Giardia lamblia   C. Trichomonas hominis
    B. Iodamoeba butschlii D. Entamoeba coli

43. Which of the illustrations above is that of the organism that is known to cause the disease commonly referred to as Montezuma's revenge?

    A. 1   C. 4
    B. 2   D. 5

Questions 44-48

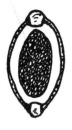 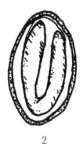 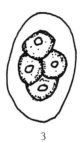 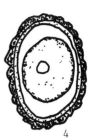

1   2   3   4

44. Which of the ova illustrated above produces the largest of the roundworms?

A. 1   C. 3
B. 2   D. 4

Match the illustrations above with their corresponding common names.

45. 1   A. pinworm
46. 2   B. microfilaria
47. 3   C. hookworm
48. 4   D. roundworm
                              E. whipworm

Questions 49-50

Directions. Select the one BEST answer for each of the following statements. Circle the appropriate response on the answer sheet.

49. Which of the following cestodes characteristically develops an ovum which has an oncosphere enveloped in a membrane with polar thickenings and polar filaments arising from these thickenings?

A. Taenia solium   C. Hymenolepsis nana
B. Taenia saginata   D. Hymenolepsis diminuta

50. Hydatid cysts are a characteristic of which of the following organisms?

A. Dipylidium canium   C. Taenia saginata
B. Echinococcus granulosa   D. Hymenolepsis diminuta

Questions 51-55

Directions. One, some, or all of the responses for each of the following statements may be correct. Indicate your response as follows:

A. if items 1 and 3 are correct
B. if items 2 and 4 are correct
C. if three of the items are correct
D. if all of the items are correct
E. if only one of the items is correct

51. Which of the following may be acquired through exposure to infected water?

    1. Schistosoma mansoni
    2. Toxocara canis
    3. Naegleria fowleri
    4. Echinococcus granulosus

52. Which of the following animal parasites may also infect humans?

    1. Toxocara canis
    2. Dirofilaria immitis
    3. Ancylostoma braziliensis
    4. Echinococcus granulosus

53. Which of the following organisms would be classified as nematodes?

    1. Entamoeba histolytica
    2. Hymenolepsis nana
    3. Ancylostoma duodenale
    4. Balantidium coli

54. Which of the following stages of development are NOT found in trematodes?

    1. miracidia
    2. sporozoites
    3. cercariae
    4. schizonts

55. Which of the following are NOT lumen dwelling protozoa?

    1. Entamoeba histolytica
    2. Acanthamoeba spp.
    3. Endolimax nana
    4. Naegleria fowleri

Questions 56-70

Directions. For each of the following numbered words or phrases listed below, select the appropriate response as follows:

A. if the item is associated with only A
B. if the item is associated with only B
C. if the item is associated with both A and B
D. if the item is associated with neither A nor B

    A. acquired through ingestion of meat or fish
    B. acquired through exposure to contaminated water

56. Naegleria infection
57. Schistosoma infection
58. Diphyllobothrium latum infection
59. Toxocara infection
60. Entamoeba histolytica infection

    A. vector borne
    B. autoinfective

61. Entamoeba histolytica
62. Naegleria fowleri
63. Babesia bigemina
64. Taenia solium
65. Trypanosoma rhodesiense

A. has a stage of development in aquatic life
B. has a stage of development in animals

66. Schistosoma haematobium
67. Toxoplasma gondi
68. Entamoeba histolytica
69. Plasmodium malariae
70. Fasciolopsis buski

Questions 71-85

Directions. The following statements contain numbered blanks. For each numbered
blank there is a corresponding set of lettered responses. Select the BEST answer
from each lettered set.

In the life cycle of Necator americanus, the adult bearing human passes the 71 which
develops in warm moist soil into the non-infective larval form known as the 72.
These larvae will grow and molt twice, developing into the infective larval form
known as the 73. When the infective stage comes in contact with the skin, the larvae
migrate through the blood stream to the 74. Final development to the mature form
takes place in the 75.

71. A. ova   C. filariform larva
    B. cercaria   D. rhabditiform larva

72. A. ova   C. filariform larva
    B. cercaria   D. rhabditiform larva

73. A. ova   C. filariform larva
    B. cercaria   D. rhabditiform larva

74. A. liver   C. lungs
    B. heart   D. small intestine

75. A. liver   C. lungs
    B. heart   D. small intestine

In the life cycle of Fasciola hepatica, the 76 are passed in the stools of infected
humans. When they reach water they release a 77 which penetrates a snail and forms
a(n) 78. This soon becomes fill with 79, which give rise to 80.

76. A. ova   C. sporocyst
    B. miracidium   D. coracidium

77. A. ova   C. sporocyst
    B. miracidium   D. coracidium

78. A. ova   C. sporocyst
    B. miracidium   D. metacercaria

79. A. miracidia   C. metacercariae
    B. rediae   D. sporocyst

80. A. miracidia   C. metacercariae
    B. cercariae   D. rediae

In the life cycle of Diphyllobothrium latum, the 81 are passed in human stools.
When these reach water they develop ciliated embryos known as 82. This stage is
then ingested by a crustacean and development to the 83 stage takes place. When
the crustacean is ingested by a fresh water fish, this stage develops into the 84.
When ingested by a human, development ot the adult stage takes place in the 85.

81. A. ova   C. coracidium
    B. miracidium   D. procercoid larva

82. A. ova   C. coracidium
    B. miracidium   D. procercoid larva

83. A. miracidium   C. procercoid larva
    B. coracidium   D. plerocercoid larva

84. A. miracidium   C. procercoid larva
    B. coracidium   D. plerocercoid larva

85. A. lungs   C. small intestine
    B. liver   D. lymphatic system

Explanatory Answers

1. (A) The characteristics stated describe the worm and ova of the organism Trichuris trichiura, the common whipworm.

2. (B) The ova of P. westermani may be confused with those of D. latum, but may be distinguished by the absence of the protruding "knob" on P. westermani.

3. (D) Naegleria produces an acute meningoencephalitis and upon examination of the CSF, the motile amoebae may be found.

4. (A) The rhabditiform larvae of the hookworm (Necator americanus) is often confused with the rhabditiform larvae of Strongyloides, but may be differentiated by the length of the buccal cavity. Hookworm larvae have the characteristic long buccal cavity.

5. (A) Sparaganosis is a condition in which man is a suitable second intermediate host for other species of Diphyllobothrium.

6. (B) The formalin-ether concentration technique is better for the recovery of the ova of the Schistosomes and operculated ova than the zinc sulfate technique.

7. (C) The description of the trophozoite is consistent with that of Balantidium coli.

8. (C) The presence of multiple infected red cells, parasites with double chromatin dots, and normal sized red blood cells all indicate that this parasite is most likely Plasmodium falciparum.

9. (D) Pneumonitis is a common symptom of Ascaris infection. Pneumonitis with associated diarrhea and rectal itching strongly suggests an Ascaris infection.

10. (D) The schizont of Plasmodium malariae will characteristically show an abundance of the malarial pigment.

11. (B) Best results are obtained from smears taken prior to the paroxysm.

12. (B) Infection with Hymenolepsis diminuta is usually the result of eating contaminated flour, since the intermediate hosts of H. diminuta are often flour moths and flour beetles.

13. (C) Infection with P. westermani is most commonly acquired in man by the ingestion of raw or improperly cooked crayfish or fresh water crabs.

14. (B) The differentiation between Ancylostoma duodenale and Necator americanus is done by examining the caudal bursa, and by the presence of teeth on A. duodenale and cutting plates instead of teeth on N. americanus.

15. (C) Parasites number 1, 3, and 4 are concentrated by the zinc sulfate technique. The operculated ova, such as that of D. latum, are usually not recovered with the zinc sulfate technique and are better recovered by the formalin-ether concentration technique.

16. (C) Enlargement of the red blood cells, Schüffner's granules, and amoeboid activity of the trophozoites are all characteristic of Plasmodium vivax, but, multiple infections of a single cell is not a finding in this infection.

17. (A) The adult worms of Ascaris lumbricoides are often found in fecal specimens and may be found in sputum, particularly after they have been aggravated by medication which makes them more motile. They are not found in urine or blood.

18. (C) Infection with E. histolytica, G. lamblia, and S. mansoni is often the result of drinking contaminated water, whereas infection with A. duodenale is often the result of skin contact with contaminated soil.

19. (B) Mosquitos are the vectors of Pl. vivax and W. bancrofti. F. hepatica is acquired through the ingestion of contaminated water vegetation and N. fowleri by exposure to stagnant swimming pools and brackish water holes.

20. (C) Parasites number 1, 3, and 4 are all capable of reinfecting the host, whereas Taenia solium requires an intermediate host, namely the pig.

21. (B) Trypanosoma cruzi, the causative agent of Chaga's disease or South American sleeping sickness, is transmitted by the Reduviid bug. The Reduviid bug is also known as the Assasin bug, the kissing bug, and triatoma.

22. (D) Trypanosoma gambiense, the causative agent of African sleeping sickness, is transmitted by the bite of the tse-tse fly.

23. (A) Leishmania donovani, the causative agent of kala-azar, is transmitted by sand flies of the genus Phlebotomus.

24. (E) Loa loa, the African eye worm, is transmitted by flies belonging to the genus Chrysops.

25. (A) Plasmodium vivax shows a preference for young red cells or reticulocytes. This is a diagnostic characteristic, because Plasmodium malariae displays a preference for older red cells, whereas Plasmodium falciparum attacks any red blood cell.

26. (B) Plasmodium ovale, characteristically is found in oval red blood cells. These oval red cells are very often fimbrinated, that is they have ragged edges.

27. (D) One of the characteristics of Plasmodium malariae is that the trophozoite form is often band shaped.

28. (C) Plasmodium falciparum is the only species of Plasmodium which has a sausage shaped gametocyte.

29. (D) Illustrations 3 and 6 depict the scolex and gravid proglottid of Diphyllobothrium latum, the broad or fish tapeworm which may produce a pernicious anemia-like anemia by selective absorption of vitamin B_{12}.

30. (B) Illustrations 2 and 5 depict the scolex and gravid proglottid of Taenia solium. Cysticercosis is a condition in which man serves as the intermediate host of Taenia solium. In this disorder, man harbors the larval form, Cysticercus cellulosae.

31. (B)   Illustrations 2 and 5 depict the scolex and gravid proglottid of Taenia solium, also known as the pork tapeworm.

32. (A)   The illustrations labeled 1 and 4 depict the scolex and gravid proglottid of the organism known as Taenia saginata. Taenia saginata is also known as the beef tapeworm; man acquires the infection by ingesting raw or improperly cooked beef.

33. (D)   Illustration 4 is that of the ova of Paragonimus westermani, the lung fluke. The ova of Paragonimus westermani very closely resembles that of Diphyllobothrium latum. Differentiation can be made by observing a knob-like projection on the ovum of Diphyllobothrium latum at the end of the ovum opposite the operculum.

34. (B)   Illustration 2 is that of the ova of Schistosoma hematobium which lives in the vesical and pelvic plexi. Schistosoma hematobium females deposit eggs which work their way through the urinary bladder, consequently, the ova are found in the urine.

35. (D)   The ovum illustrated is that of Schistosoma mansoni. Schistosoma mansoni is a blood fluke which is also known as Manson's bilharziasis.

36. (C)   The ovum illustrated in #2 is that of Schistosoma hematobium, also known as urinary schistosomiasis because it affects the urinary bladder and the ova are found in urine.

37. (B)   The ovum illustrated as #3 is that of Opistorchis sinensis or Clonorchis sinensis. This organism is commonly referred to as the oriental liver fluke.

38. (A)   The ovum illustrated in #4, is that of Paragonimus westermani, whose common name is the lung fluke.

39. (A)   Illustrations 1 and 2 are those of Schistosoma mansoni and Schistosoma hematobium respectively. Both of these organisms are blood flukes, and the adults would be found in the blood stream.

40. (B)   Illustrations 1 and 6 depict the cyst of Entamoeba histolytica and the trophozoite of Giardia lamblia respectively. Both of these organisms are pathogenic to man. Entamoeba histolytica is the causative agent of amoebic dysentery and Giardia lamblia is the causative agent of giardiasis.

41. (B)   Illustration #4 is that of Trichomonas hominis. Trichomonas hominis does not have a cyst stage, and is therefore evidence of direct fecal contamination when found in a stool specimen.

42. (B)   The cyst form of Iodamoeba butschlii characteristically displays a large glycogen vacuole which will stain yellow-brown when Iodine is added to the preparation.

43. (A)   Illustration #1 is that of the cyst form of Entamoeba histolytica, the causative agent of amoebic dysentery. Amoebic dysentery is often referred to as Montezuma's revenge.

44. (D)   Illustration #4 is that of the ova of Ascaris lumbricoides. Ascaris lumbricoides is also known as the large intestinal roundworm. These worms grow as adults to lengths of up to 35 cm or more.

45. (E)   The ova represented in illustration #1 is that of Trichuris trichiura which, because of its adult form, is more commonly known as the whipworm.

46. (A)   The ova represented in illustration #2 is that of Enterobius vermicularis which is more commonly referred to as the pinworm.

47. (C) The ova represented in illustration #3 is that of either Ancylostoma duodenale or Necator americanus, both of which are known as hookworms.

48. (D) The ova represented in illustration #4 is that of Ascaris lumbricoides which is more commonly referred to as the large intestinal roundworm.

49. (C) The cestode Hymenolepsis nana has an ovum that characteristically shows a six hooked oncosphere that is enveloped in a membrane that has polar thickenings and polar filaments arising from those polar thickenings.

50. (B) Echinococcus granulosa in man characteristically develops hydatid cysts, since man is the intermediate host for Echinococcus infection.

51. (A) Both Schistosoma mansoni and Naegleria fowleri infections may be acquired by exposure to contaminated water. Schistosoma cercariae will penetrate the skin, while Naegleria trophozoites may penetrate the nasal mucosa of a swimmer.

52. (D) All of the organisms listed may infect humans. Toxocara canis, a dog round worm, may cause visceral larva migrans. Dirofilaria immitis, the dog heart worm, may cause a microfilaria to be found in humans. Ancylostoma braziliensis, a dog hookworm, may cause cutaneous larva migrans. Echinococcus granulosus may cause hydatid cysts in humans.

53. (E) Only Ancylostoma duodenale is classified as a nematode. Entamoeba histolytica is classified as an amoeba, Hymenolepsis nana is classified as a cestode, and Balantidium coli is classified as a ciliate.

54. (B) Sporozoites and schizonts are stages of development found in those organisms classified as sporozoans. Miracidia and cercariae are stages of development in trematodes.

55. (B) Acathamoeba spp. and Naegleria are listed as extraintestinal protozoa and are most often found in cerebrospinal fluid. Entamoeba histolytica and Endolimax nana are lumen dwelling protozoa.

56. (B) Naegleria fowleri is acquired through the penetration of the trophozoites into the nasal mucosa of swimmers and is not acquired through the ingestion of meat or fish.

57. (B) Schistosoma infections are acquired through the penetration of the infective cercariae into the skin of humans when said skin is placed in contaminated water. It is not acquired through the ingestion of meat or fish.

58. (C) Diphyllobothrium latum infection is acquired through the ingestion of improperly cooked fresh water fish bearing the infective larvae. Sparganosis, which is the development of the larva of D. latum may be acquired through the ingestion of the first intermediate host, the cyclops, in contaminated water.

59. (D) Toxocara infections are acquired through the ingestion of fully embryonated larva usually found in the soil.

60. (C) Entamoeba histolytica infection may be acquired via contaminated food and drink through the ingestion of cysts.

61. (C) Entamoeba histolytica infections may be acquired through self, or autoinfection, or, the infectious agent may be vector borne. Unlike other vector borne parasites, the transferance of Entamoeba histolytica via vectors is usually a mechanical function that is the

cysts are borne on the legs of flies and cockroaches from one source of infection to another.

62. (D) Infection with Naegleria fowleri is neither vector borne nor autoinfective. Infection with Naegleria fowleri is through swimming in contaminated water.

63. (A) Babesia bigemina infections are vector borne. The organism is carried by a tick which is endemic to the southwest and Nantucket Island in New England.

64. (B) Although primary infections with Taenia solium are neither vector borne nor autoinfective, the possibility of self infection is possible in terms of the development of cysticercosis. Cysticercosis develops when humans infest the ova of Taenia solium.

65. (A) Trypanosoma rhodesiense is a vector borne parasite. The parasite is the causative agent of African Sleeping Sickness and is carried by the Tse-tse fly.

66. Schistosoma haematobium has, as its intermediate host, a snail involved in its life cycle. When ova are passed into the water, a miracidium hatches and enters the appropriate species of snail for further development.

67. (B) Toxoplasma gondii has a typical coccidian life cycle in animals, particularly mice and cats.

68. (D) Entamoeba histolytica, while being capable of infecting water and being mechanically transmitted by flies and roaches, does not have a stage of development that takes place in aquatic life or in animals.

69. (D) Plasmodium malariae does not have a stage of development in either aquatic life or animals,

other than humans. The life cycle is confined to humans and mosquitos.

70. (A) Fasciolopsis buski has crustaceans as intermediate hosts.

71. (A) In the life cycle of Necator americanus, the adult bearing human passes the ova.

72. (D) The ova, in the soil develop into the rhabditiform larva which is non-infective to humans.

73. (C) As the rhabditiform larva develops, it will molt twice and become an infective larva which is known as the filariform larva.

74. (C) As the larva enters the blood stream, it will be carried to the lungs. At the lungs, the larva will enter the air sacks (alveoli) and then progress to migrate up the bronchial tree.

75. (D) After migration up the bronchial tree, the larva will be swallowed and develop to adulthood in the small intestine.

76. (A) In the life cycle of Fasciola hepatica, the ova are passed in the stools and are deposited in water.

77. (B) When these eggs are hatched, they release a ciliated embryo known as a miracidium.

78. (C) When the miracidium penetrates the snail, it forms a sporocyst.

79. (B) The maturation of the miracidium in the snail gives rise to rediae which fill the sporocyst.

80. (B) These rediae ultimately give rise to the form of the organism known as the cercariae. The cercariae will ultimately encyst on fresh water vegetation in the infective form known as metacercariae.

81. (A) The life cycle of Diphyllobothrium latum involves the passage of ova in the stools of infected humans.

82. (C) When these ova reach the water they release a ciliated embryo known as a coracidium.

83. (C) When the coracidium is ingested by the appropriate crustacean it develops into the procercoid larval stage.

84. (D) When the crustacean bearing the procercoid stage is ingested by the appropriate species of fresh water fish, further development takes place resulting in the development of the plerocercoid larval stage.

85. (C) When humans ingest improperly cooked fish bearing the plerocercoid larval form, development to the adult stage takes place in the small intestine of the now infected human.

Bibliography and Recommended Readings

Beck, J. W. and J. E. Davies. Medical Parasitology. Third Edition. 1981. The
    C. V. Mosby Company. St. Louis.

Desowitz, R. S. Ova and Parasites. 1980. J. B. Lippincott Company. Philadelphia.

Faust, E. C., Russell, P. F. and R. C. Jung. Craig and Fuast's Clinical Parasitology.
    Eight Edition. 1970. Lea and Febiger. Philadelphia.

Henry, J. B. Todd-Sanford-Davidsohn Clinical Diagnosis and Management by Laboratory
    Methods. Sixteenth Edition. 1979. W. B. Saunders Company. Philadelphia.

Markell, E. K. and M. Voge. Medical Parasitology. Fifth Edition. 1981. W. B.
    Saunders Company. Philadelphia.

Noble, E. R. and G. A. Noble. Parasitology: The Biology of Animal Parasites.
    Fourth Edition. 1976. Lea and Febiger. Philadelphia.

Raphael, S. S. (Senior Author). Lynch's Medical Laboratory Technology. Volume I.
    Third Edition. 1976. W. B. Saunders Company. Philadelphia.

CHAPTER 7

Virology

Directions. Select the one BEST answer for each of the following statements. Circle the appropriate response on the answer sheet.

1. The etiologic agent of chickenpox is:

   A. herpes
   B. variola
   C. varicella

   D. rubella
   E. rubeola

2. Because viruses are obligate intracellular parasites, they have not been propagated:

   A. in chick embryos
   B. in genetically sensitive mouse strains
   C. on cell-free media
   D. in kidney cells
   E. in liver cells

3. All animal viruses contain:

   A. RNA only
   B. DNA only

   C. a polypeptide capsid only
   D. either RNA or DNA

4. All plant viruses contain:

   A. RNA only
   B. DNA only

   C. RNA and DNA
   D. a polypeptide capsid only

5. Electron microscopy has provided information regarding the structure of viruses. However, with a good light microscope and the proper illumination, a researcher could see some details of the following viruses:

   A. adenoviruses
   B. herpetoviruses
   C. picornaviruses

   D. poxviruses
   E. none of the above

6. The etiological agent of infectious mononucleosis is a herpetovirus now referred to as:

    A. SV 40   D. LCM
    B. HSV   E. EBV
    C. HZV

7. An intracellular DNA virus which gives rise to latent infections that may last the life span of the host is:

    A. herpes-zoster   D. rubeola
    B. verruceae   E. none of the above
    C. variola

8. Varicella, EBV and the human cytomegalovirus each have:

    A. a single serotype   C. three serotypes
    B. two serotypes   D. multiple serotypes

9. The clinical expression "acute respiratory disease" (ARD) is most frequently used to designate:

    A. a poxvirus infection   D. a cytomegalovirus infection
    B. a herpes-simplex infection E. an adenovirus infection
    C. a herpes-zoster infection

10. Chickenpox, "shingles", infectious mononucleosis, genital herpes and fever blisters are all caused by:

    A. poxviruses   D. picornaviruses
    B. herpetoviruses   E. paramyxoviruses
    C. adenoviruses

11. In 1953, Rowe and his colleagues found the adenovirus in tissue fragments of the:

    A. kidneys   D. lungs
    B. liver   E. intestine
    C. adenoids

12. The possible causative agent of a genital chancroid may be:

    A. herpes-zoster   C. herpesvirus 2
    B. herpesvirus 1   D. all of the above

13. Herpes-zoster occurs only in people who have exposure to or a history of:

    A. variola   D. herpes simplex
    B. rubella   E. varicella
    C. rubeola

14. The Paul-Bunnell test for heterophil agglutinins is a test frequently used in clinical laboratories to diagnose for:

    A. infectious hepatitis   D. shingles
    B. mumps   E. measles
    C. infectious mononucleosis

15. The polioviruses, coxsackieviruses and echoviruses belong to the genus:

    A. rhinovirus
    B. poxvirus
    C. arbovirus
    D. enterovirus
    E. paramyxovirus

16. It is difficult to differentiate Variola major from Variola minor, however one significant mode of differentiation is by:

    A. disease symptoms
    B. viral biochemical characteristics
    C. target tissue
    D. CAM of chick embryos incubated at 39°
    E. nucleic acid type

17. Hepatitis A usually enters the host by:

    A. blood transfusion
    B. skin lesion
    C. ingestion
    D. all of the above

18. There are more than 100 rhinovirus serotypes. The rhinoviruses are responsible for:

    A. mumps
    B. measles
    C. common cold
    D. chickenpox
    E. cold sores

19. A person may contact Herpes virus B as a result of a bite from an infected:

    A. chick
    B. dog
    C. monkey
    D. rabbit
    E. cat

20. Marek's disease of chickens is a disease of the lymphatic system whereby malignant cells invade the nerve cells of the chicken. A virus has been isolated from the tumors of chickens having Marek's disease. When reinoculated into healthy chickens this isolated virus induced lymphatic tumors similar to that of Marek's disease. The etiologic agent of Marek's disease is believed to be a(n):

    A. enterovirus
    B. arbovirus
    C. adenovirus
    D. reovirus
    E. herpesvirus

21. Which of the following tissues is most susceptible to the respiratory syncytial virus and is most useful when isolating this virus from a clinical specimen?

    A. chick embryos
    B. susceptible kidney cells
    C. suckling mice
    D. HEp #2 cells

22. At least 12 of the 33 types of human adenoviruses have been found to cause malignant carcinomas to:

    A. newborn mice
    B. baby hamsters
    C. baby rabbits
    D. young monkeys
    E. all of the above

23. Some adenoviruses are more oncogenic than others. Those which are more highly oncogenic have been found to contain the following pair arrangement in their DNA:

    A. low guanine and low cytosine content
    B. high guanine and high cytosine content
    C. no change in either guanine or cytosine content
    D. low guanine but high cytosine content
    E. high guanine but low cytosine content

24. The smallest icosahedral virus found in vertebrates which contains single stranded DNA, is resistant to treatment with either ether or chloroform and is believed to be the causative agent of the Norwalk disease and hepatitis A is a(n):

    A. papillomavirus   D. poxvirus
    B. polyomavirus   E. parvovirus
    C. adenovirus

25. These are structurally large, oval and complex animal viruses made up of double stranded DNA which characteristically form lesions on the host tissues. These are most probably:

    A. parvoviruses   D. poxviruses
    B. papillomaviruses   E. adenoviruses
    C. arboviruses

26. Smallpox may be diagnosed on the basis of lesion appearance and clinical symptoms. However, presumptive diagnosis may be obtained by the presence of characteristic cytoplasmic inclusions referred to as:

    A. Negri bodies   D. Nissl bodies
    B. Guarnieri bodies   E. Marchal bodies
    C. Councilman bodies

27. To date, the causative agents of viral hepatitis have:

    A. been isolated in chick embryos only
    B. been isolated in rhesus monkey kidney cells only
    C. been isolated in suckling mice only
    D. been isolated in liver cells only
    E. not been grown in cell cultures at all

28. Hepatitis A is most frequently spread by:

    A. injection of blood or serum from an infected person
    B. fecal-oral contamination
    C. infection with the Dane particle
    D. e antigen

29. Yellow fever, dengue fever and eastern and western equine encephalitis are arthropod-borne viruses which may ultimately infect individuals who come in contact with the infected mosquitoes. The etiologic viral agents of these diseases are:

A. poxviruses   D. arenaviruses
B. echoviruses   E. none of the above
C. togaviruses

30. The presence of HB_SAg in the blood, urine or feces of individuals confirms the diagnosis of:

A. viral hepatitis   D. herpes simplex type 2
B. hepatitis B   E. none of the above
C. herpes simplex type 1

31. Yellow fever is an acute infectious disease which severely damages the liver. However, a single vaccine is effective against yellow fever because:

A. the etiologic agent is mildly infectious
B. the yellow fever virus is non-resistant
C. there is only one yellow fever virus strain
D. the yellow fever virus is a weak antigen
E. none of the above

32. Eradication of the Aedes mosquito effectively controls the spread of:

A. yellow fever   D. Colorado fever
B. dengue shock syndrome   E. Norwalk disease
C. both A and B

33. The Salk and Sabin vaccines are vaccines which are effective against polioviruses. How many polioviruses are there?

A. one   D. four
B. two   E. five
C. three

34. Individuals suffering with Hodgkins disease generally demonstrate high antibody titers to the following virus:

A. Epstein and Barr (EB) virus   D. adenovirus
B. cytomegalovirus (CMV)   E. herpesvirus 1
C. herpesvirus 2

35. At one time certain viruses were frequently isolated from feces and were known to produce cytopathic changes in tissue cultures but were not known to produce any disease. Some workers referred to these as "viruses in search of disease." These viruses are now referred to as:

A. coxsackieviruses   D. reoviruses
B. hepatitis B viruses   E. echoviruses
C. rhinoviruses

36. Viruses of this family are RNA viruses which cause leukemia and sarcomas in many species of animals:

    A. Coronaviridae
    B. Paramyxoviridae
    C. Picornaviridae
    D. Retroviridae
    E. Reoviridae

37. The majority of the common cold viruses are classified as:

    A. echoviruses
    B. coronaviruses
    C. rotaviruses
    D. rhinoviruses
    E. reoviruses

38. A virus was implicated with an acute infectious diarrhea which resulted in the death of many newborn and young children. A "wheel" shaped virus was isolated from the feces of about half of the children. For lack of a better name, the virus implicated with this condition is referred to as a(n):

    A. rotavirus
    B. reovirus
    C. rhinovirus
    D. coronavirus
    E. orbivirus

39. The influenza viruses are also designated as:

    A. rhinoviruses
    B. echoviruses
    C. orthomyxoviruses
    D. paramyxoviruses
    E. coronaviruses

40. In 1976, millions of Americans were immunized against the swine influenza. However, some people experienced an ascending paralysis a few days after immunization with the swine influenza vaccine. This ascending paralysis condition is:

    A. Creutzfeldt-Jacob disease
    B. Parkinson's disease
    C. Guillain-Barre syndrome
    D. multiple sclerosis

41. Other than serological tests, early diagnosis of this disease, prior to the formation of the characteristic rash, may be made by observing small bluish-yellow Koplik spots on the mucosa of the mouth and so called giant cells in nasal secretions. This disease is most likely:

    A. chickenpox
    B. smallpox
    C. measles
    D. human herpesvirus 1
    E. "shingles"

42. The viruses, which would be most resistant to proteolytic enzymes, and would demonstrate a fairly long survival time in sewage polluted water even after chlorination, are members of the:

    A. poxviruses
    B. paramyxoviruses
    C. hepatitis A viruses
    D. arboviruses
    E. enteroviruses

43.   A virus, when recovered from respiratory secretions and grown in cell cultures, produced giant multinucleated cells within a few weeks. This virus is most likely:

A. mumps virus   D. respiratory syncytial virus
B. chickenpox virus   E. echovirus
C. rubella virus

44.   Rabies is clinically diagnosed by the presence of inclusions in the cytoplasm of infected cells. These inclusions are called:

A. Nissl bodies   C. Guarnieri bodies
B. Negri bodies   D. polar bodies

45.   The best specimen source for the recovery of the hepatitis B virus is:

A. blood   D. cerebrospinal fluid
B. urine   E. none of the above
C. feces

46.   The best specimen to obtain for the clinical diagnosis of measles is:

A. feces   D. cerebrospinal fluid
B. urine   E. throat swab
C. blood

47.   Which of the following specimens would be best to isolate the cytomegalovirus?

A. urine   D. feces
B. throat swab   E. cerebrospinal fluid
C. both A and B

48.   The etiologic agent of mumps is a(n):

A. respiratory syncytial virus   D. paramyxovirus
B. reovirus   E. orthomyxovirus
C. picornavirus

49.   Characteristically the reoviruses are unique by the fact that:

A. they are present in sewage polluted water
B. they are resistant to chloroform
C. they are resistant to chlorine
D. their RNA is double stranded
E. their DNA is single stranded

50.   The presence of HB_SAg confirms the diagnosis of hepatitis B. The serological identification of HB_SAg is routinely performed in blood banks and clinical laboratories. Of all the methods available to detect HB_SAg, which is most sensitive?

A. radioimmunoassay (RIA)   D. immunodiffusion
B. complement fixation (CF)   E. none of the above
C. counter-immunoelectrophoresis (CIEP)

51. To date, viral and rickettsial infections are most reliably diagnosed by:

    A. phage typing   C. serologic tests
    B. electron microscopy   D. all of the above

52. Using proper cultures, rhinovirus, mycoplasma, parainfluenza, and Epstein-Barr viruses may be recovered from:

    A. feces   C. throat swab or nasal secretions
    B. urine   D. spinal fluid and urine

53. The routine serological test for mycoplasma is:

    A. complement fixation   C. fluorescent antibody
    B. hemagglutination fixation   D. immunoeletron microscopy

54. Hepatitis A virus (HAV) causes:

    A. infectious hepatitis   C. infectious and serum hepatitis
    B. serum hepatitis   D. murine hepatitis

55. The Epstein-Barr virus is serologically tested for by employing the following:

    A. complement fixation   C. immunoelectrophoresis
    B. fluorescent antibody   D. neutralization

56. Using the proper cultures, rubella may be isolated primarily from specimen collected from:

    A. throat   C. CSF
    B. urine   D. all of the above

57. With the proper cultures, the mumps virus may be isolated primarily from:

    A. throat swabs only   C. throat swabs and CSF
    B. throat swabs and urine   D. throat swabs and nasal secretions

58. The lytic action of viruses on cells may be inhibited by:

    A. certain fatty acids   C. certain hormones
    B. interferons   D. vitamins

59. The mumps vaccine is:

    A. generally ineffective
    B. protects only 5%-10% of those vaccinated
    C. protects about 50% of those vaccinated
    D. protects about 90% of those vaccinated.

60. Smears of cells infected with herpes simplex reveal:

    A. anucleated giant cells   C. multinucleated giant cells
    B. multinucleated shrivelled cells D. no morphological changes

61. Infection with rubella usually confers a:

A. lifeflong immunity   C. 5-10 year immunity period
B. 2-3 year immunity period   D. 20 year immunity period

Questions 62-70

Directions. Match the item in Column A with the most closely related item in Column B. There is only one correct response.

Column A   Column B

62. poliomyelitis   A. JC virus
63. measles   B. rubeola
64. rabies   C. rhabdovirus
65. infectious mononucleosis   D. Epstein-Barr virus
66. progressive multifocal leukoence-   E. enterovirus
        phalopathy (PML)

67. subacute sclerosing panencephalitis   A. rubella
        (SSPE)   B. orthomyxoviruses
68. influenza   C. paramyxovirus
69. German measles   D. XLD
70. virus detection technique   E. ELISA

Explanatory Answers

1. (C) Varicella is the viral agent responsible for chickenpox. Chickenpox begins with fever followed by a sudden eruption of characteristic skin lesions found primarily on the body trunk.

2. (C) Viruses are obligate intracellular parasites, which have not yet been propagated on cell-free media.

3. (D) All animal viruses contain either RNA or DNA.

4. (A) Plant viruses contain only RNA.

5. (D) The poxviruses are barely large enough to be observed with a light microscope, but proper lighting is essential. Electron microscopy, however provides best results.

6. (E) The EBV or Epstein-Barr virus is the etiologic agent of infectious mononucleosis.

7. (A) Herpes-Zoster is the virus responsible for shingles. This virus may remain quiescent or inactive in the host until the proper conditions cause it to be reactivated. This may occur anytime during the life of the host.

8. (A) Varicella, EBV and cytomegalovirus each have a single serotype.

9. (E) Acute respiratory diseases (ARD) are generally associated with adenovirus infections.

10. (B) Chickenpox, "shingles", infectious mononucleosis, genital herpes and fever blisters are caused by varicella, herpes-zoster, EB virus, herpes simplex type 2 and herpes simplex type 1 viruses respectively. These are all herpetoviruses.

11. (C) While attempting to isolate the "cold" virus, Rowe and his colleagues found a new virus, the adenovirus, which appeared to be latent in adenoid and tonsil tissue.

12. (C) Herpes simplex type 2 is usually referred to as genital herpes and may be implicated in chancroid formation.

13. (E) Resistance to a second infection of varicella is lifelong. However, the resulting antibody level is not sufficient to eliminate the virus from the dorsal ganglia of some hosts prone to herpes-zoster.

14. (C) The Paul-Bunnell test is possibly one of the most common serological procedures used to diagnose infectious mononucleosis.

15. (D) The polioviruses, coxsackieviruses and echoviruses belong to the genus Enterovirus and are considered primarily as intestinal viruses.

16. (D) Variola major produces pocks on CAM of chick embryos incubated at 39°C while Variola minor fails to produce the pocks.

17. (C) Ingestion of contaminated food is the general mode of hepatitis A infection.

18. (C) The rhinoviruses are the major etiological agents of the common cold.

19. (C) Herpes B virus, also referred to as herpesvirus simiae, is a latent virus in monkeys and is an occupational hazard to laboratory workers handling infected monkeys or contaminated monkey tissue cultures.

20. (E) A herpesvirus seems implicated in Marek's disease in chickens.

21. (D) HEp #2 cells are highly susceptible to respiratory syncytial viruses and these are therefore beneficial in isolating the viruses from laboratory specimens.

22. (B) When injected into baby hamsters, at least 12 of the 33 types of human adenoviruses were found to produce malignant carcinomas.

23. (A) Those adenoviruses which are highly oncogenic do contain a low guanine and low cytosine content in their DNA. This may be a factor contributing to the oncogenic nature of certain adenoviruses, however simian viruses are highly oncogenic and they contain a high guanine and cytosine content. This finding may lead researchers to reconsider the role of the guanine and cytosine content in oncogenicity.

24. (E) Human volunteers injected with a parvovirus demonstrated the same gastroenteritis symptoms as those associated with the Norwalk disease. Since this virus is extremely difficult to isolate sufficient evidence is lacking to link this virus to the Norwalk disease and hepatitis A. However, the viral structure and resistance to ether and chloroform are established.

25. (D) Poxviruses are structurally the most complex of the animal viruses. The DNA is surrounded by a dense dumbbell-shaped core. Dense structures called lateral bodies are contained in the core and little is known about the composition or the role of the lateral bodies.

26. (B) Identification of the smallpox virus may be obtained by treating the viruses isolated from a chick embryo with known neutralizing antiserum and by inoculating more embryos with the treated specimen. However, presumptive diagnosis may be obtained by the presence of cytoplasmic inclusions referred to as Guarnieri bodies.

27. (E) Although thousands of cases of infectious hepatitis are recorded annually, to date, the etiologic agents of this disease have not been grown in cell cultures.

28. (B) Hepatitis A is mainly contracted after drinking water which is fecally contaminated or by eating food which has been prepared by a person who may be subclinically infected. Consumption of uncooked foods harvested from fecally-contaminated waters also accounts for many cases of Hepatitis A.

29. (C) The togaviruses are arthropod-borne viruses and are the etiologic agents of yellow fever, dengue fever, eastern equine and western equine encephalitis.

30. (B) The presence of HB_sAg in the blood, urine, feces or other body fluids confirms the diagnosis of hepatitis B. Treatment of the Dane particles induces their breakdown or formation into HB_sAg and HB_cAg particles.

31. (C) The yellow fever virus is a togavirus. Since there is only one yellow fever virus strain, a single vaccine is effective against the disease.

32. (C) Eradication of the Aedes mosquito will limit and control the spread of yellow fever and dengue shock syndrome since the Aedes mosquito is the vector for both diseases.

33. (C) Three serotypes of the poliovirus have been identified.

34. (A) Patients suffering with either Hodgkins disease or with acute lymphocytic leukemia have high EB virus antibody titers. However, the EB virus does not appear to be implicated with either of these diseases.

35. (E) Echoviruses were isolated from the feces of people who demonstrated no ill effects as a result of the viruses. These viruses were once called enteric cytopathogenic human orphan viruses from which was derived the name echovirus.

36. (D) RNA viruses of the family Retroviridae cause leukemia and sarcomas in many species of animals.

37. (D) Many viruses may be etiologic agents of the common cold. However, most of the common cold viruses are now grouped and classified as rhinoviruses.

38. (A) The rotaviruses cause severe diarrhea and vomiting. The newborn and young children seem most susceptible. Death is frequently due to electrolyte loss and dehydration due to diarrhea and vomiting. The double walled capsid of these viruses gives the appearance of a wheel and thus these are referred to as rotaviruses.

39. (C) The International Committee on Viral Nomenclature classify the influenza viruses as belonging to the family Orthomyxoviridae and to the genus orthomyxovirus or the genus influenzavirus. These two genera are frequently used to designate influenza viruses.

40. (C) Although the Guillain-Barre syndrome cannot be directly connected to the swine influenza vaccine, many people did demonstrate this syndrome following inoculation with the swine influenza vaccine. More must be known about the Guillain-Barre syndrome to specifically correlate it with the swine influenza vaccine.

41. (C) The measles virus has spikes protruding from its envelope. The spikes cause cell fusion and therefore giant cells may be detected in nasal secretions. Also the Koplik spots may often be seen in the mucosa of the mouth.

42. (E) The enteroviruses are particularly resistant in sewage polluted water, even chlorinated sewage water.

43. (D) The respiratory syncytial virus (RSV) causes respiratory diseases and also causes the virus infected cells to merge to form giant multinucleated cells from which the term syncytial has been derived.

44. (B) Negri bodies are characteristically found in the cytoplasm of infected cells of rabies victims. The presence of the Negri bodies is the basis for laboratory diagnosis of rabies.

45. (E) To date the hepatitis B virus has not been isolated in tissue cultures.

46. (E) Measles is an acute and highly infectious disease which is disseminated via respiratory secretions or droplets. Since the rubeola virus replicates in the upper respiratory tract, throat swabs would provide the best results for clincial diagnosis of the etiologic agent.

47.   (C)   Urine specimens and throat swabs would be good sources to recover and isolate the cytomegalovirus since it is believed that CMV is excreted in the urine and saliva for a length of time.

48.   (D)   Mumps is the infection and inflammation of the parotid glands. A paramyxovirus is the etiologic agent of mumps and it is disseminated via respiratory secretions.

49.   (D)   Reoviruses are made of double stranded RNA. They are the only RNA viruses to be double stranded.

50.   (A)   Of the techniques indicated to detect the presence of HB_SAg, counter-immunoelectrophoresis is the fastest, but radioimmunoassay is the most sensitive and yields more satisfactory results than CF, CIEP or immunodiffusion.

51.   (C)   Currently, serologic tests provide the most accessible and reliable tool for diagnosing viral and rickettsial infections.

52.   (C)   Rhinovirus, mycoplasma, parainfluenza and Epstein-Barr cause upper respiratory tract infections and are usually isolated with throat swabs or nasal secretions.

53.   (A)   Complement fixation is the usual serological test used to identify the mycoplasmas.

54.   (A)   Hepatitis A virus (HAV) causes infectious hepatitis.

55.   (B)   Fluorescent antibody is the serological test used to identify the Epstein-Barr virus.

56.   (D)   Rubella may be isolated primarily from throat, urine or CSF specimen.

57.   (B)   The mumps virus may be isolated primarily from throat swabs and urine.

58.   Interferons protect cells from the lytic action of viruses.

59.   (D)   Serologic studies usually show the mumps vaccine to induce antibody production in more than 90% of the recipients. Since antibody production is generally correlated with protection, the mumps vaccine is considered highly effective.

60.   (C)   Cells infected with herpes simplex viruses (HSV) are giant multinucleated cells. Cowdry type A intranuclear inclusion bodies may also be found in the cells.

61.   (A)   Infection with measles (rubella) confers a lifelong immunity.

62.   (E)   Poliomyelitis (Heine-Medin disease) is caused by viruses which belongs to the genus Enterovirus.

63.   (B)   Rubeola, often referred to as the 14-day measles, is an acute and highly communicable disease. A paramyxovirus is the causative agent.

64.   (C)   Rabies (also called hydrophobia) is highly neurotropic and fatal. A rhabdovirus is the causative agent of rabies. All mammals are susceptible to viral infection.

65.   (D)   The Epstein-Barr virus is the causative agent of infectious mononucleosis. The EB virus is often associated with Burkett's lymphoma.

66.   (A)   The JC virus has been frequently removed from the brain tissue of people with progressive multifocal leukoencephalopathy (PMC). This evidence supports the fact that JCV causes PML. The JC virus (JCV) is a papovavirus.

67.   (C)   A paramyxovirus is a causative agent of the central nervous system disease referred to as subacute sclerosing panencephalitis (SSPE).

68. (B) The orthomyxovirus causes viral influenza.

69. (A) German measles or rubella is frequently clinically referred to as the three day measles. A togavirus is the causative agent.

70. (E) ELISA, is a viral detection technique.

Bibliography and Recommended Readings

Dulbecco, R. and H. Ginsberg. Virology. 1980. J. B. Lippincott. Philadelphia.

Freeman, B. A. Burrow's Textbook of Microbiology. Twenty-first Edition. 1979. W. B. Saunders Company. Philadelphia.

Koneman, E., et.al. Color Atlas and Textbook of Microbiology. Second Edition. 1983. J. B. Lippincott. Philadelphia.

Luria, S. E., Darnell, J. E., Baltimore, D. and A. Campbell. General Virology. Third Edition. 1978. John Wiley and Sons, Inc. New York.

Volk, W. A. Essentials of Medical Microbiology. Second Edition. 1982. J. B. Lippincott. Philadelphia.

CHAPTER 8

Immunology/Serology

Directions. Select the one BEST answer for each of the following statements. Circle the appropriate response on the answer sheet.

1. Placental transfer routinely occurs with:

    A. IgA   D. IgG
    B. IgD   E. IgM
    C. IgE

2. Less antigen is needed to precipitate a given amount of antibody when antigen is added in small doses than when added all at once. This is known as:

    A. Danysz phenomenon   D. Arthus phenomenon
    B. Coomb's phenomenon   E. Prozone phenomenon
    C. Oudin phenomenon

3. C-reactive protein (CRP) may be anticipated in all but one of the following conditions:

    A. rheumatic fever   D. localized infection
    B. carcinoma   E. pneumonia
    C. streptococcal infection

4. False positives may occur with the VDRL slide test in all of the following conditions except:

    A. malaria   D. tuberculosis
    B. leprosy   E. lymphogranuloma venerum
    C. disseminated lupus erythematosus

5. Which of the following statements regarding the agglutinin reaction is not true:

    A. agglutination is more sensitive than precipitation
    B. agglutination usually involves IgG
    C. agglutination antigens are part of insoluble particles
    D. agglutination requires a short reaction time
    E. agglutination requires a small volume of serum

6. The Weil-Felix reaction is useful in detecting all of the following except:

   A. epidemic typhus
   B. scrub typhus
   C. Rocky Mountain spotted fever
   D. Q fever
   E. murine typhus

7. Titers of cold agglutinins are consistently elevated in:

   A. hemolytic anemias
   B. malaria
   C. atypical viral pneumonia
   D. all of the above
   E. none of the above

8. A substance capable of specific binding with antibody but incapable of stimulating antibody formation is:

   A. hapten
   B. adjuvant
   C. opsonin
   D. reagin
   E. toxoid

9. The "prozone phenomenon" is due to:

   A. extensive antigen-antibody complex formation
   B. excess antigen
   C. blocking antibody
   D. neutralizing antibody
   E. cross reactivity

10. The immunoglobulin found in the highest concentration in normal adults is:

    A. IgG
    B. IgM
    C. IgA
    D. IgD
    E. IgE

11. The Davidsohn differential test distinguishes:

    A. Forssman antigen
    B. infectious mononucleosis
    C. serum sickness
    D. all of the above
    E. none of the above

12. The most abundant component of complement in the serum of normal adults is:

    A. C1
    B. C3
    C. C5
    D. C7
    E. C9

13. Serological pregnancy tests are designed to detect urine concentrations of:

    A. human choriogonadotrophin
    B. estrogen
    C. progesterone
    D. A and B
    E. B and C

14. The method of choice in determining immunity to rubella is the:

    A. neutralization test
    B. fluorescent antibody test
    C. complement fixation test
    D. hemagglutination inhibition test
    E. agglutination test

15. The class of 19S immunoglobulins includes:

    A. IgA   D. IgG
    B. IgD   E. IgM
    C. IgE

16. The cold agglutination titer is significant when it reaches:

    A. 1:8   D. 1:64
    B. 1:16   E. 1:128
    C. 1:32

17. Which of the following statements regarding the complement fixation test is not true?

    A. patient's serum is inactivated for 30 min. at 56°C
    B. complement is usually obtained from guinea pig serum
    C. sheep red blood cells are usually used
    D. the test reactants are usually incubated at 22°C for 30 min.
    E. red blood cells are sensitized with hemolysin

18. The hemagglutination inhibition test is used to detect antibodies against:

    A. fungi   D. amebae
    B. bacteria   E. viruses
    C. nematodes

19. Passive immunity may be achieved by using:

    A. toxoids   D. all of the above
    B. immunoglobulins   E. none of the above
    C. heat-killed bacteria

20. The components of complement are:

    A. lipids   D. mucopolysaccharides
    B. proteins   E. lipopolysaccharides
    C. carbohydrates

21. The most sensitive test available for detecting Hepatitis B surface antigens (HB$_S$Ag) and anti-HB$_S$ is:

    A. radioimmunoassay   D. rheophoresis
    B. counterelectrophoresis   E. agar gel diffusion
    C. complement fixation

22. The highest titer of streptococcus MG agglutinin considered normal is:

    A. 1:5   D. 1:40
    B. 1:10   E. 1:80
    C. 1:20

23. Rheumatoid factor is usually detected by:

    A. hemagglutination test   D. neutralization test
    B. complement fixation test   E. flocculation test
    C. passive agglutination test

24. Which of the following statements about syphilis is true?

    A. serum tests for syphilis are usually positive 1-3 weeks after the
        appearance of a chancre
    B. reagin titer increases rapidly during the primary stage of syphilis
    C. reagin is usually not detectable during the secondary stage of syphilis
    D. statements A and B
    E. statements A and C

25. The most sensitive method of detecting antibody is:

    A. hemolysis
    B. bacterial agglutination
    C. virus neutralization
    D. immunoelectrophoresis
    E. precipitation

26. Antibacterial substances normally found in sera include:

    A. complement
    B. properdin
    C. β-lysin
    D. all of the above
    E. none of the above

Directions. The column on the left contains 3 scientifically related categories while the column on the right contains 4 items which may illustrate scientific phenomena or processes. Three of the items in the column on the right relate to only one of the categories in the column on the left. FIRST, indicate the category in which the 3 processes or phenomena belong. SECOND, indicate the one process or phenomenon which is not related to that category.

Category

Phenomenon

27. A. diphtheria
    B. scarlet fever
    C. typhoid fever

28. A. Schultz-Charlton phenomenon
    B. Dick test
    C. β-hemolytic streptococcus
    D. Schick test

29. A. Oudin
    B. Ouchterlony
    C. Elek

30. A. immunodiffusion
    B. diphtheria
    C. agar
    D. electrophoresis

31. A. anaphylaxis
    B. serum sickness
    C. transfusion reactions

32. A. antibody-mediated allergic reaction
    B. hay fever
    C. asthma
    D. Arthus reaction

33. A. B cells
    B. T cells
    C. macrophages

34. A. lymphocytes
    B. cell-mediated immunity
    C. antibody secreting cells
    D. highly susceptible to inactivation by ALS

Questions 35-44

Directions. The following statements contain numbered blanks. For each numbered blank there is a corresponding set of lettered responses. Select the BEST answer from each lettered set.

Bacteria may contain poisonous substances, __35__, in their cell walls, or may release harmful substances into the surrounding medium. The latter, called __36__, may be transformed into __37__ by formalin or may be neutralized by __38__ produced by the host.

35. A. endotoxins
    B. toxoids
    C. antitoxins

    D. antiglobulins
    E. exotoxins

36. A. endotoxins
    B. antitoxins
    C. toxoids

    D. exotoxins
    E. antiglobulins

37. A. antitoxins
    B. immunogens
    C. toxoids

    D. endotoxins
    E. exotoxins

38. A. immunogens
    B. toxoids
    C. antitoxins

    D. antigens
    E. endotoxins

The complement fixation test utilizes the ability of __39__ to prevent complement from reacting with subsequently added __40__. __41__ indicates a negative complement fixation test.

39. A. antigens
    B. antibodies
    C. antigen-antibody complexes

    D. sensitized red blood cells
    E. agglutinins

40. A. reagin
    B. sensitized red blood cells
    C. fixed complement

    D. guinea pig serum
    E. immunogen

41. A. agglutination
    B. precipitation
    C. flocculation

    D. hemeadsorption
    E. hemolysis

In the precipitation reaction, the zone of antigen excess is called the __42__ and the zone of antibody excess is called the __43__. The "prozone phenomenon" can be avoided by using the __44__ test.

42. A. prozone
    B. inhibition zone
    C. equivalence zone

    D. postzone
    E. precipitation zone

43. A. prozone
    B. postzone
    C. equivalence zone

    D. precipitation zone
    E. enhancement zone

44. A. agglutination
    B. complement fixation
    C. ring

    D. flocculation
    E. neutralization

Questions 45-64

Directions. For each of the numbered words or phrases listed below, select the appropriate response as follows:

A. if the item is associated with A only
B. if the item is associated with B only
C. if the item is associated with both A and B
D. If the item is associated with neither A nor B

          A. IgG
          B. IgM

45. atopic response
46. incomplete antibodies
47. complement fixation
48. opsonization

        A. somatic antigen - O
        B. flagellar antigen - H

49. thermolabile
50. Salmonella
51. Pasteurella tularensis
52. Widal test

        A. Direct Coomb's test
        B. Indirect Coomb's test

53. detects anti-erythrocyte antibodies
54. detects cell-bound antibody
55. detects IgA
56. detects serum levels of incomplete antibody

        A. precipitation reaction
        B. agglutination reaction

57. requires complement
58. involves soluble antigen
59. involves multivalent antibody
60. nonspecific

        A. opsonin
        B. reagin

61. antigenic
62. immunoglobulins
63. increase phagocytosis
64. cytotropic

Questions 65-76

Directions. One, some or all of the responses for each of the following statements
may be correct. Indicate your response as follows:

A.   if items 1 and 3 are correct
B.   if items 2 and 4 are correct
C.   if three of the items are correct
D.   if all of the items are correct
E.   if only one of the items is correct

65. Activity associated with the C3 component of complement includes:

1.   anaphylaxis   3.   hemolysis
2.   immune adherence   4.   chemotaxis

66. All flocculation tests for syphilis require:

1.   cardiolipin   3.   inactivated T. pallidum
2.   lecithin   4.   cholesterol

67. The patient's serum should be inactivated for:

1.   VDRL test   3.   hemagglutination inhibition test
2.   Coomb's test   4.   CRP test

68. The antistreptolysin O titer will be high in:

1.   rheumatic fever   3.   glomerulonephritis
2.   typhoid fever   4.   diphtheria

69. The alternative complement pathway can be activated by:

1.   phospholipids   3.   histamine
2.   endotoxin   4.   polysaccharides

70. Passive agglutination may involve the use of:

1.   polystyrene   3.   red blood cells
2.   latex   4.   bentonite

71. Adjuvants are used to:

1.   prolong retention of antigen in the body
2.   increase the distribution of antigen in the body
3.   decrease the inflammatory response of the body to antigen
4.   decrease the hypersensitivity of the body to antigen

72. Amboceptors are:

1.   exotoxins   3.   endotoxins
2.   lysins   4.   antibodies

73. The extent of agglutination is influenced by:

    1. salt concentration   3. aggitation
    2. temperature   4. pH

74. Antibodies and antigens are bound by:

    1. hydrophobic forces   3. Van der Waals forces
    2. covalent bonds   4. Coulomb forces

75. Heat-inactivated complement may be partially reactivated by:

    1. shaking   3. bile salts
    2. fresh complement   4. standing at room temperature

76. Haptens are:

    1. antigenic
    2. capable of reacting specifically with antibody
    3. immunogenic
    4. usually lipids

Questions 77-92

Directions. For each of the numbered items select the appropriate lettered response.
Do not use the same letter more than once.

77. Schick test   A. tuberculosis
78. Dick test   B. scarlet fever
79. Kahn test   C. tularemia
80. Vollmer test   D. diphtheria
                         E. syphilis

81. Wasserman   A. neutralization test
82. VDRL   B. precipitation test
83. TPI   C. complement fixation test
84. Oudin test   D. flocculation test
                         E. hemagglutination test

85. IgA   A. produced early during bacterial
86. IgM   infection
87. IgE   B. blocking antibody
88. IgG   C. present in colostrum
                         D. nonspecific antibody
                         E. characteristic of allergic response

89. Sabin-Feldman   A. in vivo anaphylaxis
90. Prausnitz-Küstner   B. in vitro anaphylaxis
91. Schultz-Dale   C. toxoplasmosis
92. Paul-Bunnell   D. rickettsia
                         E. infectious mononucleosis

Questions 93-100

Directions. Select and circle the one BEST answer for each of the following statements utilizing the information presented in either the following graph, tracing,
table or laboratory data.

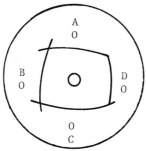

The central reservoir contains antibodies to two dissimilar antigens. One or both
antigens are present in each surrounding well.

93. Wells containing identical antigens are:

    A. A and B   D. D and A
    B. B and C   E. B and D
    C. C and D

94. Wells containing totally dissimilar antigens are:

    A. A and B   D. D and A
    B. B and C   E. A and C
    C. C and D

95. Antigens in wells B and D would react like:

    A. A and B   D. D and A
    B. B and C   E. C and A
    C. C and D

96. More than one antigen is contained in:

    A. A   D. D
    B. B   E. B and C
    C. C

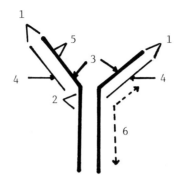

97. The part of the immunoglobulin molecule responsible for differences among classes is:

    A. 1   D. 4
    B. 2   E. 6
    C. 3

98. The region of the immunoglobulin molecule responsible for activating complement is:

    A. 1   D. 4
    B. 2   E. 5
    C. 3

99. The region of the immunoglobulin molecule which binds antigen is:

    A. 1   D. 4
    B. 2   E. 6
    C. 3

100. The constant or polymerizing region of the immunoglobulin molecule is:

    A. 1   D. 5
    B. 3   E. 6
    C. 4

Questions 101-125

Directions. Select the one BEST answer for each of the following statements. Circle the appropriate response on the answer sheet.

101. Which of the following is a synonym for IgE?

    A. hapten   C. opsonin
    B. adjuvant   D. reagin

102. A substance which enhances an antibody-antigen reaction is called a(n):

    A. hapten   C. reagin
    B. adjuvant   D. toxoid

103. An immunoglobulin that may occur in a wide variety of forms (monomers, dimers etc.) is:

    A. IgA
    B. IgE
    C. IgD
    D. IgG

104. A substance which is capable of rendering immunity without harming the patient is:

    A. reagin
    B. opsonin
    C. toxoid
    D. adjuvant

105. Penicillin is a typical example of which of the following?

    A. reagin
    B. opsonin
    C. toxoid
    D. hapten

106. Which of the following Complement components requires calcium ions to maintain its stability?

    A. C1
    B. C42
    C. C3
    D. C5a

107. Which of the following types of rosette formation is typical of T-lymphocytes?

    A. E rosettes
    B. EA rosettes
    C. EAC rosettes
    D. none of the above

108. The immunoglobulin that is most frequently found in agglutination reactions is:

    A. IgG
    B. IgM
    C. IgE
    D. IgA

109. The immunoglobulin most frequently encountered in secretions, such as tears and breast milk, is:

    A. IgG
    B. IgM
    C. IgE
    D. IgA

110. According to the Gell and Coombs classification of hypersensitivity, which of the following is predominantly mediated by IgE?

    A. anaphylactic or immediate type hypersensitivity
    B. cytotoxic type hypersensitivity
    C. immune complex type hypersensitivity
    D. cell mediated type hypersensitivity

111. The transplantation of immunocompetent lymphocytes into an immunoincompetent person is known as:

    A. nonsusceptibility
    B. active immunity
    C. passive immunity
    D. adoptive immunity

112. Which of the following is NOT true concerning cell mediated hypersensitivity?

    A. mediated by T-cells and macrophages
    B. important in immunity against viruses
    C. specific for large molecules
    D. evolves rapidly after a primary challenge

113. Which of the following immunoglobulins activates the alternative (Properdin) complement pathway?

    A. IgG   C. IgA
    B. IgM   D. IgE

114. Which of the following subclasses if IgG does not fix complement?

    A. IgG1   C. IgG3
    B. IgG2   D. IgG4

115. Which of the following immunoglobulins is most frequently found bound to mast cells?

    A. IgA   C. IgD
    B. IgE   D. IgM

116. In Waldenstrom's macroglobulinemia, which of the following immunoglobulins is found in excess?

    A. IgA   C. IgD
    B. IgG   D. IgM

117. Which of the following procedures is used for the detection of specific IgE?

    A. crossed immunoelectrophoresis   C. RAST (radioallergosorbent test)
    B. RIST (radioimmunosorbent test)   D. rocket immunoelectrophoresis

118. Chemiluminescence is a procedure used for which of the following?

    A. measurement of chemotaxis
    B. measurement rate of phagocytic ingestion
    C. measurement of metabolic burst
    D. measurement of particle ingestion

119. Which of the following is considered to be a major chemotactic factor?

    A. actin binding globulin   C. lactoferrin
    B. C5a   D. nitroblue tetrazolium

120. In phagocytosis, which of the following is NOT involved in protecting the cell?

    A. myeloperoxidase   C. catalase
    B. superoxide dismutase   D. the glutathione system

121. The test used for the detection of cell bound IgG is:

    A. direct antiglobulin test   C. nitroblue tetrazolium test
    B. indirect antiglobulin test   D. Ouchterlony double diffusion test

122. Precipitation tests use which of the following?

    A. antigens bound to red cells
    B. antigens bound to bentonite particles
    C. antigens bound to latex particles
    D. soluble antigens

123. Which of the following immunglobulins, in normal individuals, is found in the lowest concentrations?

    A. IgA   C. IgD
    B. IgG   D. IgE

124. In the evaluation of drug induced autoimmune anemias, which of the following procedures is of greatest value?

    A. indirect antiglobulin test   C. complement fixation test
    B. direct antiglobulin test   D. Boyden chamber

125. In phagocytosis, which of the following is NOT involved in metabolic stimulation and killing?

    A. catalase   C. singlet oxygen
    B. hydrogen peroxide   D. hydroxyl radicals

Questions 126-150

Directions. For each of the following numbered words or phrases listed below, select the appropriate response as follows:

A. if the item is associated with A only
B. if the item is associated with B only
C. if the item is associated with both A and B
D. if the item is associated with neither A nor B

                        A. decreased C3
                        B. decreased C4

126. coagulation associated Complement consumption
127. active systemic lupus erythematosus
128. acute glomerulonephritis
129. immune complex disease
130. hereditary angioedema

                        A. J chain
                        B. kappa chains

131. IgM molecules
132. IgG molecules
133. IgA molecules
134. gamma markers
135. Km markers

    A.   increased serum IgG
    B.   increased serum IgM

136. light chain disease
137. nephrotic syndrome
138. IgG myeloma
139. IgM myeloma
140. actinomycosis

    A.   systemic lupus erythematosus
    B.   rheumatoid arthritis

141. antinuclear antibody present
142. rheumatoid factor present
143. positive LE-prep
144. anti-smooth muscle antibody
145. high concentration of anti-native DNA

    A.   found normally in a monomeric form
    B.   found normally in a polymeric form

146. IgA
147. IgD
148. IgE
149. IgG
150. IgM

Explanatory Answers

1. (D) IgG is capable of crossing the placenta because it is a monomer, the smallest antibody.

2. (A) This is known as the Danysz phenomenon.

3. (D) CRP is an indicator of inflammation and is found in illnesses accompanied by inflammation and tissue breakdown.

4. (D) All of the conditions listed may give false positives with the VDRL test with the exception of tuberculosis.

5. (B) IgG is monomeric and does not agglutinate well. IgM is characteristic of agglutination reactions.

6. (D) The Weil-Felix test is used to detect rickettsial disease, with the exception of Q fever.

7. (C) Cold agglutinins may be elevated in all conditions listed, but are consistently elevated in atypical viral pneumonia.

8. (A) Haptens will only stimulate antibody production when they are attached to larger molecules.

9. (C) The "prozone phenomenon" results from an excess of antibody or blocking antibody such that each antigen is saturated with antibody, and the lattice required for precipitation fails to form.

10. (A) IgG constitutes almost 80% of the total circulating antibodies in the normal adult.

11. (D) The Davidsohn differential test distinguishes between types of heterophil antibody on the basis of absorption patterns using guinea pig kidney cells and beef erythrocytes.

12. (B) C3 is the most abundant component of complement in normal serum, possibly in part due to the fact that properdin helps to stabilize C3.

13. (A) Serological pregnancy tests detect HCG in the urine.

14. (D) Hemagglutination inhibiting antibody persists for years after exposure to rubella and therefore is the best antibody to test for.

15. (E) IgM is the largest immunoglobulin; all of the other classes of immunoglobulins sediment between 6-12S.

16. (C) Cold agglutination titer is considered normal at 1:16 and less.

17. (D) The reactants are usually incubated at 37°C for 30 min.

18. (E) Certain viral infections result in viral antigens being inserted into the membranes of infected cells. The antigens cause hemagglutination of certain red blood cells. HAI can be used to determine the immune status of individuals against these viruses.

19. (B) Toxoids and heat-killed bacteria are used to stimulate active antibody production.

20. (B) Complement is a group of 11 serum proteins.

21. (A) Radioimmunoassay is the most sensitive test for HB_SAg and anti-HB_S; the most widely used types are solid phase and radioimmunoprecipitation.

22. (B) Titers of streptococcus MG agglutinin higher than 1:10 are not considered normal.

23. (C) Particulate carriers are usually used to provide an agglutination reaction between rheumatoid antigen and IgG.

24. (D) The reagin titer rises rapidly during the primary stage of syphilis and remains elevated for about 6 months.

25. (C) Virus neutralization can detect antibodies in concentrations as low as 10^{-5} µg per ml or less; the other tests listed have a sensitivity limit of 10^{-3} µg per ml or less.

26. (D) All substances listed are proteins found in normal serum.

27. (B) Scarlet fever is caused by β-hemolytic streptococcus; the Dick test detects susceptibility to scarlet fever; the Shultz-Charlton phenomenon detects the presence of scarlet fever in a patient.

28. (D) The Schick test is for diphtheria.

29. (C) Elek's diffusion test is a modification of the agar diffusion test of Ouchterlony. It is used to determine the toxigenicity of strains of diphtheria.

30. (D) None of the methods listed utilize electrophoresis.

31. (A) All reaction types listed are antibody-mediated. Hayfever and asthma are anaphylactic reactions.

32. (B) Arthus reaction is a serum sickness.

33. (B) T-cells are lymphocytes involved in cell-mediated immunity. They are highly susceptible to inactivation by ALS.

34. (C) B cells secrete antibody.

35. (A) Endotoxins are contained in the cell bodies of bacteria and are only given off after the bacterium dies.

36. (D) Exotoxins are soluble toxins released by bacteria into the surrounding medium.

37. (C) Toxoids may be produced by formalin treatment of exotoxins; they are antigenic, but have lost their toxicity.

38. (C) Antibodies produced in response to toxins are called antitoxins.

39. (C) Antigen-antibody complexes fix complement so that it is not free to lyse subsequently added sensitized red blood cells.

40. (B) Sensitized red blood cells will be lysed by any free complement.

41. (E) If complement has not been fixed by antibody-antigen complexes in the initial step of the complement fixation test, then free complement lyses sensitized red blood cells in the second step.

42. (D) The zone of antigen excess is called the postzone.

43. (A) The zone of antibody excess is called the prozone.

44. (C)   The ring test is usually performed by layering antigen on antiserum in a test tube. Diffusion results in an area of optimal antigen-antibody concentration resulting in a ring of precipitation.

45. (D)   Atopy is associated with IgE.

46. (A)   Certain antibodies are incapable of agglutination because their length is insufficient to build antibody bridges between molecules. These are incomplete antibodies, members of the class IgG.

47. (C)   Both immunoglobulins are capable of fixing complement.

48. (C)   Both immunoglobulins are capable of opsonization.

49. (B)   Somatic antigen is heat stable.

50. (C)   Salmonella contains both O and H antigens.

51. (A)   Tularemia is detected by its somatic, O, antigen; it does not contain H antigen.

52. (C)   The Widal test is for typhoid fever; it detects both O and H antigens.

53. (C)   The purpose of the Coomb's test is to detect non-agglutinating anti-erythrocyte antibodies.

54. (A)   The direct Coomb's test detects incomplete antibody bound to erythrocytes.

55. (D)   Neither test detects IgA; incomplete antibodies belong to the class, IgG.

56. (B)   The indirect Coomb's test involves _in vitro_ sensitization of test cells with patient's serum, to detect the presence of incomplete antibody.

57. (D)   Neither reaction requires complement.

58. (A)   Insoluble antigen when reacted with antibody results in agglutination.

59. (C)   Both reactions require a valence greater than 1.

60. (D)   All antibody-antigen reactions are specific.

61. (C)   Since both are proteins, each is capable of inducing antibody formation in organisms other than the one in which it was produced.

62. (C)   Both opsonin and reagin are immunoglobulins.

63. (A)   Opsonins are antibodies which react with surface antigens of bacteria, making them more susceptible to phagocytosis.

64. (C)   Reagin is homocytotropic, and opsonin is bacteriotropic.

65. (C)   Anaphylaxis, immune adherence and chemotaxis are associated with C3; hemolysis is associated with C8 and C9.

66. (C)   Cardiolipin, lecithin and cholesterol are all reagents in the flocculation tests for reagin, an antibody produced upon exposure to T. pallidum.

67. (E)   The patient's serum should be inactivated for the VDRL test by heating for 30 min. at 56°C.

68. (A)   Streptolysin O is produced by Streptococcus pyogenes; the measurement of anti-streptolysin O is a reliable indicator of such streptococcal infections as rheumatic fever and glomerulonephritis.

69. (B)   Certain bacterial endotoxins and polysaccharides can activate the complement system by bypassing components C1, C2 and C4.

70.   (D)   All are large, insoluble particles to which antigens may be attached to achieve passive agglutination.

71.   (E)   Adjuvants are used to prolong the retention of antigen and thereby increase the amount and duration of antibody production.

72.   (B)   Amboceptors are antibodies with lytic properties usually requiring the presence of complement.

73.   (D)   Changes in any of the physical parameters listed will result in a change in the extent of the agglutination reaction.

74.   (C)   Antibody-antigen complexes are held together by weak, non-specific forces, hydrophobic, Van der Waals, and Coulomb, not by covalent bonds.

75.   (B)   Aggitation and bile salts inactivate complement.

76.   (E)   Haptens are incapable of independently eliciting an antibody response, but are capable of reacting specifically with antibody. Haptens are most often protein.

77.   (D)   The Schick test is a skin test for immunity to diphtheria toxin.

78.   (B)   The Dick test is a skin test for immunity to scarlet fever toxin.

79.   (E)   The Kahn test is a flocculation test for reagin, produced during syphilis infection.

80.   (A)   The Vollmer test is a skin test for tuberculin immunity.

81.   (C)   The Wasserman test for syphilis is a complement fixation test.

82.   (D)   The VDRL screening test for syphilis is a flocculation test in which the nonspecific protein reagin reacts with antigen containing cardiolipin and lecithin.

83.   (A)   TPI - Treponema pallidum inhibition is a test in which the activity of T. pallidum spirochetes is inhibited in the presence of specific antibody.

84.   (B)   The Oudin test is for precipitation antibodies performed using agar gels.

85.   (C)   IgA, produced by secretory cells, is present in colostrum.

86.   (A)   IgM is the first class of antibody produced during bacterial infection.

87.   (E)   IgE has skin-sensitizing properties and is responsible for a number of allergic reactions.

88.   (B)   Blocking antibodies belong to the class, IgG.

89.   (C)   Sabin-Feldman is a dye test in which neutralizing antibodies prevent the uptake of methylene blue by toxoplasma.

90.   (A)   Prausnitz-Küstner- is an intradermal test for measuring anaphylactic hypersensitivity.

91.   (B)   Schultz-Dale test is an _in vitro_ test for anaphylaxis.

92.   (E)   Paul-Bunnell test is an agglutination test for heterphil antibody produced during infectious mononucleosis.

93.   (D)   The fused precipitation band between A and D is characteristic of reactions of identity.

94.   (A)   When antigens are totally dissimilar, precipitation bands are independent of one another and therefore cross.

95.   (A)   Since A is identical to D, B would react with D exactly as it does with A.

96.   (C)   The antigen in C is partially
identical to both B and D. B and
D are not identical. Therefore, C
must contain more than one antigen.

97.   (C)   The heavy chains are responsible for class distinctions.

98.   (B)   The complement activating
region of the immunoglobulin
molecule is located in the middle
of the heavy chain.

99.   (A)   The amino terminal is where
immunoglobulins bind antigens.

100.   (E)   The majority of the immunoglobulin is constant, starting with
the carboxyl terminal.

101.   (D)   The term reagin is used
synonymously with IgE.

102.   (B)   An adjuvant is a substance
that enhances or improves an
immune response.

103.   (A)   IgA antibodies may be found
as monomers, dimers, or multimers.
IgG, IgD, and IgE antibodies are
normally found only as monomers.

104.   (C)   Toxoids are, essentially,
toxins that have been rendered
harmless or avirulent. Although
they are considered harmless, they
are capable of eliciting an immune
response, thereby providing the
individual with immunity without
harming him/her.

105.   (D)   Penicillin is a typical hapten.
Haptens are molecules which cannot
elicit an immune response by themselves, however, when they are
coupled to a larger carrier
molecule, they are capable of acting as immunogens.

106.   (A)   The complement component Cl,
which is made up of Clq, Clr, and
Cls is dependent on the presence
of calcium ions for its formation.

107.   (A)   E rosettes are characteristically formed by T-lymphocytes.
When T-lymphocytes are incubated
with sheep red blood cells, the
receptors on the T-lymphocytes
bind the red cells forming rosettes.
EA rosettes and EAC rosettes are
formed by B-lymphocytes.

108.   (B)   The antibody most frequently
encountered in agglutination
reactions are IgM molecules.

109.   (D)   The immunoglobulin most
frequently encountered in secretions is IgA. Not all IgA molecules are found in secretions,
since they must have the requisit
secretor fragment which is not
found on all IgA molecules.

110.   (A)   According to the Gell and
Coombs classification of hypersensitivities, the anaphylactic
or immediate type hypersensitivities are mediated by IgE. The
cytotoxic type hypersensitivities
are mediated by antigen-antibody-
complement, the immune complex
type hypersensitivities are
mediated by antigen-antibody complexes, and the cell mediated type
hypersensitivities are mediated
by sensitized T-lymphocytes.

111.   (D)   Adoptive immunity, which is
still considered to be experimental, consists of the transplantation of immunocompetent cells,
lymphocytes, into an immunoincompetent individual in an attempt
to provide the individual with
a proper immune response.

112.   (D)   Cell mediated immunity is
mediated by T-lymphocytes and
macrophages, is important in
immunity against various bacteria,
fungi and viruses, is specific
for large molecules, but is not
rapidly evolving. After a secondary challenge, cell mediated
immunity requires 24 to 48 hours
to evolve.

113. (C) Aggregated IgA activites the alternative (Properdin) pathway.

114. (D) IgG4 does not fix Complement in the classical complement pathway, all of the other isotypes of IgG do fix Complement.

115. (B) IgE, which is associated with immediate type hypersensitivity reactions is most frequently found bound to mast cells.

116. (D) Waldenstrom's macroglobulinemia is the result of an IgM producing tumor.

117. (C) The test of choice for specific IgE is the RAST (radioallergosorbent test). RIST measures total IgE while RAST measures specific IgE.

118. (C) Chemiluminescence is a testing procedure that measures the ability of the excited, singlet, oxygen to produce light as it comes back to ground state and is a measurement of the metabolic burst in phagocytosis.

119. (B) C5a, a Complement fraction, is considered to be the primary chemotactic factor in the immunologic response to infection.

120. (A) Myeloperoxidase is a major source of the production of singlet oxygen, which is involved in the killing process of phagocytosis. Superoxide dismutase, catalase, and the glutathione system are involved in the overall protection of the cell from the killing activities utilized in phagocytosis.

121. (A) The direct antiglobulin test, or, direct Coomb's test, is utilized for the detection of cell bound IgG. The indirect antiglobulin test is utilized for the detection of circulating antibody, the nitro-blue tetrazolium test is utilized for the measurement of metabolic burst associated with phagocytosis, and the Ouchterlony double diffusion test is utilized for the detection and/or identification of soluble antigens and antibodies.

122. (D) Precipitation test employ soluble antigens and antibodies. All of the other choices are utilized in agglutination techniques.

123. (C) IgD, about which little is known, is the immunoglobulin found in lowest concentrations in normal individuals.

124. (B) In the evaluation of auto-immune anemias, which are drug induced, the direct antiglobulin test is the most useful of tests listed in response to this question. The antiglobulin test measures the presence of cell bound antibody.

125. (A) Catalase is utilized by the cell as a protective mechanism to prevent the cell from being destroyed by the hydrogen peroxide produced as a killing mechanism. Singlet oxygen, hydrogen peroxide and hydroxyl radicals are all potent killing products produced as the result of the phagocytosis of a foreign particle.

126. (D) In coagulation associated Complement consumption, both the C3 and C4 levels are normal.

127. (C) In active systemic lupus erythematosus, both the C3 and the C4 levels will be decreased.

128. (A) In post-streptococcal acute glomerulonephritis, the C3 level will be decreased while the C4 level will remain normal.

129. (C) In immune complex diseases both the C3 and C4 levels will be decreased.

130. (B) In hereditary angioedema, the C3 level will remain normal while the C4 level will decrease.

131. (C) IgM molecules have both J chains and kappa light chains.

132. (B) IgG molecules may have kappa light chains, but, they do not have a J chain.

133. (C) IgA molecules may have both a J chain and kappa light chains.

134. (D) Gamma markers are allotypic determinants on gamma heavy chains and have nothing to do with J chains or kappa light chains.

135. (B) Km markers are allotypic determinants on kappa chains and have nothing to do with J chains.

136. (D) In light chain disease, neither the serum IgG nor the serum IgM levels will be increased. In light chain disease, the levels of both IgG and IgM will either be normal or markedly decreased.

137. (D) In nephrotic syndrome, as in the previous case of light chain disease, the levels of IgG and IgM will be normal or decreased, but will not be elevated.

138. (A) In a case of IgG type myeloma, the IgG level will be increased, while the IgM, and probably other immunoglobulins, will be decreased.

139. (B) In a case of IgM type myeloma, the IgG level will be decreased, while the IgM levels will be markedly elevated.

140. (D) In cases of actinomycosis, neither IgG nor IgM levels will be increased, rather, they will both be normal.

141. (C) In cases of systemic lupus erythematosus and in cases of rheumatoid arthritis, anti-nuclear antibodies may be found. While they are more commonly associated with SLE, approximately 30% of patients having rheumatoid arthritis will have a positive ANA.

142. (C) While more commonly associated with rheumatoid arthritis, the rheumatoid factor may be found in approximately 20 to 30% of patients having SLE.

143. (C) Once again, even though this procedure is commonly associated with SLE patients, it may be positive in patients with rheumatoid arthritis as well.

144. (D) Neither SLE nor RA patients will have an anti-smooth-muscle antibody, unless they also have some concurrent liver problem.

145. (A) High concentrations of anti-native (double stranded) DNA are associated with patients having active lupus erythematosus.

146. (C) IgA molecules are found in monomeric, dimeric or polymeric forms.

147. (A) IgD is found in a monomeric form.

148. (A) IgE is found in a monomeric form.

149. (A) IgG is found in a monomeric form.

150. (B) IgM is normally found in a polymeric form. IgM is normally a pentamer, however, in IgM myelomas, monomers of IgM, or IgM heavy chains alone, may be found.

Bibliography and Recommended Readings

Bach, Jean-Francoise. Immunology. 1982. John Wiley and Sons., Inc. New York.

Belanti, J. Immunology II. 1978. W. B. Saunders Company. Philadelphia.

Cooper, E. L. General Immunology. 1982. Pergamon Press, Inc. Elemsford, New York.

Eisen, H. N. Immunology. Second Edition. 1980. J. B. Lippincott Company. Philadelphia.

Fudenberg, H. H., et. al. (Editors). Basic and Clinical Immunology. Third Edition. 1980. Lange Medical Publications. Los Altos, California.

Hudson, L. and F. C. Hay. Practical Immunology. Second Edition. 1981. The C. V. Mosby Company. St. Louis.

Kimball, J. W. Introduction to Immunology. 1983. Macmillan Publishing Company. New York.

Myrvik, W. N. and R. S. Weiser. Fundamentals of Immunology. 1983. Lea and Febiger. Philadelphia.

Peacock, J. E. and R. H. Tomar. Manual of Laboratory Immunology. 1980. Lea and Febiger. Philadelphia.

Roitt, I. M. Essential Immunology. 1981. The C. V. Mosby Company. St. Louis.

Rose, N. and P. E. Bigazzi. Methods in Immunodiagnosis. Second Edition. 1980. John Wiley and Sons., Inc. New York.

Rose, N. R. and H. Friedman (Editors). Manual of Clinical Immunology. Second Edition. 1980. American Society for Microbiology. Washington, D. C.

CHAPTER 9

Immunohematology

Directions. Select the one BEST answer for each of the following statements. Circle the appropriate response on the answer sheet.

1. Which of the following is the usual order of reactivity with anti-H?

   A. $O > A_2 > A_2B > A_1 > A_1B$
   B. $O > A_1 > A_1B > A_2 > A_2B$
   C. $A_1B > A_1 > A_2B > A_2 > O$
   D. $A_2B > A_2 > A_1B > A_1 > O$

2. Which of the following blood types may be the result of the union of two AB parents?

   A. A, B, and AB
   B. A and B only

   C. AB only
   D. A and AB only

3. A patient was typed for ABO blood group and the following results were obtained:

   Forward Grouping
   Anti-A   Anti-B   Anti-AB
    Pos.   Neg.   Pos.

   Reverse Grouping
   A_1 Cells   B Cells
    Pos.   Pos.

   Which of the following is the most probable reasons for these results?

   A. the patient is blood group O, the forward typing sera is contaminated
   B. the patient is blood group A_1, the A_1 cells are contaminated
   C. the patient is blood group A_2 with an anti-A_1 antibody
   D. the patient is an A_1B, the forward typing sera is contaminated

4. The serum of patients with group AB blood normally contains which of the following?

   A. only anti-A
   B. only anti-B
   C. both anti-A and anti-B
   D. neither anti-A nor anti-B

5. A person who is typed in the Rh grouping system is classified in the Fisher-Race nomenclature as dce; the Weiner nomenclature would be:

   A. Rh_1 C. rh
   B. Rh_2 D. rh"

6. In the Duffy blood group system, which of the following is true?

   A. Fy^a genes are dominant

   B. Fy^b genes are dominant

   C. Fy^a genes are recessive

   D. Fy^a and Fy^b genes are codominant

7. The Duffy blood group system gene appears to be on the same chromosome as the genes of which of the following blood group systems?

   A. ABO blood group system   C. Kell blood group system
   B. Rh blood group system   D. Kidd blood group system

8. The MNS_s blood group system was discovered by:

   A. Landsteiner and Levine
   B. Coombs, Mourant and Race
   C. Landsteiner and Weiner
   D. Levine and Stetson

9. Anti-s antibody is usually which of the following types of immunoglobulin?

   A. IgG   C. IgD
   B. IgM   D. IgA

10. Which of the following is a cold reacting antibody?

    A. anti-A   C. $anti-P_1$
    B. anti-Rh   D. anti-Kell

11. The blood component of choice for hemophilic patients is:

    A. cryoprecipitate   C. packed red blood cells
    B. serum albumin (5%)   D. platelet concentrates

12. Which of the following lectins is used for the detection of T cells?

    A. Dolichas bifloris   C. Iberis amara
    B. Vicia graminae   D. Arachis hypogea

13. In the process of deglycerolizing thawed red blood cells, the first wash is done with 50% dextrose solution. What is the reason for using a 50% dextrose solution?

    A. to increase the ionic strength of the solution
    B. to increase the pH of the blood
    C. to crenate the red blood cells
    D. none of the above

14. Which of the following proteolytic enzymes is NOT derived from plants?

    A. bromelin
    B. ficin
    C. pepsin
    D. trypsin

15. Which of the following antibodies is inactivated or destroyed by enzyme treatment?

    A. anti-Jk^a
    B. anti-I
    C. anti-M
    D. anti-P_1

Questions 16-25

Directions. One, some or all of the responses for each of the following statements may be correct. Indicate your response as follows:

A. if items 1 and 3 are correct
B. if items 2 and 4 are correct
C. if three of the items are correct
D. if all of the items are correct
E. if only one of the items is correct

16. The antibody anti-Le^a is which of the following?

    1. usually IgM
    2. able to bind complement
    3. occurs in people with the phenotype Le(a⁻B⁻)
    4. reacts with approximately 50% of the adult population

17. Which of the following substances will NOT be found in the saliva of a person with blood group B?

    1. A substance
    2. B substance
    3. O substance
    4. H substance

18. Which of the following could result in erroneous results in ABO blood grouping?

    1. recent transfusion of blood of another ABO blood group
    2. chimeras
    3. acute leukemia
    4. Tn cells

19. If two homozygous A adults were to have offspring, what blood types might those offspring be?

    1. A
    2. B
    3. O
    4. AB

20. A technologist believes that he is dealing with a patient who has a subgroup of A_1 or an A variant. He has narrowed the probabilities down to A_m and A_x. Which of the following tests will tell him which of the variants of A his patient has?

    1. patient's cells, with anti-A
    2. patient's cells, with anti-B
    3. patient's serum, with A_1 cells
    4. patient's serum, with B cells

21. Which of the following cold agglutinins are considered to be isoagglutinins?

    1. anti-M
    2. anti-P_1
    3. anti-Le^a
    4. anti-H

22. Which of the following drugs are known to cause incompatibilities in the major crossmatch?

    1. L-dopa
    2. keflin
    3. penicillin
    4. lasix

23. Which of the following may produce false negative Coombs tests?

    1. inadequate washing procedure
    2. cell suspensions
    3. inactive antiglobulin serum
    4. under centrifugation

24. Which of the following may result in a false positive Coombs test?

    1. Wharton's jelly
    2. aldomet
    3. over centrifugation
    4. under centrifugation

25. What are the probable blood types of the union of two people who have the following blood groups:

    mother: heterozygous group A
    father: heterozygous group B

    1. group A
    2. group B
    3. group O
    4. group AB

Questions 26-44

Directions. Select the one BEST answer for each of the following statements. Circle the appropriate response on the answer sheet.

26. What is the correct sequence of attachment of complement factors to the sensitized red blood cell?

    A. C_1, C_2, C_3, C_4
    B. C_1, C_4, C_2, C_3
    C. C_1, C_3, C_2, C_4
    D. C_1, C_4, C_3, C_2

27. The basic antibody unit is composed of four polypeptide chains, two light chains and two heavy chains. Immunoglobulins of the IgM class have which of the following types of heavy chains?

    A. alpha chains
    B. gamma chains
    C. delta chains
    D. mu chains

28. The major crossmatch utilizes:

    A. the patient's serum and the donor's cells
    B. the patient's cells and the donor's serum
    C. both of the above
    D. neither of the above

29. Why can't the IgM type of antibody cross the placental barrier?

    A. it is too big
    B. the Fc portion of the antibody is bound
    C. both of the above
    D. neither of the above

30. Cellano is the name given to which of the following antigens?

    A. C   C. K
    B. c   D. k

31. The antigens Js^a and Js^b belong to which of the following blood group systems?

    A. Kidd   C. Jensen
    B. Kell   D. Jobbins

32. Which of the following antigens will NOT cause hemolytic disease of the newborn?

    A. Kell (K)   C. Rh (D)
    B. Kidd (Jk^a)   D. Lewis (Le^a)

33. Copper sulfate solutions are often used to screen the hemoglobin concentration of prospective donors. What is the specific gravity of the copper sulfate solution used to screen potential male donors?

    A. 1.035   C. 1.055
    B. 1.045   D. 1.065

34. The usual interval between blood donations is:

    A. 4 weeks   C. 12 weeks
    B. 8 weeks   D. 16 weeks

35. The proper temperature for the performance of the tube test anti-Rho (D) test is:

    A. 4°C   C. 37°C
    B. 18°C   D. 56°C

36. A crossmatch will provide which of the following?

    A. detect all errors in ABO grouping
    B. prevent immunization of the recipient
    C. detect Rh typing errors
    D. detect some ABO errors in grouping

37. According to Landsteiner's Law:

    A. antibodies are present in plasma only when the corresponding antigen is not present on the erythrocytes
    B. antibodies are present in plasma only when the corresponding antigen is present on the erythrocytes
    C. both A and B
    D. neither A nor B

38. Antigens of A, B, and H cannot be demonstrated on the red blood cells of:

    A. chimeras   C. AB individuals
    B. Oh individuals   D. Rh negative individuals

39. Which of the following would produce a positive saline crossmatch?

    A. Rouleaux formation   C. both A and B
    B. cold agglutinins   D. neither A nor B

40. The symbol used to indicate the Duffy blood group is:

    A. D^u C. Fy
    B. D   D. Js

41. Which of the following is commonly known as an incomplete antibody?

    A. IgG   C. both A and B
    B. IgM   D. neither A nor B

42. Which of the following is the reason for the 21 day outdate on stored blood?

    A. the anticoagulent deteriorated
    B. the blood is easily contaminated after 21 days
    C. the blood bank would rather use it for components
    D. less than 70% of the red cells will be viable

43. Why aren't reverse blood groupings reliable on serum from newborn infants?

    A. because Wharton's jelly interferes
    B. because the infant's antibodies are not well developed
    C. because antigens of the infant are ill defined
    D. because the I antigen interferes with the reaction

44. Which of the following antigens is considered to be a sex linked antigen?

    A. Yt^a C. S^b
    B. Xg^a D. Di^a

Questions 45-52

Directions. The column on the left contains 3 scientifically related categories while the column on the right contains 4 items which may illustrate scientific phenomena or processes. Three of the items in the column on the right relate to only one of the categories in the column on the left. FIRST, indicate the category in which the 3 processes or phenomena belong. SECOND, indicate the one process or phenomena which is not related to that category.

Category

Phenomenon

45. A. IgA
     B. IgG
     C. IgM

46. A. placental transfer
     B. hemolysis in vitro
     C. optimum temperature 37°C
     D. primary reponse

47. A. anti-Le^a
     B. anti-K
     C. anti-D

48. A. naturally occurring
     B. usually IgM
     C. originally called anti-X
     D. lele phenotype

49. A. T activated cells
     B. Tn activated cells
     C. cad polyagglutination

50. A. polybrene test negative
     B. Arachis hypogea positive
     C. anti-A lectin negative
     D. inherited characteristic

51. A. anti-I
     B. anti-i
     C. anti-H

52. A. enhanced with enzymes
     B. reacts with cord cells
     C. reacts with all rbc's
     D. reacts weakly or not at all
          with adult O cells

Questions 53-76

Directions. For each of the numbered items select the appropriate lettered response. Do not use the same letter more than once.

53. positive direct Coombs
54. **rouleaux** formation
55. albumin crossmatch
56. erythroblastosis fetalis

A. dispersed by adding saline
B. most commonly associated with anti-D
C. associated with anti-Le^a
D. detects most IgG antibodies
E. associated with acquired hemolytic anemia

57. Group A blood
58. Group B blood
59. Group AB blood
60. Group O blood

A. serum contains anti-A
B. serum contains anti-O
C. serum contains anti-B
D. serum contains anti-A and anti-B
E. serum contains no antibodies

61. Kell system
62. ABO system
63. Duffy system
64. Rh system

A. anti-H
B. Weiner nomenclature
C. Sutter antigen
D. most common phenotype is Jk (a$^+$b$^+$)
E. appears to be on the same gene as the Rh system

65. Rh$_o$
66. rh'
67. hr"
68. hr'

A. C
B. D
C. c
D. E
E. e

69. CPD
70. ACD
71. EDTA
72. Heparin

A. strong chelating agent
B. better post-transfusion survival of cells
C. neutralizes thrombin
D. coagulates blood
E. 2,3-DPG less than 10% after 2 weeks

73. saline agglutination 22°C
74. albumin agglutinations 4°C
75. enzyme agglutinations
76. all techniques and temperatures

A. anti-Jk^a
B. anti-P$_1$
C. anti-A$_1$
D. anti-p^k
E. anti-D

Questions 77-78

Directions. One, some or all of the responses for each of the following statements may be correct. Indicate your response as follows:

A. if items 1 and 3 are correct
B. if items 2 and 4 are correct
C. if three of the items are correct
D. if all of the items are correct
E. if only one of the items is correct

77. Cells that are coated with antibody in vivo are found in which of the following instances?

    1. hemolytic disease of the newborn
    2. autoimmune hemolytic anemia
    3. incompatible transfused blood
    4. enhancement of subgroups of A

78. Which of the following are reasons for rejections of a potential donor?

    1. ear piercing   3. tattoos
    2. birth control pill   4. vitamins

Questions 79-93

Directions. For each of the numbered words or phrases listed below, select the appropriate response as follows:

A. if the item is associated with A only
B. if the item is associated with B only
C. if the item is associated with both A and B
D. if the item is associated with neither A nor B

A. plasma protein fraction
B. fresh frozen plasma

79. used as a plasma volume expander
80. used in factor IX deficiencies
81. used in thrombocytopenia

A. T activated cells
B. Tn activated cells

82. activated in vivo and in vitro
83. have reduced electrophoretic mobility
84. permanent condition

A. low glycerol method for freezing red cells
B. high glycerol method for freezing red cells

85. fast freezing required
86. maintained at -196°C
87. maintained at temperatures below -65°C

A. Rouleaux formation
B. mixed field agglutination

88. associated with multiple myeloma
89. associated with "acquired B"
90. associated with Tn activated cells

A. causes hemolytic reactions in vitro
B. causes agglutination reactions in vitro

91. Kell antibodies in saline at 22°C
92. Rh antibodies in saline at 22°C
93. M antibodies in saline at 22°C

Questions 94-106

Directions. Select the one BEST answer for each of the following statements. Circle the appropriate response on the answer sheet.

94. Which of the following is the recommended concentration of red blood cells for crossmatching?

    A. 2% suspension   C. 7% suspension
    B. 5% suspension   D. 10% suspension

95. The usual albumin concentration used in blood banking procedures is:

    A. 10-20%   C. 30-40%
    B. 20-30%   D. 40-50%

96. Which of the autosomal chromosomes has been associated with the HLA antigens?

    A. chromosome 1   C. chromosome 4
    B. chromosome 2   D. chromosome 6

97. The removal of antibodies from red blood cells is accomplished through which of the following techniques?

    A. elution   C. agglomeration
    B. agglutination   D. none of the above

98. Which of the following procedures is used to inactivate complement?

    A. freezing red cells at -20°C
    B. store the blood at 4°C for 4 hours
    C. leave the blood at room temperature for 3 hours
    D. incubate the serum at 56°C for 30 minutes

99. A patient who is classified as Rh positive for donor purposes but Rh negative as a recipient is most likely to have which of the following?

    A. the genotype cDe/cde
    B. the phenotype Rho^D negative D^u positive
    C. anti D
    D. anti E

100. The concentration of copper sulfate used in screening female donors for hemoglobin content is:

    A. specific gravity 1.052   C. specific gravity 1.054
    B. specific gravity 1.053   D. specific gravity 1.055

101. If the mother and child are both group O, the father cannot be group:

    A. A   C. O
    B. B   D. AB

102. In a life threatening situation when there is no time for a crossmatch, the blood of choice would be:

    A. AB negative whole blood
    B. O negative whole blood
    C. AB negative red blood cells
    D. O negative red blood cells

103. Which of the following techniques is used to remove antibodies from red blood cells?

    A. elution
    B. agglutination
    C. adsorption
    D. sensitization

104. Albumin is useful in blood bank testing because it:

    A. decreases the dielectric constant and decreases the zeta potential and allows the RBC's to come closer together.
    B. decreases the dielectric constant which increases the zeta potential and allows the RBC's to come closer together
    C. cleaves sialic acid which decreases the zeta potential and allows the RBC's to come closer together
    D. increases the dielectric constant which decreases the zeta potential which allows the RBC's to come closer together

105. The single most important aspect of compatibility testing is:

    A. major crossmatch
    B. minor crossmatch
    C. antibody screen
    D. absolute patient identification

106. Mr. G.I. Bleeder is type A, Rh negative and has never received a blood transfusion. When performing a standard major and minor crossmatch using A, Rh positive units of blood, you would expect:

    A. agglutination in the minor, and not the major crossmatch
    B. agglutination in neither the major nor the major crossmatch
    C. agglutination in the major, and not the minor crossmatch
    D. agglutination in both the major and minor crossmatch

Questions 107-114

Directions. For each of the numbered phrases listed below, select the appropriate response as follows:

A. if the item is associated with A only
B. if the item is associated with B only
C. if the item is associated with both A and B
D. if the item is associated with neither A nor B

    A. direct antiglobulin test
    B. indirect antiglobulin test

107. investigates antibody coating the red blood cells
108. washing intended to remove unbound globulin from solution
109. searching for sensitization in vivo
110. searching for sensitization in vitro
111. most useful in diagnosing HDN

112. essential in detecting the D^u antigen
113. useful in detecting drug-induced hemolysis
114. useful in detecting autoimmune hemolytic anemia

Questions 115-120

Directions. One, some or all of the responses for each of the following statements may be correct. Indicate your response as follows:

A. if items 1 and 3 are correct
B. if items 2 and 4 are correct
C. if items 1, 2 and 3 are correct
D. if all of the items are correct
E. if only one of the items is correct

115. A positive direct antiglobulin test can be found in a person:

1. with no resultant hemolysis
2. whose eluate shows no antibody activity
3. due to complement components only
4. who has a negative antibody screen

116. Rh null cells are known to:

1. have an increased osmotic fragility
2. show dosage effect
3. exhibit an abnormal Na^+ and K^+ exchange
4. are affected by the inheritance of the Se gene

117. Which of the following persons can be accepted as a blood donor?

1. a 19 year old sailor: pulse 75; B/P 150/80; Hgb 14 gms; tattooed 4 months ago
2. 49 year old nurse: pulse 85; B/P 170/90; Hgb 23.8 gms; recovering from mono
3. 62 year old male: pulse 80; B/P 170/90; Hgb 15 gms; good health
4. 20 year old female: pulse 60; B/P 120/80; Hgb 12.8; tooth extracted yesterday

118. Exchange transfusion in an infant with hemolytic disease of the newborn is undertaken to:

1. reduce the bilirubin level in the infant
2. replace the sensitized baby cells with donor cells
3. increase the RBC oxygen carrying capacity in the infant
4. reduce the maternal antibody level in the child

119. Mrs. T.J. has been typed as an A Rh negative. Her husband has been typed as an A Rh positive. She has had 3 previous Rh negative children. She is now 7 months pregnant and has an anti-Rh_o(D) antibody present in her serum with a rising titer which is currently 1:64. Which of the following are <u>possible</u> conclusions?

1. she did not receive a large enough dose of Rh_o immune globulin following her last pregnancy
2. her husband is heterozygous for the D antigen
3. Mrs. T.J. may have had an undetected antigen
4. the fetus is Rh positive

120. Passive Rh immunization (Rh Immune Globulin) is intended to:

1. compensate for failure to produce antibodies in hypogammaglobulinemia
2. prevent transplacental passage of fetal cells during delivery
3. stimulate production of antibodies during pregnancy
4. prevent Rh immunization by pregnancy

Explanatory Answers

1. (A) Although reactivity varies considerably, the usual order of reactivity is O > A_2 > A_2B > A_1 > A_1B.

2. (A) Since either parent could only give an A gene or a B gene, their offspring could be AA, BB, or AB.

3. (C) The most probable reason for these results is that the patient is an A_2 blood group with an anti-A_1 antibody.

4. (D) The serum of patients with blood group AB will contain neither anti-A nor anti-B substances.

5. (C) The Weiner nomenclature for dce is rh. Rh_1 would be DCe, Rh_2 would be DcE, and rh" would be dcE.

6. (D) Fy^a and its allele Fy^b are codominant.

7. (B) The Duffy and Rh blood group systems genes appear to be on the same chromosome, but apparently they are far enough apart so as not to be inherited together.

8. (A) The MNS_s blood group system was first described in 1928 by Landsteiner and Levine.

9. (A) Anti-s antibody is a rare antibody which is most usually an immune IgG.

10. (C) Anti-P_1 is a cold reacting antibody which reacts best at 4°C

while anti-Rh and anti-Kell anti- bodies are best demonstrated at 37°C.

11. (A) The main component of cryoprecipitate is Factor VIII, and hemophilia is due to Factor VIII deficiency. Cryoprecipitate may also be used in the treatment of von Willebrand's disease and fibrinogen deficiency.

12. (D) Arachis hypogea, a lectin made from raw peanuts is used for the detection of T cells. Dolichos bifloris is used for the detection of blood group A or Tn-activated cells. Vicia graminae and Iberis amara are used for the detection of M and N blood groups.

13. (C) 50% dextrose is used to crenate the red blood cells to expel the intracellular glycerol, and to crenate them to the point that they will be normocytic after all of the washing process is completed.

14. (D) Trypsin is obtained from hog intestine; each of the others listed are plant proteases.

15. (C) Anti-M antibody is one of many antibodies that are destroyed or inactivated by proteolytic enzymes.

16. (C) Anti-Le^a is usually IgM, occurs in people who do not have the Lewis antigen, therefore are $Le(a^-b^-)$, and are all able to bind complement. It reacts with approxi- mately 20% of the adult population.

17. (A) The substances found in the saliva of group B people are B substances and H substances.

18. (D) All of the answers listed can result in erroneous blood groupings. Recent transfusions of blood groups of another ABO group may give positive reactions for the patient's blood group and that of the transfused blood. Chimeras will result in mixed field reactions. Acute leukemias may depress red cell antigens, and Tn cells will give positive reactions with lectins regardless of ABO group.

19. (E) Two people who are homozygous for blood group A could only give their offspring A genes, therefore, their offspring could only be type A.

20. (E) Differentiations between patients with A_m blood and A_x blood is best accomplished by their reactions with A_1 cells. A_m variants will have negative results when their serum is mixed with known A_1 cells while A_x patients will display a weakly positive reaction when their serum is mixed with A_1 cells.

21. (C) The cold agglutinins anti-M, anti-P_1, and anti-Le^a are all isoagglutinins, while anti-H is considered to be an autoagglutinin.

22. (D) All of the drugs listed are known to cause incompatabilities in the major crossmatch.

23. (D) Inadequate washing procedure may leave free protein which could neutralize the Coombs sera; cell suspensions that are too heavy or too weak will not permit adequate coating of the antigen by the antibody; and under centrifugation will not allow for the formation of a proper cell button.

24. (C) Cord blood samples with Wharton's jelly, Aldomet and several other drugs, and over

centrifugation, may all result in false positive Coombs tests.

25. (D) All of the blood groups listed are possible. Heterozygous parents of group A and B would have an A gene and an O gene, and a B gene and an O gene respectively. Therefore, all of the combinations are possible.

26. (B) Complement attaches to the sensitized red cell in the following manner: C_1 attaches to the bound antibody, followed by C_4 attachment either to the antibody-antigen complex itself or to the red cell. Once the C_4 attaches, C_2 will then form a complex with C_4 forming an activated C_{42} complex which activates C_3 molecules to attach to the red blood cell.

27. (D) Immunoglobulin M is made up of 20 polypeptide chains, 10 of these chains are "heavy" chains of the mu type, the remaining are "light" chains of either the kappa or lambda type.

28. (A) The major crossmatch is performed using the patient's serum and the donor's cells.

29. (B) IgM antibodies have a pentameric structure which involves the binding of the Fc fragments of the antibody.

30. (D) The antigen k of the Kell blood group system is known as Cellano

31. (B) Js^a and Js^b or the Sutter and Matthews antigens are a part of the Kell blood group system.

32. (D) Lewis antibodies are IgM antibodies. IgM antibodies cannot cross the placental barrier, therefore, they cannot cause a hemolytic disease of the newborn.

33. (C) The copper sulfate solution used to screen prospective male donors has a specific gravity of 1.055. Blood samples having a hemoglobin concentration of 13.5 gm/dl or greater will sink in this solution; those of less

than 13.5 gm/dl will not sink to the bottom.

34. (B) Except under unusual conditions, where the donor has the written permission of a physician, the donor should have an interval of 8 weeks between donations.

35. (C) These antisera react best to directly agglutinate Rho (D) positive cells, at 37°C.

36. (D) No crossmatch can detect all errors of ABO grouping, prevent immunizations of the recipient, or detect Rh typing errors (unless the patient has been sensitized), but, the crossmatch may detect some errors in ABO grouping.

37. (A) Landsteiner's law states that antibodies are present in plasma only when the corresponding antigen is not present on the erythrocytes.

38. (B) Group 0 indicates the absence of either A or B antigens, while h denotes the absence of the H antigen.

39. (B) Cold agglutinins may produce a positive reaction in a saline crossmatch since saline crossmatches are designed to detect IgM antibodies which react at room temperature or lower.

40. (C) The symbols used to indicate the Duffy antigens are Fy^a and Fy^b.

41. (A) IgG antibodies are warm reacting or so called incomplete antibodies.

42. (D) Blood stored beyond 21 days will normally have less than 70% viable red blood cells.

43. (B) Reverse blood grouping is not reliable on the serum of newborn infants because the infant's antibodies are not well developed.

44. (B) The Xg^a antigen is considered to be a sex linked antigen having a frequency of approximately 90% in females and 66% in males.

45. (B) Placental transfer, in vitro hemolysis, and an optimum temperature of 37°C are all characteristics of IgG.

46. (D) Primary response is a characteristic of IgM, not of IgG.

47. (A) Anti-Le^a is naturally occurring, usually IgM, and occurs in people with the phenotype lele.

48. (C) The antibody that was originally called anti-X is anti-Le^x.

49. (A) T activated cells will be negative when tested with polybrene and anti-A lectin, and positive when tested with the lectin made from peanuts, Arachis hypogea.

50. (D) T activated cells are not inherited, whereas, cad polyagglutinable cells are inherited.

51. (B) Anti-i reacts with cord blood cells, is enhanced with the use of enzymes, and reacts weakly or not at all with adult group 0 cells.

52. (C) Anti-i does not react with all cells, rather it reacts only with red cells having i antigen, i.e., cord cells and genetic i cells.

53. (E) Acquired hemolytic anemias will give a positive result with the direct Coombs test.

54. (A) The addition of saline to cells showing Rouleaux formation will cause the cells to disperse.

55. (D) The albumin crossmatch presents ideal conditions for the detection of most IgG antibodies.

56. (B) Erythroblastosis fetalis or hemolytic disease of the newborn is most commonly associated with anti-D and other Rh antibodies.

57. (C) People with blood group A have the corresponding anti-B antibody in their serum.

58. (A) People with blood group B have the corresponding anti-A antibody in their serum.

59. (E) People with blood group AB will have neither anti-A nor anti-B in their serum.

60. (D) People with blood group O will have both anti-A and anti-B in their serum.

61. (C) The Sutter antigen, Js^a, is a part of the Kell blood group system.

62. (A) Anti-H is associated with the ABO blood group system.

63. (E) The Duffy blood group system has its genetic information on the same gene as that of the Rh system.

64. (B) The Weiner nomenclature is one of the nomenclatures used in the Rh blood group system.

65. (B) Rho is the Weiner nomenclature for the D factor, the D being the Fisher-Race nomenclature.

66. (A) rh' is the Weiner nomenclature for the C factor, the C being the Fisher-Race nomenclature.

67. (E) hr" is the Weiner nomenclature for the e factor, the e being the Fisher-Race nomenclature.

68. (C) hr' is the Weiner nomenclature for the c factor, the c being the Fisher-Race nomenclature.

69. (B) CPD anticoagulant has been shown to have a better post-transfusion survival of red blood cells than other anticoagulants.

70. (E) The 2,3-DPG levels of cells maintained in ACD solution have been shown to be less than 10% after 2 weeks of storage.

71. (A) EDTA is a strong chelating agent, which is not commonly used as a blood preservative except for hematological procedures.

72. (C) Heparin acts as an anti-coagulant by neutralizing thrombin.

73. (C) Anti-A_1, like other antibodies of the ABO system, are best detected in saline techniques at 22°C.

74. (B) Anti-P_1 as well as the Lewis antibodies and anti-M are detected at 4°C in albumin.

75. (E) Anti-Rh antibodies are enhanced in enzyme treated solutions of red blood cells.

76. (D) Anti-p^k will agglutinate in all techniques and at all temperatures.

77. (C) Hemolytic disease of the newborn, autoimmune hemolytic anemia, and incompatible transfused blood are all cases in which the red blood cells have been coated with antibody in vivo.

78. (A) Ear piercing and tattoos, if they are relatively recent, should be rejected for at least 6 months in case hepatitis develops. Birth control pills and vitamins are not usually cause for rejections or deferment of donors.

79. (C) Fresh frozen plasma and plasma protein fraction are two blood components that are used as plasma volume expanders.

80. (B) Fresh frozen plasma is the component of choice when treating factor IX deficient patients.

81. (D) Neither of these blood components is of value in the treatment of thrombocytopenia.

82. (A) T activation of red blood cells can occur in vivo or in vitro; Tn activation of red blood cells cannot be reproduced in vitro.

83. (C) Both T and Tn activated red blood cells have decreased electrophoretic mobility.

84. (B) Tn activation is permanent while T activation is transient.

85. (A) Low glycerol methods for freezing red blood cells must be frozen rapidly. If the freezing is too slow, intracellular ice forms and hemolysis occurs.

86. (A) Low glycerol methods must be frozen quickly and be maintained at -196°C.

87. (B) Low glycerol methods for freezing red blood cells require lower temperatures for both freezing and maintenance. Cells frozen by the high glycerol method are usually maintained at -65°C or lower.

88. (A) Rouleaux formation is associated with multiple myeloma as well as other conditions associated with increased serum proteins.

89. (B) Mixed field agglutination is seen in "acquired B," where a group B like polysaccharide adsorbs onto the red blood cells.

90. (B) Mixed field polyagglutination is a characteristic of Tn activation of red blood cells. Tn activation is often referred to as PMFP, permanent mixed field polyagglutination.

91. (D) Kell antibodies usually do not cause hemolytic or agglutination reactions in vitro at 22°C.

92. (D) Rh antibodies usually do not cause hemolytic or agglutination reactions in vitro at 22°C.

93. (B) M antibodies will cause agglutination reactions in vitro at 22°C.

94. (B) The recommended cell suspension for compatibility testing is a 5% solution of red blood cells.

95. (B) The albumin solution normally used in blood banking procedures is between 20 and 30%. Most techniques employ either 22% bovine albumin or 30% bovine albumin.

96. (D) The HLA immunogenetic system is apparently associated with the autosomal chromosome #6.

97. (A) The removal of antibodies from red blood cells is called elution.

98. (D) Incubation of the serum at 56°C for 30 minutes inactivates complement.

99. (B) This patient most likely has the Rho (D) variant D^u. Because D^u is essentially a weak D antigen, these individuals must be classified as Rh positive as donors. Because these individuals may produce antibodies against Rho (D), they must be classified as Rh negative for transfusion purposes.

100. (B) A solution of copper sulfate of specific gravity 1.053 is used to screen the hemoglobin content of the blood of prospective female donors. Copper sulfate with a specific gravity of 1.053 will allow a drop of blood with a hemoglobin concentration of 12.5 gm to sink to the bottom.

101. (D) For a person to be group O, the person would have to be homozygous for the O antigen. This would mean he/she would have to inherit one O gene from each parent, therefore, neither parent could be an AB.

102. (D) Group O blood should be given in an emergency case because it does not have any ABO antigens to react with the recipient's anti-A or anti-B or anti-A,B. The plasma should be removed and red blood cells transfused because there

could be a "minor" incompatibility with the donor's anti-A,B and the recipient's RBC's.

103. (A) Elution is the removal of antibody from red blood cells. Agglutination refers to the clumping of red cells caused by the formation of antibody bridges between antigens on different cells. Adsorption refers to the uptake of antibody onto the antigen binding site. Sensitization is the initial exposure of an individual to a specific antigen resulting in an immune response.

104. (D) The use of bovine albumin in the indirect antiglobulin technique will decrease the incubation time because it will increase the dielectric constant which decreases the zeta potential. This allows the RBC's to come closer together. The use of enzymes also will enhance the agglutination of some antigen-antibody reactions, cleave the sialic acid from the RBC membranes, which lowers the zeta potential and allows the RBC's to come closer together.

105. (D) Absolute patient identification is the most important aspect of any laboratory test. Over 90% of all transfusion accidents are caused by clerical error.

106. (B) Because Mr. G.I. Bleeder has never been exposed to Rh positive RBC's, it would be unlikely that he would possess an anti-D, therefore, Rh positive RBC's would be compatible.

107. (A) The direct antiglobulin test is used to demonstrate an antibody which is already coating the RBC.

108. (C) Red blood cells must be washed 3-4 times with large volumes of normal saline before the adding antihuman globulin serum. This washing step is essential because the slightest amount of unwashed

protein will neutralize the antiglobulin serum and cause a "false negative" result.

109. (A) In vivo sensitization would result in a positive direct antiglobulin test.

110. (B) In vitro sensitization would require the use of the indirect antiglobulin test where the antibody would be bound to reagent RBC's in vitro.

111. (A) The direct antiglobulin test is used to diagnose HDN since one is looking for maternal antibody, which is bound to the infant's RBC's in vivo.

112. (B) The D^u antigen requires the use of the indirect antiglobulin technique for its identification.

113. (A) Drug-induced hemolysis may be a result of a positive direct antiglobulin reaction causing premature lysis of the sensitized RBC's by the RE system.

114. (A) In autoimmune hemolytic anemia, the person has an auto-antibody which binds to his/her own RBC's. This causes a positive direct antiglobulin.

115. (D) A positive direct antiglobulin test can be caused by IgG or complement components binding to the red blood cells. The sensitized red blood cells may be prematurely cleared by the RE system causing increased hemolysis, but in some cases of drug induced positive direct antiglobulin tests this premature removal of RBC is not noticed. The eluate may not show antibody activity especially in drug related antibody sensitization. The indirect antiglobulin test may or may not be positive depending on the cause of the positive direct antiglobulin test.

116. (A) Rh null cells have a weakened cell membrane. The weakened membrane will cause an increased osmotic fragility and an abnormal Na^+ and K^+ exchange.

117. (E) Requirements for blood donors are as follows: 1) age: 17-66; 2) hemoglobin: male - 13.5; female - 12.5; 3) hematocrit: male - 41%; female - 38%; 4) pulse: 50-100 and regular; 5) temperature: must not exceed 37.5°C; 6) B/P: systolic 90-180mm diastolic 50-100mm

118. (C) Exchange transfusion for the treatment of HDN will: 1) remove sensitized RBC's from fetal circulation; 2) reduce the bilirubin level; 3) remove unbound maternal antibody; and 4) provide compatible donor RBC's with a good oxygen carrying capacity and relieve the anemia.

119. (B) A rising titer of anti-D in an Rh negative pregnant women indicates current stiumulation by the fetus's Rh positive red blood cells. In order for the fetus to be Rh positive, the father would have to posses the D gene. Because the other 3 children are Rh negative, the father must be heterozygous for the D gene.

120. (E) Rh immune globulin is given to Rh negative women who deliver an Rh positive child. The Rh immune globulin will bind to the Rh positive fetal cells which will enter the maternal circulation during delivery. This will prevent the maternal immune system from recognizing the "foreign" Rh positive fetal cells.

Bibliography and Recommended Readings

American Association of Blood Banks. <u>Technical Manual</u>. Eighth Edition. 1981.
AABB. Washington, D. C.

Bryant, Neville J. <u>An Introduction to Immunohematology</u>. Second Edition. 1982.
W. B. Saunders Company. Philadelphia.

Issitt, P. O. and C. Issitt. <u>Applied Blood Group Serology</u>. Second Edition. 1979.
Sprectra Biologicals. Oxnard, California.

Todd, J. C. <u>Clinical Diagnosis and Management by Laboratory Methods</u>. Sixteenth
Edition. 1979. W. B. Saunders Company. Philadelphia.

CHAPTER 10

Hematology

Directions. Select the one BEST answer for each of the following statements. Circle the appropriate response on the answer sheet.

1. The immediate precursor of the mature neutrophil is:

    A. myelocyte   C. promyelocyte
    B. metamyelocyte   D. band cell

2. The following results were obtained on analysis of an anemic patient:

    MCV = 115   MCH = 50   MCHC = 34

    Which of the following conditions would produce these results?

    A. acute blood loss   C. iron deficiency
    B. aplastic anemia   D. pernicious anemia

3. The term that indicates a variation in the shape of red blood cells is:

    A. anisocytosis   C. macrocytosis
    B. poikilocytosis   D. hypochromia

4. Which of the following hemoglobins is NOT found in normal adult blood?

    A. HbA   C. HbF
    B. HBA_2 D. HBC

5. Which of the following amino acid substitutions is responsible for hemoglobin C?

    A. lysine for glutamine in the sixth position on the beta chain
    B. glutamine for lysine in the sixth position on the alpha chain
    C. lysine for glutamine in the sixth position on the alpha chain
    D. glutamine for lysine in the sixth position on the beta chain

6. Which of the following conditions will usually result in leukopenia?

    A. measles   C. appendicitis
    B. tonsillitis   D. peritonitis

7. Upon examination of a peripheral blood smear, a technologist finds 8 nucleated
    red blood cells per 100 white blood cells. The white blood cell count is found
    to be 15,500. Which of the following is the next step to be taken?

    A. report the 15,500 white blood cell count
    B. report the 15,500 white blood cell count and make note of the nucleated red
        blood cells
    C. correct the white blood cell count for the nucleated red blood cells present
    D. none of the above

8. The normal white blood cell count is:

    A. 3,500-7,000/c. mm   C. 8,000-12,000/c. mm
    B. 5,000-10,000/c. mm   D. 10,000-15,000/c. mm

9. Which of the following would indicate a macrocytic anemia?

    A. MCV = 83 fl   C. MCV = 94 fl
    B. MCV = 87 fl   D. MCV = 103 fl

10. Which of the following hemoglobin values would be considered abnormal in a male
    patient?

    A. 12.5 gm/dl   C. 15.5 gm/dl
    B. 13.5 gm/dl   D. 17.5 gm/dl

11. Normal hemoglobin A is made up of which of the following?

    A. 2 alpha chains and 2 beta chains
    B. 2 alpha chains and 2 delta chains
    C. 2 alpha chains and 2 gamma chains
    D. none of the above

12. Which of the following cells shows an affinity for the acid dyes?

    A. eosinophils   C. neutrophils
    B. basophils   D. monocytes

13. What is the normal daily requirement for folic acid?

    A. 50 μg/day   C. 200 μg/day
    B. 100 μg/day   D. 400 μg/day

14. Which of the following hemoglobins is an abnormal hemoglobin composed of four
    beta globin chains?

    A. hemoglobin F   C. hemoglobin H
    B. hemoglobin G   D. hemoglobin S

15. Which of the following hemoglobins characteristically resists alkali denaturation?

    A. hemoglobin A   C. hemoglobin C
    B. hemoglobin F   D. hemoglobin S

16. Which of the following criteria should be used when attempting to identify cells?

    A. cell size   C. cytoplasmic characteristics
    B. nuclear characteristics   D. all of the above

17. An increase in the total white blood cell count is known as:

    A. leukopenia   C. lymphocytosis
    B. leukocytosis   D. eosinophilia

18. Which of the following conditions is NOT a cause of eosinophilia?

    A. trichinosis   C. skin disease
    B. asthma   D. appendicitis

19. The normal range for a platelet count is:

    A. 5,000-10,000   C. 150,000-400,000
    B. 50,000-100,000   D. 1,000,000-3,500,000

20. What is the chief use of the osmotic fragility test?

    A. detection of hereditary spherocytosis
    B. detection of paroxysmal nocturnal hemoglobinuria
    C. detection of chronic lymphocytic leukemia
    D. detection of sickle cell anemia

21. Which of the following is the structure of hemoglobin F, fetal hemoglobin?

    A. 2 alpha chains and 2 beta chains
    B. 2 alpha chains and 2 delta chains
    C. 2 alpha chains and 2 gamma chains
    D. 4 beta chains

22. Beta thalassemia, or thalassemia major, is also known as:

    A. Cooley's anemia   C. sickle cell trait
    B. sickle cell anemia   D. none of the above

23. The Philadelphia chromosome is associated with which of the following disorders?

    A. chronic granulocytic leukemia
    B. chronic lymphocytic leukemia
    C. acute granulocytic leukemia
    D. acute lymphocytic leukemia

24. Which of the following terms is used to indicate a variation of size in red blood cells?

    A. anisocytosis   C. hypochromia
    B. poikilocytosis   D. polychromasia

25. Which of the following is NOT one of the Romanowsky's stains?

    A. Giemsa's stain
    B. May-Grünwald stain
    C. Pappenheim's stain
    D. new methylene blue

26. Which of the following structures is that of hemoglobin A_2?

    A. 2 alpha chains and 2 beta chains
    B. 2 alpha chains and 2 delta chains
    C. 2 alpha chains and 2 gamma chains
    D. 4 alpha chains

Questions 27-29

Directions. One, some or all of the responses for each of the following statements may be correct. Indicate your response as follows:

A. if items 1 and 3 are correct
B. if items 2 and 4 are correct
C. if three of the items are correct
D. if all of the items are correct
E. if only one of the items is correct

27. Which of the following diseases may exhibit drepanocytes?

    1. Hb SC disease
    2. Hb S disease
    3. Hb S-thalassemia syndrome
    4. Hereditary spherocytosis

28. The prothrombin time test will be prolonged in which of the following cases?

    1. factor V deficiency
    2. factor VII deficiency
    3. factor X deficiency
    4. factor VIII deficiency

29. Which of the following may result in a vitamin B_{12} deficiency?

    1. defective production of Intrinsic Factor
    2. infection with the fish tapeworm
    3. total gastrectomy
    4. strict vegetarian diet

Questions 30-38

Directions. For each of the numbered words or phrases listed below, select the appropriate response as follows:

A. if the item is associated with A only
B. if the item is associated with B only
C. if the item is associated with both A and B
D. if the item is associated with neither A nor B

A.   absolute increase
B.   relative increase

30. WBC count of 3,000/c. mm with 60% lymphocytes
31. WBC count of 12,500/c. mm with 78% lymphocytes
32. WBC count of 12,500/c. mm with 40% neutrophils
33. WBC count of 4,000/c. mm with 90% neutrophils

A.   hereditary condition
B.   acquired condition

34. Pelger-Huet anomaly
35. May-Hegglin anomaly
36. Chediak-Higashi anomaly
37. Spherocytosis
38. Paroxysmal nocturnal hemoglobinuria

Questions 39-40

Directions. The column on the left contains 3 scientifically related categories while the column on the right contains 4 items which may illustrate scientific phenomena or processes. Three of the items in the column on the right relate to only one of the categories in the column on the left. FIRST, indicate the category in which the 3 processes or phenomena belong. SECOND, indicate the one process or phenomenon which is not related to that category.

	Category		Phenomenon	
39.	A. iron deficiency anemia	40.	A. MCV	99
	B. pernicious anemia		B. MCHC	30
	C. sickle cell anemia		C. MCH	25
			D. B_{12} deficiency	

Questions 41-44

Directions. Select and circle the one BEST answer for each of the following statements utilizing the illustrations found on page 167.

41. Which of the following cells are found in hereditary conditions?

    A. 2, 3, and 7
    B. 5, 6, and 7

    C. 2, 4, and 6
    D. 4, 6, and 8

42. Which of the illustrated cells are found commonly in hemolytic disease of the newborn?

    A. 2 and 3
    B. 4 and 5

    C. 5 and 7
    D. 2 and 6

43. Which of the illustrations demonstrates a degenerating cell?

    A. 6
    B. 2

    C. 8
    D. 4

44. Which of the illustrations is that of a cell commonly found in vitamin B_{12} deficiency?

    A. 4
    B. 7

    C. 6
    D. 8

Questions 45-100

Directions. For each of the numbered items select the appropriate lettered response. Do not use the same letter more than once.

45. Hemoglobin C
46. Hemoglobin S-C
47. Hemoglobin D
48. Hemoglobin E

    A. migrates like hemoglobin S but non-sickling
    B. decreased osmotic fragility
    C. at pH 6.5 moves slower than hemoglobin S
    D. heterozygous state with 2 abnormal alleles
    E. increased red blood cell survival

49. Gower's solution
50. Drabkin solution
51. Isoton
52. ammonium oxalate, 1%

    A. eosinophils
    B. white blood cells
    C. red blood cells
    D. platelets
    E. hemoglobin

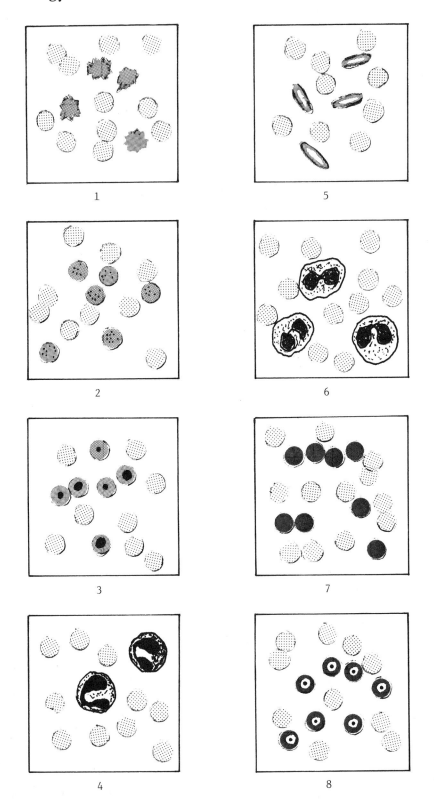

1

5

2

6

3

7

4

8

Term	Red Blood Cells
53. polychromatophilia	A. larger central pale area
54. hypochromia	B. coarse blue-black granules
55. basophilic stippling	C. blue-gray tint
56. Howell-Jolly bodies	D. loop shaped structures
	E. smooth round, dark granule

57. azurophilic granules	A. eosinophil
58. large red granules	B. monocyte
59. large purple granules	C. plasma cell
60. bluish gray cytoplasm	D. neutrophil
	E. basophil

61. hypersegmented neutrophils	A. two-lobed nuclei
62. Barr body	B. folic acid deficiencies
63. Pelger-Huet anomaly	C. found normally in females
64. toxic granulation	D. dark blue-black cytoplasmic granules
	E. darkly stained lymphocytes

Test

Formula

65. mean corpuscular volume (MCV)
66. mean corpuscular hemoglobin (MCH)
67. mean corpuscular hemoglobin concentration (MCHC)
68. corrected reticulocyte count

A. $\dfrac{\text{absolute percentage}}{\text{maturation time}}$

B. $\dfrac{\#\text{ counted}}{\#\text{ of red cells} \times 10} \times 100$

C. $\dfrac{\text{hematocrit (percent)} \times 10}{\text{red cell count (millions/ml)}}$

D. $\dfrac{\text{hemoglobin (gm/dl)} \times 100}{\text{hematocrit (percent)}}$

E. $\dfrac{\text{hemoglobin (gm/dl)} \times 10}{\text{red cell count (millions/ml)}}$

69. leptocytes	A. cigar shaped red cells
70. acanthocytes	B. red cells with thorn-like projections
71. elliptocytes	C. target cells
72. schistocytes	D. crescent shaped cells
	E. red cell fragments

73. Factor I	A. calcium
74. Factor IV	B. Hageman factor
75. Factor VIII	C. fibrinogen
76. Factor XII	D. prothrombin
	E. antihemophilic factor

77. Hemophilia
78. Christmas disease
79. Stuart factor deficiency
80. Hageman trait

A. Factor I deficiency
B. Factor VIII deficiency
C. Factor XII deficiency
D. Factor IX deficiency
E. Factor X deficiency

81. Gaucher's disease
82. Myelogenous leukemia
83. Lead poisoning
84. Di Guglielmo's disease

A. proliferative disorder of the erythrocyte precursors
B. WBC's contain fat
C. Auer bodies
D. Basophilic stippling
E. Dohle's inclusion bodies

85. Burr cell
86. Tart cell
87. Stomatocyte
88. L. E. cell

A. hematoxylin bodies
B. red blood cells with slit-like areas of pallor
C. knobby projections on red cell surface
D. nucleophagocytosis
E. red cell with dark center

Substance

89. complex carbohydrates
90. iron
91. monocytes
92. lipids

Stain

A. Gomori's method
B. Leukocyte Alkaline Phosphatase
C. Peroxidase stain
D. Periodic Acid-Schiff stain
E. Sudan Black B

Anticoagulant

93. EDTA
94. Ammonium potassium oxalate
95. Sodium citrate
96. Heparin

Mode of action

A. inactivates calcium ions
B. anti-thrombin and anti-thromboplastin
C. chelating agent
D. forms insoluble calcium
E. neutralizes fibrinogen

97. granulocyte
98. erythrocyte
99. platelet
100. lymphocyte

A. B cell
B. promyelocyte
C. promonocyte
D. megakaryocyte
E. basophilic normoblast

Questions 101-126

Directions. Select the one BEST answer for each of the following statements. Circle the appropriate response on the answer sheet.

101. The mobilities obtained on hemoglobin electrophoresis at pH 8.6 show:

A. HbS moves faster than HbA
B. HbC moves faster than HbA
C. HbA moves slower than HbC or HbS
D. HbS moves faster than HbC but more slowly than HbA

102. Schumm's test is used to identify:

A. methemoglobin   C. oxyhemoglobin
B. sulfhemoglobin   D. methemalbumin

103. Which of the following would give a reliable hematocrit determination?

A. collect 1 ml of blood in a 5 ml EDTA tube
B. perform fingerstick and squeeze finger to fill the capillary tube
C. omit the buffy coat from the measurement of the cell column height
D. centrifuge the hematocrit until you think the RBC are well packed

104. Which of the following needles has the largest berul?

A. 18 gauge   C. 21 gauge
B. 20 gauge   D. 22 gauge

105. Erythropoietin is produced in man primarily in the:

A. pancreas   C. kidney
B. small intestine   D. pituitary

106. The initial step in the biosynthesis of heme is the combination of glycine and succinyl CoA to form:

A. protoporphyrin IX   C. uroporphyrin III
B. coproporphyrin III   D. delta-aminolevulinic acid

107. Which of the following is the average red blood cell survival time?

A. 1-5 days   C. 60 days
B. 9-10 days   D. 120 days

108. Consider the following indices:

MCV = 60.6 cu microns   MCH = 25μμg, MCHC - 15.1%

Which of the following would you expect to find on the differential blood smear evaluation of red blood cell morphology?

A. normothromic red blood cells
B. hypochromic, macrocytic red blood cells
C. hypochromic microcytic red blood cells
D. macrocytic red blood cells

109. Hemoglobinopathies such as Hgb S and C have abnormalities occurring in their:

    A. alpha chains of globin
    B. beta chains of globin
    C. heme
    D. pyrrole ring structure

110. An eosinophil count of 800 cells/cu. mm. could be indicative of which of the following?

    A. a normal finding
    B. the patient is suffering from an allergic reaction
    C. the patient has adrenal gland disease
    D. the patient is harboring a virus

111. L. E. "factor" is:

    A. a component of serum gamma globulin
    B. a nucleoprotein
    C. a phagocytic neutrophil
    D. a lyzed neutrophilic leukocyte

112. Excessive denaturation of hemoglobin within the red blood cell is characteristic of the formation of which of the following?

    A. Heinz bodies
    B. Howell-Jolly bodies
    C. Dohle bodies
    D. siderocytic granules

113. A large cell, prone to developing multiple and bizarre nuclei characteristics of Hodgkin's disease is:

    A. histiocyte
    B. Ferrata cell
    C. Reed-Sternberg cell
    D. mast cell

114. In the adult, lymphocytes are principally produced in the:

    A. bone marrow
    B. liver
    C. lymphoid tissue
    D. pancreas

115. According to the laboratory procedure manual at "Hospital X", hematocrits are to be spun at 10,000 RPM for 4 minutes. A new employee centrifuged the hematocrits for only 2 minutes at 5,000 RPM. The hematocrit value may be:

    A. falsely decreased
    B. falsely increased
    C. both of the above
    D. neither of the above

116. Hemolysis in acidified serum and sugar water is evidenced in patients with:

    A. multiple myeloma
    B. Hodgkin's disease
    C. paroxysmal nocturnal hemoglobinuria
    D. iron deficiency anemia

117. A positive peroxidase stain will be seen in:

    A. lymphocytes
    B. promyelocytes
    C. myeloblasts
    D. lymphoblasts

118. The Price-Jones curve gives which of the following?

    A. an analysis of hemoglobin pigments at various wavelengths
    B. the distribution of red cell size in quantitative terms
    C. the rate of hemoglobin degredation
    D. the rate of hemoglobin synthesis

119. The inherited variation in neutrophils which is characterized by dumbbell or spectacle-like nuclei of only two lobes is:

    A. May-Hegglin anomaly
    B. Dohle body
    C. Pelger Huet anomaly
    D. Chediak Higashi anomaly

120. Acute myelogenous leukemia:

    A. has an age incidence similar to chronic lymphocytic leukemia
    B. is never preceded by a preleukemia state
    C. is often related to immunoglobulin abnormalities
    D. can be differentiated from acute lymphocytic leukemia (ALL) because blasts usually contain auer rods

121. DiGuglielmo's syndrome is a condition characterized in the blood smear by:

    A. immature, atypical, nucleated red blood cells
    B. the presence of "hairy cells"
    C. plasma cells
    D. mast cells

122. The Ehlers-Danlos syndrome is a bleeding abnormality associated with:

    A. platelet dysfunction
    B. connective tissue disorders
    C. immunologic vascular injury
    D. infectious purpura

123. There may be a prolonged bleeding time in many patients taking aspirin because it interferes with:

    A. platelet factor 3 production
    B. clot retraction
    C. vascular constriction
    D. platelet aggregation

124. Which of the following represent the end products of the breakdown of the fibrin (ogen) monomer?

    A. Fragment X
    B. Fragments Y and D
    C. Fragment D
    D. Fragments D + E + D

125. The activated substance responsible for lysis of the fibrin clot is called:

    A. actomysin
    B. plasminogen
    C. plasmin
    D. thromboplastin

126. The most valuable test in differentiating fibrinolysis from consumption
      coagulopathy is the:

    A. Thrombin time   C. clot solubility test
    B. Factor V, VIII assay   D. platelet count

Questions 127-132

Directions. The column on the left contains 3 scientifically related categories while
the column on the right contains 4 items which may illustrate scientific phenomena
or processes. Three of the items in the column on the right relate to only one of
the categories in the column on the left. FIRST, indicate the category in which the
3 processes or phenomena belong. SECOND, indicate the one process or phenomenon
which is not related to that category.

Category	Phenomenon
127. A. calcium	128. A. EDTA
B. thrombin	B. potassium oxalate
C. thromboplastin	C. heparin
	D. sodium citrate
129. A. Factor XII	130. A. Factor VII: Tissue complex
B. Factor X	B. Russell's Viper Venom
C. Factor V	C. Factor IXa, Factor VIII, Ca^{++}, Platelet factor 3
	D. Factor Xa, Factor V, Ca^{++}, Platelet factor 3
131. A. Neutrophils	132. A. Russell bodies
B. Lymphocytes	B. Dohle bodies
C. Plasma cells	C. Mott cells
	D. Flame cells

Questions 133-163

Directions. One, some, or all of the responses for each of the following statements
may be correct. Indicate your response as follows:

A. if items 1 and 3 are correct
B. if items 2 and 4 are correct
C. if three of the items are correct
D. if all of the items are correct
E. if only one of the items is correct

133. Phloxine B in the eosinophil diluting fluid functions in:

    1. staining eosinophils
    2. rendering red blood cells non-refractile
    3. hemolyzing red blood cells
    4. hemolyzing WBC other than eosinophils

134. In the fetus, hematopoiesis takes place in the:

   1. yolk sac
   2. liver
   3. bone marrow
   4. spleen

135. Which of the following statements are true about HbA, HbA₂, and HbF?

   1. are all normal hemoglobins
   2. are present in equal amounts at birth
   3. each have a pair of alpha chains
   4. each have a pair of beta chains

136. As the red blood cell matures, which of the following changes occur?

   1. cell becomes smaller
   2. nucleus becomes denser and smaller and is finally extruded
   3. the amount of hemoglobin increases in the cytoplasm
   4. cytoplasm progresses from blue to orange with Wright's stain

137. Examples of microcytic hypochromic anemias include which of the following?

   1. iron deficiency anemia
   2. sideroblastic anemia
   3. thalassemia
   4. folic acid deficiency

138. The Hema Tek automated slide stainer will automatically perform which of the following?

   1. fixes blood smears
   2. stains smears
   3. rinses smears
   4. air dries stained smears

139. Which of the following statements are accurate for both the Coulter model Fn and the Coulter model S?

   1. indices are calculated
   2. 1/50,000 dilution for RBC
   3. 1/500 dilution for WBC
   4. operation is based upon electronic particle counting

140. Wright's stain consists of:

   1. eosin
   2. janus green
   3. methylene blue
   4. safranin

141. Which of the following statements concerning capillary specimens are NOT true:

   1. milking or squeezing the finger dilutes the specimen with tissue juices
   2. for most determinations, the first drop is acceptable
   3. with capillary smears, platelets are clumped
   4. smears can be made from heparinized hematocrit capillary tubes

142. A patient has been diagnosed as having myelofibrosis with myeloid metaplasia. Which abnormalities would you expect to see on the blood smear?

   1. teardrop shaped red blood cells
   2. nucleated red blood cells
   3. variable WBC count
   4. decreased platelets with some giant forms

143. Which of the following values would be increased from a patient with hereditary spherocytosis?

    1. reticulocyte count   3. autohemolysis
    2. osmotic fragility   4. MCHC

144. You have been asked to collect a CBC blood sample from a patient. Upon entering the room you notice the patient has IV solutions in both arms. It would be acceptable to do which of the following?

    1. draw blood from a vein 8-10 cm below the IV
    2. disconnect the IV and draw a sample from the IV connection with a syringe
    3. collect a capillary specimen
    4. draw the specimen from a femoral vein

145. Which of the following will cause erroneous results with the Coulter Model S?

    1. WBC count greater than 50,000
    2. cold agglutinin titer 1:500
    3. erythroblastosis fetalis with significant nucleated red blood cells
    4. WBC counts less than 1000

146. Autoimmune hemolytic anemia may be seen in patients with which of the following?

    1. lupus erythematosus   3. granulomas
    2. neoplasms   4. no signs of disease

147. A newborn has a hemoglobin of 10 gm/dl, a reticulocyte count of 12%, 25 normoblasts per 100 WBC, marked polychromasia and is jaundiced. What additional tests should be done on the child?

    1. direct Coombs test   3. ABO group and Rh
    2. bilirubin   4. hemoglobin electrophoresis

148. Which of the following will be increased in a patient with hereditary spherocytosis?

    1. MCV   3. red cell count
    2. MCHC   4. osmotic fragility

149. Which of the following are examples of normochromic, normocytic anemias?

    1. hemolytic anemias   3. pernicious anemia
    2. acute blood loss   4. myelophthisic anemia

150. Sideroblastic anemia is characterized by which of the following?

    1. hypochromia and microcytosis
    2. increased iron stores in the bone marrow
    3. significant ring sideroblasts
    4. X-linked recessive trait found mainly in males

151. In the granulocytic maturation series nucleoli will be visible with light microscopy in which of the following?

    1. promyelocytes
    2. myelocytes
    3. myeloblasts
    4. metamyelocytes

152. Which of the following findings are common in chronic granulocytic leukemia?

    1. peripheral blood basophilia
    2. all stages of myeloid maturation present in the peripheral blood
    3. a low leukocyte alkaline phosphatase
    4. a distinctive small chromosome (Ph) present in granulocytes and erythroid precursors

153. With infectious mononucleosis, the patient will have which of the following?

    1. an absolute lymphocytosis with atypical lymphocytes
    2. a positive heterophil agglutinin test
    3. antibodies to the Epstein Barr virus
    4. cytomegalovirus in the urine

154. Which of the following represent malignant lymphoma(s)?

    1. Hodgkin's disease
    2. DiGuglielmo's syndrome
    3. Burkitt
    4. Schilling

155. Which of the following laboratory tests are useful in diagnosing an abnormality in platelet function?

    1. template bleeding time
    2. platelet aggregation
    3. platelet adhesion
    4. clot retraction

156. Platelet function includes which of the following?

    1. formation of a platelet plug
    2. release of phospholipid (Pf$_3$)
    3. maintenance of vascular integrity
    4. release of thromboplastin for proper clot retraction

157. Which of the following factors does NOT have an enzymatically active form?

    1. Factor XII
    2. Factor VIII
    3. Factor X
    4. Factor V

158. If a patient has a factor VIII deficiency which of the following are true?

    1. the APTT will be prolonged and corrected with adsorbed plasma
    2. the APTT will be prolonged and corrected with aged serum
    3. the PT will be prolonged and corrected with adsorbed plasma
    4. the PT will be prolonged and corrected with aged serum

159. If a patient has a Factor X deficiency which of the following are true?

    1. the APTT will be prolonged
    2. the PT will be prolonged
    3. aged serum will correct abnormal results
    4. adsorbed plasma will correct abnormal results

160. Blood coagulation is controlled and confined to the immediate area of tissue damage by means of which of the following?

    1. natural inhibition such as anti-thrombins
    2. platelets which act as sponges to adsorb excess thrombin
    3. the fibrinolytic mechanisms
    4. action of Factor XIII

161. In severe liver disease, all coagulation factors may be depressed except which of the following?

    1. Factor V   3. Factor VIII
    2. Factor VII   4. Factor X

162. Overall competence of the coagulation system is assessed by performing which of the following tests?

    1. prothrombin time   3. fibrinogen level
    2. partial thromboplastin time   4. clot solubility test

163. A patient with macroglobulinemia of Waldenström will have which of the following?

    1. large amounts of monoclonal IgM globulin
    2. cryoglobulins
    3. a proliferation of plasma-cytoid lymphocytes
    4. anemia

Questions 164-177

Directions. The following statements contain numbered blanks. For each numbered blank there is a corresponding set of lettered responses. Select the BEST answer from each lettered set.

Platelets play an initial role in arresting bleeding by formation of a platelet plug. Within 1-2 seconds platelet 164 occurs followed by a release of 165 . The next stage is platelet 166 and 167 is released to form the platelet plug. 168 is then released and is essential for consolidation of the plug and proper clot retraction.

A. aggregation   D. ADP
B. thrombosthenin   E. adhesion
C. thrombin

The normal adult contains __169__ gms or iron. __170__ % is incorporated into hemoglobin and __171__ % into the storage form as ferritin and hemosiderin. Normally __172__ mg of iron is ingested in the diet per day with __173__ mg/day absorbed in the duodenum and upper jejunum.

A. 66
B. 10-25
C. 3-4

D. 0.5-1.6
E. 29

With Wright's stain, the nuclei of white cells will appear pale grey and the erythrocytes bright red if there is __174__. Excess blue coloration of nuclei and gray eosinophilic granules will result in __175__ and __176__. Pale nuclei, granules, and cytoplasm result from an __177__.

A. excessive decoloration
B. very acid pH

C. a very alkaline pH
D. overstaining

Questions 178-179

Directions. Select the one BEST answer for each of the following statements. Circle the appropriate response on the answer sheet.

178. When performing a manual red blood cell count, 370 cells were counted on side #1 of the hemocytometer, 396 cells on side #2. A 1/200 dilution of Hayem's solution was used and the area counted on each side was 1/5 sq. mm. The correct RBC count per cu mm is:

A. 7,660,000
B. 3,830,000

C. 766,000
D. 383,000

179. When performing a manual white blood cell count, 136 cells were counted on side #1 of the hemocytometer, 144 cells on side #2. A 1/20 dilution of 1% HCl was used and the area counted on each side was 4 mm. The correct WBC count per cu mm is:

A. 28,000
B. 70,000

C. 2,800
D. 7,000

Questions 180-185

Directions. One, some, or all of the responses for each of the following statements may be correct. Indicate your response as follows:

A. if items 1 and 3 are correct
B. if items 2 and 4 are correct
C. if three of the items are correct
D. if all of the items are correct
E. if only one of the items is correct

180. An increased erythropoietin level is seen in which of the following:

1. secondary erythrocytosis
2. polycythemia vera

3. rheumatoid arthritis
4. cancer

181. The erythrocyte sedimentation rate (ESR) will be increased in the following situations:

    1. increased room temperature
    2. anemia
    3. ESR tube is not exactly vertical
    4. increased red cell mass

182. The Coulter Model S-Plus directly measures which of these parameters?

    1. MCV
    2. RBC
    3. WBC
    4. PLT
    5. HCT

183. What tests would be helpful in confirming the diagnosis of paroxysmal nocturnal hemoglobinuria?

    1. ferritin assay
    2. Ham's test
    3. bone marrow
    4. sugar water test

184. What diagnostic criteria can be used to identify myelofibrosis in a patient?

    1. tear drop shaped and nucleated red cells
    2. immature granulocytes
    3. marrow fibrosis
    4. splenomegaly

185. As the red cell matures, which of the following changes occur?

    1. cell becomes smaller
    2. nucleus becomes denser and smaller and is finally extruded
    3. the amount of hemoglobin increases in the cytoplasm
    4. cytoplasm progresses from blue to red with Wright's stain

Questions 186-197

Directions. Select the one BEST answer for each of the following statements. Circle the appropriate response on the answer sheet.

186. The bleeding time is a test for:

    A. factor VIII deficiency
    B. fibrin formation
    C. contact factor activation
    D. platelet and vascular function

187. If a differential has 10-20 white blood cells per high power field, what would be the patient's estimated white cell count?

    A. 8,000-12,000/cu.mm.
    B. 13,000-18,000/cu.mm.
    C. 25,000-30,000/cu.mm.
    D. 35,000-40,000/cu.mm.

188. Megaloblastic anemias are characterized by:

    A. hypochromic red cells
    B. defective DNA synthesis
    C. toxic granulation
    D. acanthocytes

189. A patient with the following indices could be said to have what type of anemia?

MCV--71   MCH--22   MCHC--31

A. hypochromic, normocytic   C. hypochromic, microcytic
B. normochromic, microcytic   D. normochromic, normocytic

190. Which of the following is produced by the first stage of coagulation?

A. thrombin   C. plasmin
B. fibrin   D. thromboplastin (plasma)

191. The F.A.B. classification is used in which group of disorders?

A. anemias   C. leukemias
B. hemoglobinopathies   D. disorders of hemostasis

192. Which disorder is characterized by increased levels of sphingomyelin in the
      tissues?

A. Niemann-Pick disease   C. Pelger-Huet anomaly
B. Gaucher's disease   D. chloroma

193. The Kleihauer-Betke technique can be used for:

A. counting white cells
B. detection of fetal cells in maternal blood
C. detecting the presence of HgbS
D. estimating a platelet count

194. An increased erythropoietin level is seen in which of the following?

A. secondary erythrocytosis   C. rheumatoid arthritis
B. polycythemia vera   D. cancer

195. Esterase stains are used for what purpose?

A. to identify lymphocytic leukemias
B. to differentiate reactive lymphs
C. to distinguish between granulocytic and monocytic precursors
D. to differentiate pro-megakaryocytes from myeloblasts

196. The most common type of leukemia in four year old children is:

A. acute lymphoblastic leukemia   C. acute myelogenous leukemia
B. chronic lymphocytic leukemia   D. myelomonocytic leukemia

197. An increased reticulocyte count would be characteristic of which disorders?

A. immune hemolytic anemia   C. leukemia
B. aplastic anemia   D. Hodgkin's disease

Explanatory Answers

1. (D) The band cell is the immediate precursor of the mature neutrophil; each of the other cells listed are precursors to the band cell.

2. (D) Pernicious anemia is a macrocytic normochromic anemia, which the results indicate. Acute blood loss and aplastic anemia would produce a normocytic normochromic anemia, and iron deficiency would result in a microcytic hypochromic anemia.

3. (B) Poikilocytosis is the term applied to red cells that show a variation in shape.

4. (D) Hemoglobin A is the major normal hemoglobin found in normal adult blood. Hemoglobin A_2 is found normally in small amounts as is hemoglobin F. Hemoglobin C is an abnormal hemoglobin.

5. (A) Hemoglobin C is formed when lysine is substituted for glutamine in the sixth position of the beta globin chain in hemoglobin.

6. (A) Measles, as well as rubella, influenza, infectious hepatitis, and Colorado tick fever which are caused by viral and rickettsial organisms usually result in leukopenia. All of the other items listed will result in a neutrophilic leukocytosis.

7. (C) Because the immature red blood cells are not destroyed by lysing agents, they are counted as white blood cells. If more than 5 nucleated red blood cells are found per 100 white blood cells, the white blood cell count should be corrected.

8. (B) The normal white blood cell count is generally accepted to be 5,000-10,000/c. mm. White blood cell counts that are significantly below 5,000 or above 10,000 are considered abnormal.

9. (D) The normal range for the mean corpuscular volume (MCV) is 82-98 fl. MCV values of over 98 fl. indicate a macrocytic condition.

10. (A) The normal range for hemoglobin concentration in an adult male is 13.5-18.0 gm/dl. Therefore, a 12.5 gm/dl hemoglobin would indicate an anemic condition in a man.

11. (A) Normal adult hemoglobin, HbA, is composed of 2 alpha chains and 2 beta chains. HbA_2 is made up of 2 alpha chains and 2 delta chains, and HbF, fetal hemoglobin, is made up of 2 alpha chains and 2 gamma chains.

12. (A) Eosinophils display an affinity for the acid dyes. Eosin, normally found in the Wright's stain, is an acid dye.

13. (A) The normal daily requirement for folic acid is 50 μg/day. In pregnancy, the daily requirement may be as high as 400 μg/day.

14. (C) Hemoblogin H is an abnormal hemoglobin composed of four beta globin chains. It is unstable and found in alpha thalassemia as well as in hemoglobin H diseases.

15. (B) Hemoglobin F, fetal hemoglobin, characteristically resists alkali denaturation providing a good diagnostic tool for the estimation of hemoglobin F levels.

16. (D) All of the criteria listed, cell size, nuclear characteristics, and cytoplasmic characteristics are important in the identification of cells.

17. (B) Leukocytosis is the term applied to an increase of white blood cells above 10,000 per c. mm.

18. (D) Appendicitis usually results in a marked neutrophilic leuko-cytosis, while each of the other conditions listed will often result in eosinophilia.

19. (C) The normal platelet count is 150,000-400,000; 95% of the healthy controls fall within this range.

20. (A) The chief value of the osmotic fragility test is for the diagnosis of hereditary spherocytosis.

21. (C) Hemoglobin F, fetal hemoglobin, is made up of 2 alpha globin chains and 2 gamma globin chains.

22. (A) Beta thalassemia, or thal-assemia major, is also known as Cooley's anemia. This is charac-terized by a hypochromic and microcytic, hemolytic disease, reticulocytosis, and extreme poikilocytosis.

23. (A) The Philadelphia chromosome, a 22 chromosome with part of the long arm deleted, is found in cells of patients with chronic granulocytic leukemia.

24. (A) Anisocytosis is the term used to designate an abnormal variation in the size of the red blood cells.

25. (D) New methylene blue is a supravital stain used for staining reticulocytes.

26. (B) Hemoglobin A_2 is comprised of 2 alpha globin chains and 2 delta globin chains.

27. (C) Drepanocytes are cells that are produced by deoxygenation. Hb SC disease, homozygous Hb S disease, and HbS-thalassemia syndrome are all conditions in which drepanocytes may be found.

28. (C) Deficiencies of Factors V, VII or X or a combination of these factor deficiencies will result in a prolonged prothrombin time.

29. (D) All of the conditions listed may result in a vitamin B_{12} deficiency. Defective production of Intrinsic Factor is the most common cause of vitamin B_{12} deficiency; infection with the fish tapeworm, Diphyllobothrium latum, may cause a vitamin B_{12} deficiency since vitamin B_{12} is selectively absorbed by this organism; total gastrectomy may result in vitamin B_{12} deficiency because it will remove the source of production of Intrinsic Factor; and, a strict vegetarian diet which excludes all animal foods will result in an inadequate intake of vitamin B_{12}.

30. (B) The figures indicate a relative increase in the number of lymphocytes. Relative increases indicate an in-crease in the percentage of cells, not the actual number of these cells. The actual number of lymphocytes in this case is 1,800, and the normal absolute count for lymphocytes is 1,500-4,000.

31. (C) The figures in this case indicate both an absolute increase and a relative increase of lymphocytes. 78% is a relative increase, whereas the absolute count of lymphocytes is 10,600 which is an absolute increase.

32. (D) The figures here show neither an absolute nor a relative increase in the neutrophilic count.

33. (B) The figures here indicate a relative increase in neutrophils. 90% neutrophils is an increase in the percentage of neutrophils, but 90% of a 4,000 white blood cell count is 3,600 for an absolute number of neutrophils. The normal absolute count for neutrophils is 2,000-6,800.

34. (C) Pelger-Huet anomaly is a benign anomaly which may be inherited or acquired as in certain leukemias.

35. (A) May-Hegglin anomaly is an inherited anomaly affecting the neutrophils and platelets.

36. (A) Chediak-Higashi anomaly or syndrome is apparently an inherited condition.

37. (A) Spherocytosis is a hereditary condition that is characterized by spheroidal red blood cells and episodes of anemia.

38. (B) Paroxysmal nocturnal hemoglobinuria is an uncommon acquired disease which is characterized by chronic continuous intravascular hemolysis.

39. (B) Pernicious anemia characteristically shows an elevated MCV, an elevated MCHC, and is usually the result of a vitamin B_{12} deficiency.

40. (C) The mean corpuscular hemoglobin in macrocytic anemias is usually elevated, an MCH of less than 25 would more likely be found in a microcytic anemia like iron deficiency anemia.

41. (B) Figures 5, 6, and 7 are all associated with hereditary conditions. Figure 5 illustrates dense elliptocytes which are found in sickle cell anemia; figure 6 illustrates bi-lobed neutrophils of Pelger-Huet anomaly; and figure 7 illustrates spherocytes which are found in hereditary spherocytosis.

42. (A) Basophilic stippling and nucleated red blood cells are common findings in hemolytic disease of the newborn as well as in many other conditions.

43. (D) Illustration 4 represents a dying neutrophil.

44. (D) The cell illustrated is a target cell which is a common finding in pernicious anemia which is the result of vitamin B_{12} deficiency.

45. (B) Hemoglobin C disease shows decreased osmotic fragility, reduced RBC survival and an elevated reticulocyte count.

46. (D) Hemoglobin S-C disease is a heterozygous state with 2 abnormal beta globin alleles, one hemoglobin S and one hemoglobin C.

47. (A) Hemoglobin D disease is a disease with abnormal hemoglobin migrating like hemoglobin S but is non-sickling.

48. (C) Hemoglobin E when electrophoresed moves faster than hemoglobin C at pH of 8.6 and slower than hemoglobin S at a pH of 6.5.

49. (C) Gower's solution, which is composed of sodium sulfate, glacial acetic acid, and distilled water is used in red blood cell counts.

50. (E) Drabkins solution utilizes potassium cyanide and potassium ferricyanide, to form cyanmethemoglobin for the determination of the hemoglobin concentration.

51. (B) Isoton, as well as other commercially prepared solutions, is used in the automated determination of white blood cell counts.

52. (D) A 1% ammonium oxalate solution is used for platelet counts.

53. (C) Polychromatophilia is the term used for red blood cells that stain with a blue-gray tint. These are usually reticulocytes whose residual RNA has taken up the basic stain.

54. (A) Hypochromia is the term applied to those red blood cells that have a diminished amount of hemoglobin in them, and consequently have a larger central pale area than normal red blood cells.

55. (B) Basophilic stippling is the term used for red blood cells that contain coarse or fine, blue-black granules.

56. (E) Howell-Jolly bodies are actually remnants of nuclear chromatin. They are usually smooth round, and stain dark blue to black.

57. (D) Neutrophils characteristically display azurophilic granules in their cytoplasm.

58. (A) Eosinophils characteristically display large red granules in their cytoplasm due to a strong affinity for acid stains such as eosin.

59. (E) Basophils characteristically display large purple granules in their cytoplasm due to their strong affinity for basic dyes.

60. (B) Monocytes have a blue gray, slate, or ground glass appearance to their cytoplasm.

61. (B) Hypersegmented neutrophils are neutrophils having 5 or more lobes. They are commonly found in pernicious anemia and folic acid deficiencies.

62. (C) A Barr body is a small knob on a lobe of the nucleus of the neutrophil. It is found normally in females.

63. (A) Pelger-Huet anomaly is a failure of the neutrophil nucleus to segment properly. All of the neutrophils have no more than a two-lobed nucleus.

64. (D) Toxic granulation shows a dark blue-black staining to the cytoplasmic granules in the neutrophil. It is found in acute infections, drug poisoning, and burns.

65. (C) The mean corpuscular volume (MCV) is a measure of the average volume of a red blood cell and is calculated by dividing the hematocrit (a measure of volume) by the number of red blood cells.

66. (E) The mean corpuscular hemoglobin is a measure of the average amount of hemoglobin in a red blood cell and is calculated by dividing the hemoglobin concentration by the number of red blood cells.

67. (D) The mean corpuscular hemoglobin concentration is a measure of the average concentration of hemoglobin in 100 ml of packed red blood cells and is calculated by dividing the hemoglobin concentration by the hematocrit.

68. (A) In order to correctly determine the rate of production of reticulocytes, the reticulocyte count must be corrected for the increased maturation time. This is done by dividing the absolute percentage of reticulocytes by the maturation time.

69. (C) Leptocytes are more commonly referred to as target cells; these cells show a centrally stained area.

70. (B) Acanthocytes are red blood cells with thorn-like projections on the outer edge of the cells.

71. (A) Elliptocytes are oval red blood cells that are more oval than ovalocytes and tend to be cigar shaped.

72. (E) Schistocytes are red blood cell fragments.

73. (C) Factor I is also known as fibrinogen.

74. (A) Factor IV is also known as calcium.

75. (E) Factor VIII is also known as antihemophilic globulin, antihemophilic factor and cryoprecipitate.

76. (B) Factor XII is also known as the Hageman factor.

77. (B) Hemophilia is a sex linked inherited defect in the production of Factor VIII.

78. (D) Christmas disease is a sex linked recessive disorder that results in a Factor IX deficiency.

79. (E) Stuart factor deficiency is an incompletely recessive autosomal disorder resulting in a Factor X deficiency.

80. (C) Hageman trait is an autosomal inherited defect resulting in a Factor XII deficiency.

81. (B) The disease entity known as Gaucher's disease is a disorder of lipid metabolism which results in an accumulation of glucocerebrocides in the white blood cells.

82. (C) Auer bodies are found in about 40% of the cases of myelogenous leukemia. Auer bodies are rod shaped, elongated, red structures formed from azurophilic granules.

83. (D) Basophilic stippling is a common finding in the red blood cells of patients suffering from lead poisoning.

84. (A) Di Guglielmo's disease is a proliferative disorder of the erythrocyte precursors.

85. (C) Burr cells are red blood cells that have knobby projections on their surface. This type of cell is produced by rupture of the cell membrane and may be found in liver diseases, hemolytic anemia, and chronic renal disease.

86. (D) A tart cell is a phagocyte, usually a monocyte, that has phagocytized a nucleus. It is of importance since it must be distinguished from the L.E. cells which contain hematoxylin bodies.

87. (B) Stomatocytes are red blood cells that have slit-like areas of pallor with a dense surrounding zone. They are associated with a marked increase in the red cell membrane's permeability.

88. (A) Hematoxylin bodies are associated with L.E. cells. The L.E. factor reacts with the DNA of the nucleus producing a round hemogenous mass called hematoxylin bodies which are later phagocytized by neutrophils or eosinophils.

89. (D) Periodic Acid-Schiff stain is used for the detection of complex carbohydrates. Periodic acid reacts with the hydroxyl groups of carbohydrates to form aldehydes which react with the Schiff reagent to produce a magenta color.

90. (A) Gomori's method is a staining procedure for iron. Ferric ions react with acid ferrocyanide to form ferric ferrocyanide which has a Prussian blue color.

91. (C) Peroxidase stain is used in the differentiation between acute granulocytic leukemia and acute lymphocytic leukemia. Peroxidase in the cytoplasm of WBC's transfers hydrogen from benzidine to hydrogen peroxide resulting in a blue-brown color. Monocytes react positively with this stain, although the granules of stain are few and faint.

92. (E) Sudan Black B stains lipids, including neutral fat, phospho-lipids, and sterols which are found in granulocytes.

93. (C) EDTA, Ethylenediamine tetraacetic acid is a chelating agent which combines with calcium thereby preventing coagulation.

94. (D) Ammonium potassium oxalate prevents coagulation by forming insoluble salts, thereby removing the calcium.

95. (A) Sodium citrate prevents coagulation by inactivating calcium ions.

96. (B) Heparin prevents coagulation by acting as an anti-thrombin and anti-thromboplastin.

97. (B) The promyelocyte is an early precursor of the cells of the granulocytic series.

98. (E) The basophilic normoblast is the youngest recognizable precursor of the red blood cell.

99. (D) The megakaryocyte is the immediate precursor of the platelet. The number of platelets produced is directly proportional to the amount of cytoplasm in the megakaryocyte.

100. (A) B cells are a type of lymphocyte. B cells form memory cells and differentiate to plasma cells.

101. (D) HbS moves faster than HbC but slower than HbA.

102. (D) Schumm's test is used to detect methemalbumin.

103. (C) Only the statement regarding the reading of the hematocrit tubes by omitting the buffy coat is accurate.

104. (A) The smaller the gauge the larger the berul.

105. (C) Erythropoietin is produced in man primarily in the kidney.

106. (D) Glycine and succinyl CoA combine to form delta amino levulinic acid.

107. (D) Red cells have a survival time of 120 days.

108. (C) The red cells would appear hypochromic, microcytic.

109. (B) HbS represents an abnormal substitution of valine for glutamic acid in the 6th position of the beta chain. HbC represents a substitution of lysine for glutamic acid in the 6th position of the beta chain.

110. (B) The eosinophil count is elevated and may be due to an allergic reaction.

111. (A) L. E. factor is a substance present in the gamma globulin fraction of serum or plasma.

112. (A) Excessive denaturation of hemoglobin within the red blood cell is characteristic of the formation of Heinz bodies.

113. (C) A diagnostic feature of Hodgkins disease is the presence of Reed-Sternberg cells.

114. (C) In the adult, lymphocytes are produced primarily in lymphoid tissue such as lymph nodes, spleen and thymus.

115. (B) Inadequate centrifugation will give falsely elevated results.

116. (C) Paroxysmal nocturnal hemoglobinuria will hemolyze red blood cells in acidified serum and sugar water.

117. (B) A positive peroxidase stain is seen in promyelocytes and later cells in the same series. Peroxidase is not seen in lymphoblasts, myeloblasts and lymphocytes. It is seen to a small degree in monocytes.

118. (B) The Price-Jones curve gives the distribution of red cell size in quantitative terms.

119. (C) Pelger Huet anomaly is characterized by the predominance of two lobed polymorphonuclear neutrophils.

120. (D) Acute myelogenous leukemia can be differentiated from acute lymphocytic leukemia (ALL) because blasts may often contain auer rods.

121. (A) Erythroleukemia or DiGuglielmo's syndrome is a rare form of leukemia. It is characterized by the presence of immature, atypical, nucleated red blood cells.

122. (B) Ehlers-Danlos syndrome is a bleeding disorder associated with a defect in the supportive framework of connective tissue.

123. (D) Aspirin as well as other pharmacologic agents can interfere with the process of platelet aggregation, specifically inhibiting the release phenomenon.

124. (D) Fragments D + E + D represent the end products of the fibrinolytic sequence.

125. (C) Plasminogen is activated to form plasmin which is responsible for lysis of the fibrin clot.

126. (D) The platelet count is the most valuable test in differentiating fibrinolysis from consumptive coagulopathy. Consumptive coagulopathy consumes platelets while fibrinolysis does not.

127. (A) EDTA acts as a chelating agent and binds calcium, sodium citrate inactivates calcium ions and potassium oxalate absorbs calcium to prevent coagulation.

128. (C) Heparin acts as an anti-thrombin and anti-thromboplastin to prevent clotting.

129. (B) Factor X is activated by Russell's viper venom, Factor VII: Tissue complex in the Extrinsic System and Factors IXa, VII, Ca^{++}, Pf_3 in the Intrinsic System.

130. (D) Factors Xa, V, Ca^{++}, Pf_3 convert prothrombin to thrombin.

131. (C) Russell bodies, Mott cells and flame cells are morphologic variants of plasma cells.

132. (B) Dohle bodies are cytoplasmic inclusions found in neutrophils of patients with severe burns, infections, normal pregnancies and ingestion of cytotoxic agents.

133. (A) Phloxine B selectively stains eosinophils and hemolyzes red blood cells.

134. (D) In the fetus, hematopoiesis begins in the yolk sac, followed at $1\frac{1}{2}$ months by the liver and, to a limited extent, at $2\frac{1}{2}$ months by the spleen. At around four months the bone marrow begins to produce blood cells and, at birth, is the primary blood forming organ.

135. (A) HbA, A_2 and F are all normal hemoglobins. At birth, 60-65% of the hemoglobin is Hb, F; 30-35% is HbA with a small amount of HbA_2. All three hemoglobins have a pair of alpha chains but differ in their second pair of polypeptide chains.

136. (D) As the red blood cell matures, the cell becomes smaller, the nucleus is more dense, and is finally extruded, and, as hemoglobin is produced, it changes staining characteristics from deep blue to orange.

137. (C) Iron deficiency, sideroblastic anemias and thalassemias are examples of hypochromic microcytic anemias.

138. (D) The Hema Tek slide stainer automatically fixes, stains, rinses and air dries blood smears.

139. (B) Both the Coulter Model Fn and S count particles electronically and dilute specimens for RBC 1/50,000. The Coulter Model Fn dilutes WBC 1/500 while the Coulter Model S dilutes 1/250 for WBC. Only the Coulter Model S calculates indices.

140. (A) Wrights stain consists of eosin and methylene blue.

141. (B) For most determinations, the first drop is not acceptable. Usually the third drop is free flowing and approaches that of venous blood. Smears made from heparinized tubes are not acceptable since the red cells take on a sheen.

142. (D) A patient with myeloid metaplasia would have teardrop shaped red blood cells, nucleated red blood cells, a variable white blood cell count and decreased platelets with some giant forms on the blood smears.

143. (D) The reticulocyte count, osmotic fragility, auto-hemolysis and MCHC would all be increased with hereditary spherocytosis.

144. (A) It would be acceptable to draw blood 8-10 cm below the IV if there is a suitable vein. Also a CBC can be collected using the capillary method. The sample would not be accurate drawn from the IV and it is not appropriate for a technologist to draw from the femoral vein if other means are available.

145. (D) All of these clinical conditions will cause erroneous results in the Coulter Model S and should be repeated using manual methods.

146. (D) Autoimmune hemolytic anemia may be seen in patients with lupus erythematosus, neoplasms, granulomas and in idiopathic states where no disease is evident.

147. (C) Since the child probably has hemolytic disease of the newborn, the ABO Group and Rh, direct Coombs test and bilirubin should be performed. Most of the Hb at birth is HbF so that the electrophoresis will not provide useful information in this instance.

148. (B) A patient with hereditary spherocytosis will have an increased osmotic fragility and MCHC. The MCV and red cell count are decreased.

149. (C) Hemolytic anemia, acute blood loss and myelophthisic anemia are examples of normochromic, normocytic anemias. Pernicious anemia is a macrocytic, normochromic anemia.

150. (D) Sideroblastic anemias are characterized by impaired heme synthesis. A hereditary X-linked form is found mainly in males. In the circulating blood, red cells appear microcytic and hypochromic. In the bone marrow, the iron stores are increased and ring sideroblasts are present.

151. (A) Nucleoli are visible with the light microscope in myeloblasts and promyelocytes.

152. (D) With chronic granulocytic leukemia, there is bosophilia, all myeloid maturation series are present, the leukocyte alkaline phosphatase is reduced and the Philadelphia chromosome is present.

153. (C) Patients with infectious mononucleosis have an absolute lymphocytosis with atypical lymphocytes, and a positive heterophile and anti-EB virus titer. There is no cytomegalovirus found in the urine.

154. (A) Hodgkins disease and Burkitts are malignant lymphomas. Di-Guglielmo's syndrome is an erythroleukemia and Schilling is a monocytic leukemia.

155. (D) The Bleeding Time, platelet adherence and aggregation, and clot retraction are all useful in diagnosing a platelet function abnormality.

156. (D) Platelets function to form a platelet plug, release Pf_3, maintain vascular integrity and release thrombosthenin for proper clot formation.

157. (B) Factors V and VIII do not have an enzymatically active form.

158. (E) Only one statement is correct. The APTT will be prolonged and corrected with adsorbed plasma.

159. (C) With a Factor X deficiency both the APTT and PT will be prolonged and corrected with aged serum.

160. (C) Blood coagulation is confined to the immediate area of tissue damage by means of natural inhibitors, platelets to absorb excess thrombin and the fibrinolytic mechanism.

161. (E) In severe liver disease, the levels of all coagulation factors may be depressed except Factor VIII which is the only factor not synthesized in the liver.

162. (D) Overall competence of the coagulation mechanism is assessed by performing a prothrombin time to test the extrinsic system, a partial thromboplastin time to assess the intrinsic system, a fibrinogen assay, and a clot solubility test for Factor XIII.

163. (D) Pateints with Macroglobinuria of Waldenström have large amounts of monoclonal IgM globulin, cryoglobulins, a proliferation of plasmacytoid lymphocytes and usually a moderate to severe anemia.

164. (E) Adhesion.

165. (D) ADP.

166. (A) Aggregation.

167. (C) Thrombin.

168. (B) Thrombosthenin.

169. (C) 3-4 gms.

170. (A) 66%.

171. (E) 29%.

172. (B) 10-25 mg.

173. (D) 0.5-1.6 mg/day.

174. (B) A very acid pH.

175. (C) A very alkaline pH.

176. (D) Overstaining.

177. (A) Excessive decoloration.

178. (B) $383 \text{ cells} \times \dfrac{1}{\frac{1}{200}} \times \dfrac{1}{\frac{1}{10}}$

$$\frac{1}{5}$$

383 cells x 10,000 = 3,830,000/cu mm.

179. (D) Ave. # cells = 140

$$(140) \quad \times \quad \frac{1}{\frac{1}{20}} \quad \frac{1}{\frac{1}{10}} \quad mm =$$

4 sq mm

140 x 50   7,000/cu mm.

180. (E) Increased levels of erythropoie-
sis is seen in secondary erythropoie-
sis, where the body is being deprived
of sufficient oxygen for various
reasons, and this lack is being compensated by an increased production
of red cells.

181. (C) The ESR will be increased as
the room temperature is increased.
Anemia will cause an increase in
the ESR except for sickle cell
anemia. If the ESR tube is inclined,
the cells will go to the lower edge
and gradually slide down the tube,
causing a falsely increased ESR.

182. (C) The Coulter Model S-Plus uses
the classic Coulter principles of
counting particles, to directly
enumerate WBC's, RBC's and Platelets. The MCV is derived from the
mean population of red cells that
are counted.

183. (B) Both the sugar water test and
Ham's test create a situation
conducive to complement activation,
which is tolerated by normal red
cells but not by cells from patients
with paroxysmal nocturnal hemoglobinuria.

184. (D) All of these findings are
indicative of myelofibrosis. Anemia
is also present. It is presently
not known why the red cell and
white cell changes occur, and
several hypotheses have been put
forward. The splenomegaly is caused
by extramedullary hematopoiesis.

185. (D) All of the answers are correct.
As cells mature they become smaller,
both the nucleus and cytoplasm
decrease in amount. In the red cell
series hemoglobinization does not

take place until the second stage,
the prorubricyte., and the amount
of hgb increase until the mature
red cell is formed. The cytoplasm
changes from being basophilic when
it is stained to the reddish hue
seen in mature red cells. This
change in cytoplasmic staining
properties is due to a loss of DNA
synthesis, as the cell matures.
The nucleus progressively gets
smaller and denser, until it is
extruded to yield the mature
anucleate red cell.

186. (D) The proper clotting of a
small superficial wound (as is
done in a template bleeding time)
depends on the rate at which there
is a platelet plug formed, this
will thereby measure the efficiency
of the vascular and platelet phases
of hemostasis.

187. (B) A rule of thumb for correlating
the examination of a differential
smear with a white blood cell count
is that, if there are 2 to 4 WBC/
HPF the estimated WBC should be
between 4-7,000/CU.MM. 4-6 WBC/HPF
would be 7-10,000/cu.mm., 6-10 WBC/
HPF means 10-13,000 WBC and if
there are 10-20/HPF the white count
should be between 13-18,000/cu.mm.

188. (B) Defective DNA synthesis is
present in megaloblastic anemias,
this abnormality leads to a state
of asynchronous (unbalanced) cell
growth, in which DNA synthesis is
decreased, while RNA and protein
synthesis continue at a normal
rate. This leads to the formation
of an enlarged cell.

189. (C) The patient's red cells are
smaller than normal (microcytic),
and the red cells do not contain
a sufficient amount of hemoglobin
(hypochromic). The MCV is below
the normal range, the MCH and MCHC
are also below normal.

190. (D) Stage 1 is the generation of
plasma thromboplastin, the intrinsic

systems are activated and both systems via different mechanisms convert factor X to its active form Xa. This activated factor X then interacts with factor V, in the presence of calcium ions and platelets phospholipids to form plasma thromboplastin.

191. (C) The French-American-British (FAB) classification of leukemias is based upon the morphology of cells in Romanowsky-stained smears.

192. (A) Neimann-Pick disease is distinguished by the excessive levels of sphigomyelin. The catabolism of sphingomyelin requires the presence of sphingomyelase, this enzyme is deficient in this disorder thus causing the abnormal accumulation of material.

193. (B) The Kleihauer-Betke method is used to detect the presence of fetal cells (hgb F) in the maternal circulation. HgbA is eluted from red cells by an acid phosphate buffer, HgbF is resistant to this elution.

194. (A) Increased levels of erythropoietin is seen in secondary erythrocytosis, where the body is being deprived of sufficient oxygen for various reasons, and this lack is being compensated by an increased production of red cells.

195. (C) Esterase stains are used primarily to distinguish between granulocytic and monocytic precursors. The chlor-acetate esterase reacts with neutrophilic cells, while monocytes are negative. While alpha napthyl acetate can be used to identify monocytes.

196. (A) Acute lymphoblastic leukemia is most commonly seen in young children, with the mean age being four years. It is uncommon after the age of 15.

197. (A) An increased reticulocyte count is seen in immune hemolytic anemia, where red cells are being destroyed and the bone marrow is producing more red cells to compensate for the loss.

Bibliography and Recommended Readings

Brown, B. A. Hematology: Principles and Procedures. Third Edition. 1980.
    Lea and Febiger. Philadelphia.

Platt, W. R. Color Atlas and Textbook of Hematology. Second Edition. 1979.
    J. B. Lippincott Company. Philadelphia.

Williams, W. J. et. al. Hematology. Third Edition. 1983. McGraw-Hill Company.
    New York.

Wintrobe, M. W. et. al. Clinical Hematology. Eighth Edition. 1981. Lea and
    Febiger. Philadelphia.

CHAPTER 11

Nuclear Medicine

Directions. Select the one BEST answer for each of the following statements. Circle the appropriate response on the answer sheet.

1. Which of the following statements regarding isomers is true?

   A. they differ in atomic number
   B. they differ in mass number
   C. they exist in the excited state for a measurable amount of time
   D. all of the above
   E. none of the above

2. Most naturally occurring radioactive series end with the formation of:

   A. lead
   B. mercury
   C. iron
   D. uranium
   E. bismuth

3. The rate of decay of a radionuclide is affected by:

   A. temperature
   B. pressure
   C. pH
   D. all of the above
   E. none of the above

4. Radioactive decay is measured in:

   A. rads
   B. rems
   C. curies
   D. reps
   E. roentgens

5. Gamma rays are effectively shielded by:

   A. paper
   B. glass
   C. lead
   D. all of the above
   E. none of the above

6. Phosphorus compounds used for bone scanning include:

   A. stannous polyphosphate
   B. diphosphonate
   C. pyrophosphonate
   D. all of the above
   E. none of the above

7. The function of the collimator is:

   A. to shield the detector from background radiation
   B. to supply voltage to the system
   C. to record information from the detector
   D. to display data
   E. to move the detector over the organ to be scanned

8. The pulse-height analyzer selects:

   A. frequency   D. wavelength
   B. amplitude   E. all of the above
   C. voltage

9. An isotope has a half-life of six hours. If the initial dose was 40 µCi, how many µCi would be left at the end of 12 hours?

   A. 20   D. 2.5
   B. 10   E. 1.25
   C. 5

10. In areas where iodide is in the diet, an oral dosage of ^{131}I is accumulated by the normal adult thyroid to the following extent:

    A. 5-15%   D. 55-75%
    B. 15-35%   E. 75-95%
    C. 35-55%

11. Radioisotopic procedures used to test thyroid function include:

    A. Berson clearance   D. all of the above
    B. pertechnetate uptake   E. none of the above
    C. T_3 uptake

12. The total iron binding capacity of normal serum is:

    A. 100-200 µg/ml   D. 400-500 µg/ml
    B. 200-300 µg/ml   E. 500-600 µg/ml
    C. 300-400 µg/ml

13. With regard to linear energy transfer (LET):

    A. α is greater than β^- D. γ is greater than β^-
    B. β^- is greater than α E. γ is greater than α
    C. γ is greater than x-ray

14. The atomic number of an element is based upon:

    A. the number of neutrons
    B. the number of protons
    C. the number of protons plus neutrons
    D. the number of electrons plus neutrons
    E. the number of protons, neutrons and electrons

Questions 15-26

Directions. For each of the numbered items select the appropriate lettered response.
Do not use the same letter more than once.

15. α emission
16. β⁻ emission
17. γ emission
18. x-ray emission

A. high velocity electron
B. nuclear electromagnetic wave
C. helium nucleus
D. orbital electromagnetic wave
E. high velocity neutron

19. roentgen
20. rad
21. rem
22. RBE

A. a measure of radiation exposure per gram of tissue
B. a measure of human absorbed dose
C. a measure of radiation dose absorbed by any matter
D. a measure of the relative effectiveness of various radiations
E. a measure of radiation exposure

23. ¹³¹I-thyroid uptake
24. thyroid stimulating hormone
25. triiodothyronine uptake test
26. ¹³¹I-ortho-hippurate

A. administered intramuscularly
B. administered intravenously
C. in vitro test
D. administered orally
E. administered by lumbar puncture

Questions 27-35

Directions. One, some, or all of the responses for each of the following statements
may be correct. Indicate your response as follows:

A. if items 1 and 3 are correct
B. if items 2 and 4 are correct
C. if three of the items are correct
D. if all of the items are correct
E. if only one of the items is correct

27. Isotopes may have:

1. different atomic numbers
2. different mass numbers

3. different chemical properties
4. different radioactive properties

28. Isobars may have:

1. different atomic numbers
2. different mass numbers

3. different chemical properties
4. different radioactive properties

29. Nuclides may be produced by:

1. fission
2. fusion

3. neutron activation
4. transmutation

30. The harmful effects of radiation are dependent upon:

    1. energy
    2. penetrability
    3. ionizing ability
    4. half-life

31. ^{99m}Tc has a number of clinical usages because:

    1. it has a short half-life
    2. if emits a gamma which is optimal for counting
    3. it is easily separated from its parent compound
    4. it has a weak beta

32. It is important to use isotopes with short half-lives for clinical work because:

    1. it decreases the radiation exposure to the patient
    2. it increases the biological clearance rate of the compound
    3. it decreases the interference with subsequent tests
    4. it increases the effective half-life of the substance

33. Currently scintigraphic procedures are indicated in the determination of:

    1. hypothyroidism
    2. thyroid tumor
    3. hyperthyroidism
    4. ectopic thyroid tissue

34. ^{131}I taken orally may be expected to appear in:

    1. hydroiodic acid in the stomach
    2. urine
    3. saliva
    4. hydroxyapatite

35. ^{131}I-albumin is used to assay plasma volume because:

    1. it is measurable in small quantities
    2. it has a beta which is optimal for counting
    3. it leaves the blood slowly
    4. one only needs to fast for 6 hours prior to the test

Questions 36-39

Directions. Select the answer which quantitatively describes or compares the paired statements.

    A. if β^- is greater than γ
    B. if γ is greater than β^-
    C. if β^- and γ are nearly the same

36. energy
37. penetrability
38. charge
39. mass

Questions 40-55

Directions. For each of the numbered words or phrases listed below, select the appropriate response as follows:

A. if the item is associated with A only
B. if the item is associated with B only
C. if the item is associated with both A and B
D. if the item is associated with neither A nor B

A. in vitro assay
B. in vivo assay

40. T_3 uptake test
41. thyroid uptake
42. scintigraphy
43. Fe binding capacity of proteins

A. X-ray
B. γ-ray

44. mass of 1
45. negatively charged
46. may follow alpha emissions
47. electromagnetic radiation

A. β^- emitter
B. γ emitter

48. ^{32}P

49. ^{131}I

50. ^{14}C

51. ^{99m}Tc

A. dependent upon half-life of atoms in sample
B. dependent upon half-life of sample in body

52. physical half-life
53. biological half-life
54. effective half-life
55. patient dose

Questions 56-60

Directions.   Select and circle the one BEST answer for each of the following statements utilizing the information presented in either the following graph, tracing, table or laboratory data.

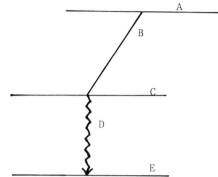

56. Alpha emission is represented by:

    A. A   D. D
    B. B   E. E
    C. C

57. Gamma emission is represented by:

    A. A   D. D
    B. B   E. E
    C. C

58. A and C would:

    A. be the same element   D. all of the above
    B. have the same mass   E. none of the above
    C. have the same atomic number

59. C and E would:

    A. be the same element   D. all of the above
    B. have the same mass   E. none of the above
    C. have the same atomic number

60. The excited state is represented by:

    A. A   D. A and B
    B. C   E. C and E
    C. E

Explanatory Answers

1. (C) Isomers are nuclides which exist in the excited state for measurable amounts of time.

2. (A) The thorium, actinium, and uranium series end with the formation of lead; the neptunium series ends with the formation of bismuth.

3. (E) Physical parameters do not alter the rate of decay of a radionuclide.

4. (C) The curie is the unit of radioactive decay, equal to 3×10^7 disintegrations per second.

5. (C) Glass and paper can effectively shield β^- and α respectively; γ are very penetrating and must be stopped by denser substances such as lead.

6. (D) All of the phosphorus compounds listed are used for bone scanning.

7. (A) The collimator shields the detector from background radiation and also limits the field to the organ being scanned.

8. (B) The pulse-height analyzer selects pulses which are over a given amplitude or which are within a given amplitude range.

9. (B) At the end of six hours, 50% or 20 µCi would be left; at the end of 12 hours, 25% or 10 µCi would be left.

10. (B) In areas where iodide is in the diet, 15-35% of ingested iodine is taken up by the thyroid; in areas where iodide is not in the diet, the values are higher.

11. (D) All of the procedures listed test thyroid function.

12. (C) Normal serum binds 300-400 µg iron/ml.

13. (A) In general the linear energy transfer of α particles exceeds that of β^- particles, and the LET of β^- particles exceeds that of γ and X-rays.

14. (B) The number of protons in the nucleus determines the atomic number.

15. (C) An alpha particle consists of two protons and two neutrons; it is equivalent to a helium nucleus.

16. (A) Beta emissions result from the conversion of a neutron into a proton and an electron. The electron escapes from the nucleus as a beta particle.

17. (B) A gamma ray is an electromagnetic wave resulting from nuclear instability.

18. (D) An X-ray is an electromagnetic wave resulting from orbital instability; in all other aspects, it is exactly like a γ ray.

19. (E) The roentgen is a measure of the total quantity of radiation emitted.

20. (C) The rad is a measure of radiation dose absorbed by any matter.

21. (B) The rem (radiation equivalent man) is a measure of the radiation dose absorbed by man.

22. (D) The RBE (relative biological effectiveness) is a measure of the effectiveness of various radiations on man.

23. (D) For thyroid uptake studies, ^{131}I is administered orally.

24. (A) Thyroid stimulating hormone is administered intramuscularly in order to determine the patient's capacity to respond to the hormone.

25. (C) The triiodothyronine (T$_3$) uptake test is an in vitro test to determine the binding capacity of thyronine-binding proteins in the patient's serum.

26. (B) ^{131}I-ortho-hippurate (OIH) is administered intravenously for renograms.

27. (B) Isotopes are different forms of the same element and must therefore, have the same atomic number and same chemical properties.

28. (C) Isobars are atoms with the same mass.

29. (D) All methods listed are capable of producing nuclides.

30. (D) The harmful effects of radiation depend upon the energy, penetrability, ability to ionize and concentration, which in turn depends upon half-life.

31. (C) ^{99m}Tc has a half-life of 6 hours, emits a o.14 Mev gamma, and is easily separated from its parent compound, molybdenum. It does not emit beta particles.

32. (A) Using isotopes with short half-lives decreases the radiation exposure of the patient and decreases interference with subsequent tests. Biological clearance rate is dependent upon the nature of the compound and not the radioactivity; effective half-life is decreased by isotopes with short half-lives.

33. (B) Scintigraphy is used in the detection of tumors and ectopic tissue; hypothyroidism and hyperthyroidism are best detected by measuring serum thyroxine and TSH levels.

34. (C) Labeled iodine will appear in stomach acid, saliva and urine; hydroxyapatite is a calcium phosphate complex and does not bind iodine.

35. (A) ^{131}I-albumin is used to assay plasma volume because it is measurable in small quantities, leaves the blood slowly, and the patient need not fast at all; beta rays are not penetrable enough to be used for scanning.

36. (C) Both β^- and γ have wide energy spectra which overlap.

37. (B) γ rays have a lower linear energy transfer than β^- and are therefore more penetrating.

38. (A) β^- has a negative charge; γ is uncharged.

39. (A) β^- has the mass of an electron; γ is without measurable mass.

40. (A) The T$_3$ uptake test measures the thyronine binding capacity of serum proteins in vitro.

41. (B) The thyroid uptake test measures the ability of the thyroid gland to accumulate radiolabeled iodine in vivo.

42. (B) Scintigraphy measures the distribution of various isotopes in organs <u>in vivo</u>.

43. (A) Fe binding capacity is performed <u>in vitro</u> to determine the transport capacity of serum proteins.

44. (D) Neither radiation has measurable mass.

45. (D) Neither radiation is charged.

46. (B) Alpha emissions are nuclear events which may be followed by γ emission.

47. (C) Both x-rays and γ-rays are electromagnetic radiations.

48. (A) ^{32}P is a β^- emitter.

49. (C) ^{131}I emits a 0.61 Mev β^- and a 0.36 Mev γ.

50. (A) ^{14}C emits a 0.71 Mev β^-.

51. (B) ^{99m}Tc emits a 0.14 Mev γ.

52. (A) The physical half-life is solely dependent upon the half-life of the atoms in the sample.

53. (B) The biological half-life is the half-life of the sample in the body.

54. (C) The effective half-life is a composite of the physical and biological half-lives.

55. (C) The patient dose is dependent upon the effective half-life of the labeled compound in the body.

56. (B) Alpha emission is represented by B.

57. (D) Gamma emission is represented by D.

58. (E) Alpha particles are the result of the emission of 2 protons and 2 neutrons from an atom. Therefore, the daughter would differ in mass and atomic number.

59. (D) C is E in the excited state. They would be the same element.

60. (C) A is the parent atom, E is the daughter atom in the ground state; i.e. nonradioactive.

Bibliography and Recommended Readings

Altman, K. I., Gerber, G. B. and S. Okada. <u>Radiation Biochemistry</u>. 1970. Academic Press. New York.

Casarett, A. P. <u>Radiation Biology</u>. 1968. Prentice-Hall, Inc. New Jersey.

Davidson, I. and J. Henry (Editors). <u>Todd-Sanford Clinical Diagnosis by Laboratory Methods</u>. Fifteenth Edition. 1974. W. B. Saunders Company. Philadelphia.

Rothfeld, B. <u>Nuclear Medicine In Vitro</u>. 1974. J. B. Lippincott Company. Philadelphia.

Shtasel, P. <u>Speak to Me in Nuclear Medicine</u>. 1976. Harper and Row Publishers, Inc. Hagerstown, Maryland.

CHAPTER 12

Clinical Chemistry

Directions. Select the one BEST answer for each of the following statements. Circle
the appropriate response on the answer sheet.

1. Which of the following is the substance used in the Jaffe reaction for serum
    creatinine?

    A. Ehrlich's reagent   C. acetic anhydride
    B. phosphomolybdate   D. alkaline picrate

2. Which of the following is the end product of purine metabolism?

    A. amino acids   C. creatinine
    B. uric acid   D. peptides

3. Which of the following reagents is used in the determination of serum phosphorus?

    A. Titan yellow   C. EDTA
    B. molybdate   D. thiocynate

4. Decreases in total serum calcium may result in:

    A. hyponatremia   C. tetany
    B. hypokalemia   D. none of the above

5. Which of the following is NOT a good source of carbohydrates?

    A. fruits   C. meat
    B. molasses   D. honey

6. Which of the following is considered to be fructosan?

    A. starch   C. inulin
    B. glycogen   D. none of the above

7. Glycogenesis means:

    A. conversion of glucose to glycogen
    B. breakdown of glycogen to glucose
    C. conversion of glucose to lactate or pyruvate
    D. formation of glucose from non-carbohydrate sources

8. Which of the following proteins has the fastest electrophoretic mobility?

    A. albumin   C. beta globulins
    B. alpha globulins   D. gamma globulins

9. Which of the following would you find in a primary hyperparathyroidism?

    A. elevated serum calcium and decreased serum phosphorus
    B. elevated serum calcium and elevated serum phosphorus
    C. decreased serum calcium and decreased serum phosphorus
    D. decreased serum calcium and increased serum phosphorus

10. Which of the following is the major intracellular cation?

    A. Na^+ C. K^+
    B. Mg^{++} D. Ca^{++}

11. Which of the following pH's is recommended for protein electrophoresis?

    A. 7.4   C. 8.4
    B. 7.8   D. 8.6

12. Which of the following substances is the most commonly found sterol in man?

    A. cholesterol   C. estriol
    B. cortisol   D. pregnanediol

13. Which of the following is the immediate precursor of porphobilinogen?

    A. coproporphyrin   C. delta-aminolevulinic acid
    B. uroporphyrin   D. heme

14. Which of the following organs is responsible for the major portion of bilirubin conjugation?

    A. kidney   C. spleen
    B. liver   D. pancreas

15. Which of the following substances is added to the "direct" bilirubin to form indirect bilirubin?

    A. ascorbic acid   C. uric acid
    B. glucuronic acid   D. tungstic acid

16. Bilirubin is the product of the breakdown of which of the following?

    A. proteins   C. cholesterol
    B. urea   D. hemoglobin

17. Which of the following is the optimal pH for alkaline phosphatase?

    A. 7.0   C. 9.0
    B. 8.0   D. 10.0

18. The chemical bond between amino acids in the primary structure of proteins is:

    A. hydrogen bonds   C. peptide bonds
    B. disulfide bonds   D. hydrophilic bonds

19. At which of the following pH's is acid phosphatase unstable?

    A. 5.2   C. 6.8
    B. 6.6   D. 7.2

20. Which of the following is used to differentiate between prostatic and non-specific acid phosphatase?

    A. carbonate ions   C. bromide ions
    B. tartrate ions   D. chloride ions

21. Glycogen is classified as:

    A. monosaccharide   C. polysaccharide
    B. disaccharide   D. none of the above

22. Which of the following is the term used to designate the formation of glucose from non carbohydrate sources?

    A. glycolysis   C. glycogenolysis
    B. glucogenesis   D. glycogenesis

23. In an enzymatic glucose determination it is necessary to use a mutarotase because:

    A. all of the glucose in serum is β-D-glucose
    B. all of the glucose in serum is α-D-glucose
    C. some of the glucose in serum is α-D-glucose
    D. none of the above

24. β-hydroxybutyric acid is formed as the result of an accumulation of which of the following?

    A. acetyl Co A   C. uric acid
    B. oxaloacetic acid   D. triglycerides

25. The enzyme aldolase has been designated by Enzyme Commission as E.C. 4.1.2.13. The 4, or first digit, indicates

    A. the class of the enzyme   C. the sub-sub class of the enzyme
    B. the sub class of the enzyme   D. the serial number of the enzyme

26. Hypernatremia is found in which of the following?

    A. Addison's disease   C. diarrhea
    B. Cushing's syndrome   D. renal tubular disease

27. Which of the following substances is required for CPK reactions?

    A. magnesium ions   C. potassium ions
    B. chloride ions   D. acetyl Co A

28. Hyperchloridia is observed in which of the following?

    A. duodenal ulcers   C. carcinoma of the stomach
    B. pernicious anemia   D. all of the above

Questions 29-45

Directions. One, some, or all of the responses for each of the following statements may be correct. Indicate your response as follows:

A. if items 1 and 3 are correct
B. if items 2 and 4 are correct
C. if three of the items are correct
D. if all of the items are correct
E. if only one of the items is correct

29. Which of the following enzymes will be elevated in acute pancreatitis?

    1. amylase   3. lipase
    2. acid phosphatase   4. cholinesterase

30. Which of the following are the end products of amylase activity on starch?

    1. glucose   3. maltose
    2. fructose   4. sucrose

31. Serum alkaline phosphatase levels are found elevated in which of the following?

    1. liver disease   3. bone disease
    2. pancreatic disease   4. stomach disease

32. Which of the following are requisites for immunogenicity?

    1. stability of structure   3. molecular mass
    2. randomness of structure   4. foreignness of structure

33. Which of the following give a positive reaction with biuret reagents?

    1. amino acids   3. dipeptides
    2. tripeptides   4. polypeptides

34. Which of the following substances may produce respiratory depression?

    1. alcohol
    2. carbon tetrachloride
    3. mercurials
    4. cyanide

35. Which of the following statements are true of carbon tetrachloride?

    1. it is toxic to the liver
    2. it is readily absorbed by the respiratory tract
    3. it is readily absorbed by the skin
    4. ethanol increases its toxicity

36. Which of the following enzymes is useful in the diagnosis of muscular dystrophy?

    1. lactic dehydrogenase
    2. lipase
    3. creatine kinase
    4. amylase

37. Which of the following substances are involved in the breakdown of dietary fats?

    1. bile
    2. amylase
    3. lipases
    4. maltase

38. Which of the following vitamins are fat soluble vitamins?

    1. B_{12}
    2. A
    3. C
    4. D

39. Which of the following ions is necessary for amylase to act at its optimum?

    1. chloride ions
    2. bromide ions
    3. sodium ions
    4. nitrate ions

40. Which of the following substances can be assayed by flame photometry?

    1. sodium
    2. potassium
    3. magnesium
    4. lithium

41. Which of the following amino acids contain sulfur in their chemical structure?

    1. valine
    2. cystine
    3. serine
    4. cysteine

42. Which of the following will result in falsely elevated inorganic phosphorus levels in serum?

    1. hemolysis
    2. bed rest
    3. lipemia
    4. oral contraceptives

43. A technologist is using the Technician Auto Analyzer II system for the measurement of serum urea nitrogen levels. The results coming out of the instrument show non-linearity. Which of the following may be the reason for this result?

    1. defective reagents
    2. incorrect pump tube size
    3. defective phototube
    4. incorrect heating bath temperature

44. Which of the following reagents is/are used in serum uric acid concentrations?

    1. phosphotungstic acid
    2. picric acid

    3. uricase
    4. urease

45. Which of the following hormones will raise blood sugar levels?

    1. epinephrine
    2. insulin

    3. glucagon
    4. hydrocortisone

Questions 46-47

Directions. Select and circle the one BEST answer for each of the following statements utilizing the information presented in either the following graph, tracing,
table or laboratory data.

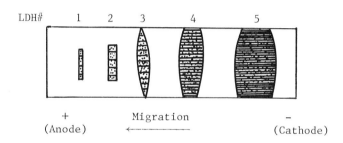

46. The LDH isoenzyme pattern shown above would most likely indicate damage to the:

    A. heart
    B. liver

    C. lung
    D. spleen

47. The elevated LDH fraction shown above would have which of the following
    tetrameric structures?

    A. H_4
    B. H_2M_2

    C. M_4
    D. HM_3

Questions 48–62

Directions. For each of the numbered words or phrases listed below, select the appropriate response as follows:

A. if the item is associated with A only
B. if the item is associated with B only
C. if the item is associated with both A and B
D. if the item is associated with neither A nor B

>   A. decreased pH and decreased pCO_2
>   B. decreased pH and elevated pCO_2

48. respiratory alkalosis
49. respiratory acidosis
50. metabolic acidosis
51. metabolic alkalosis

>   A. found elevated in hemolytic anemias
>   B. found elevated in progressive muscular dystrophy

52. serum LDH levels
53. serum CPK levels
54. bilirubin levels
55. serum potassium levels

>   A. acute hepatitis
>   B. obstructive jaundice

56. prothrombin time, increased
57. elevated serum aldolase
58. decreased serum globulins

>   A. elevated in liver disease
>   B. elevated in myocardial infarctions

59. serum LDH levels
60. serum CPK levels
61. serum alkaline phosphatase levels
62. serum acid phosphatase levels

Questions 63-72

Directions. The column on the left contains 3 scientifically related categories while the column on the right contains 4 items which may illustrate scientific phenomena or processes. Three of the items in the column on the right relate to only one of the categories in the column on the left. FIRST, indicate the category in which the 3 processes or phenomena belong. SECOND, indicate the one process or phenomenon which is not related to that category.

Category

Phenomenon

63. A. lipids
    B. proteins
    C. carbohydrates

64. A. triglycerides
    B. chilomicrons
    C. measured by the biuret method
    D. separated by electrophoresis

65. A. BUN
    B. creatinine
    C. uric acid

66. A. synthesized in the liver
    B. diacetyl monoxime method
    C. elevated in gout
    D. elevated in renal disease

67. A. glucose
    B. lactose
    C. maltose

68. A. an aldose
    B. a ketose
    C. reduces cupric ions
    D. has the basic formula $C_6H_{12}O_6$

69. A. α_1 globulins
    B. α_2 globulins
    C. β_1 globulins

70. A. haptoglobin
    B. pre-β-lipoprotein
    C. β-lipoprotein
    D. α_2-macroglobulin

71. A. CPK
    B. LDH
    C. ALP

72. A. elevated in myocardial infarctions
    B. elevated in liver diseases
    C. has 5 distinct isoenzymes
    D. elevated in patients with acute cerebrovascular disease

Questions 73-92

Directions. For each of the numbered items select the appropriate lettered response. Do not use the same letter more than once.

Common Name

73. Vitamin A
74. Vitamin B_1
75. Vitamin B_{12}
76. Vitamin B_2

Chemical Name

A. Cyanocobalamin
B. Ascorbic acid
C. Retinol
D. Thiamine
E. Riboflavin

Disorder   Enzyme

77. bone disease   A. amylase
78. pancreatic disorders   B. acid phosphatase
79. prostate disorders   C. alkaline phosphatase
80. heart disease   D. lactic dehydrogenase
                              E. lipase

Enzyme   Standard letter abbreviation

81. alanine aminotransferase A. AMS
82. aspartate transferase   B. TPS
83. lipase   C. AST
84. amylase   D. LPS
                              E. ALT

85. chromoprotein   A. hemoglobin
86. metalloprotein   B. collagens
87. glycoprotein   C. orosomucoid
88. albuminoids   D. cardiolipin
                              E. ceruloplasmin

89. rickets   A. Ca^{++} ↓, HPO_4 = ↓, alkaline phosphatase ↑
90. primary hyperparathyroidism   B. Ca^{++} N, HPO_4 = N, alkaline phosphatase ↑
91. Paget's disease   C. Ca^{++} ↑, HPO_4 = ↓, alkaline phosphatase N or ↑
92. vitamin D intoxication   D. Ca^{++} ↓, HPO_4 = ↓, alkaline phosphatase ↓
                              E. Ca^{++} ↑, HPO_4 = N, ↑, or ↓, alkaline
                                    phosphatase N

Questions 93-109

Directions. Select the one BEST answer for each of the following statements. Circle the appropriate response on the answer sheet.

93. The colligative property most commonly measured in the determination of the concentration of osmotically active particles in biological fluids is:

    A. decrease in osmotic pressure   D. decrease in vapor pressure
    B. freezing point depression   E. none of the above
    C. boiling point depression

94. The Biuret method is used for the determination of serum:

    A. creatinine   D. uric acid
    B. blood urea nitrogen   E. blood ammonia
    C. protein

95. In the manometric determination of total CO_2 in serum and plasma, CO_2 is released from the specimen by the addition of:

    A. sodium hydroxide   D. acetic acid
    B. lactic acid   E. none of the above
    C. caprylic acid

96. Electrophoretic techniques for the separation and classification of protein utilize the following protein property:

   A. differences in molecular volume and shape
   B. variation in molecular mass and shape
   C. differences in localized molecular surface structure
   D. differences in surface electrical charge density
   E. changes in solubility in the presence of charged ion

97. Standard deviation is expressed mathematically by the formula:

   A. $\sqrt{\dfrac{\Sigma(x + \bar{x})^2}{N}}$

   B. $\sqrt{\dfrac{\Sigma(x - \bar{x})}{N - 1}}$

   C. $\sqrt{\dfrac{\Sigma(x - \bar{x})^2}{N - 1}}$

   D. $\sqrt{\dfrac{\Sigma(x^2 - \bar{x})}{N - 1}}$

   E. $\sqrt{\dfrac{\Sigma(x + \bar{x})^2}{n - 1}}$

98. A normal solution is defined as:

   A. one gram equivalent weight of the solute in one deciliter of solution
   B. one gram molecular weight of the solute in one liter of solution
   C. one gram molecular weight of the solute in one deciliter of solution
   D. one gram equivalent weight of the solute in one liter of solution
   E. none of the above

99. A 1 N solution would contain:

   A. 10 milliequivalents of solute in 1 ml of solution
   B. 1 milliequivalent of solute in 1 ml of solution
   C. 1 milliequivalent of solute in 10 ml of solution
   D. 1 milliequivalent of solute in 100 ml of solution
   E. 10 milliequivalents of solute in 100 ml of solution

100. 250 mg/100 ml of Na^+ is equal to:

   A. 10.87 mEq/liter
   B. 1.087 mEq/liter
   C. 108.7 mEq/liter
   D. 217.40 mEq/liter
   E. 21.74 mEq/liter

101. Which of the following hyperlipoproteinemias is NOT usually associated with nephrotic syndrome?

   A. type I
   B. type II
   C. type IV
   D. type V

102. Which of the following protein fractions is NOT primarily produced by the liver?

   A. haptoglobin
   B. immunoglobulin
   C. C2
   D. ceruloplasmin

103. In the electrophoretic separation of proteins, which of the following will not be found in the beta bands?

    A. haptoglobin
    B. fibrinogen
    C. hemopexin
    D. transferrin

104. Which of the following statements is TRUE concerning primary hyperparathyroidism?

    A. serum calcium, phosphorous and urine calcium, phosphorous will all be elevated
    B. serum calcium, phosphorous and urine calcium, phosphorous will all be decreased
    C. serum calcium, and urine calcium, phosphorous will be elevated, but serum phosphorous will be decreased
    D. serum calcium and urine calcium will be elevated, but, serum and urine phosphorous will be decreased

105. Given that approximately 68% of the iron in the normal adult male is found in hemoglobin, which of the following has the next highest concentration of iron?

    A. myoglobin
    B. ferritin
    C. transferrin
    D. enzyme iron

106. In primary hypothyroidism, which of the following is TRUE?

    A. T4 is decreased, T3 is normal or decreased, and the TSH is normal
    B. T4 is decreased, T3 is normal or decreased, and the TSH is increased
    C. T4 is decreased, T3 is increased, and the TSH is normal
    D. T4 is increased, T3 is decreased, and the TSH is normal

107. In which of the following cases will the fasting glucose be below normal?

    A. alimentary hypoglycemia
    B. functional hypoglycemia
    C. diabetic hypoglycemia
    D. ethanol-induced hypoglycemia

108. Which of the following types of hyperlipoproteinemia may be caused by pregnancy?

    A. type I
    B. type II
    C. type III
    D. type IV

109. Which of the following protein fractions is produced primarily by the liver?

    A. C1
    B. C2
    C. C3
    D. immunoglobulin G

Questions 110-114

Directions: For each of the numbered words or phrases listed below, select the appropriate response as follows:

A. if the item is associated with A only
B. if the item is associated with B only
C. if the item is associated with both A and B
D. if the item is associated with neither A nor B

A.   increased total LD
B.   increased total CK

110.   neurogenic muscle disease
111.   acute myocardial infarction
112.   progressive muscular dystrophy
113.   megaloblastic anemia
114.   pulmonary infarction

A.   increased total CK
B.   increased CK-MB

115.   acute myocardial infarction
116.   progressive muscular dystrophy
117.   organic brain disease
118.   acute hepatitis
119.   neurogenic muscle disease

A.   myocardial infarction
B.   acute hepatitis

120.   elevated total CK activity
121.   elevated total LD activity
122.   elevated AST (SGOT) activity
123.   elevated Amylase activity
124.   elevated ALT (SGPT) activity

A.   direct (conjugated) bilirubin
B.   indirect (unconjugated) bilirubin

125.   soluble in water
126.   soluble in alcohol
127.   has an affinity for brain tissue
128.   has a tetrapyrrole structure
129.   is a polar compound

A.   increased serum iron
B.   increased total iron binding capacity

130.   iron deficiency anemia
131.   viral hepatitis
132.   thalassemia
133.   nephrosis
134.   iron poisoning

A.   decreased serum calcium
B.   decreased urine calcium

135.   primary hyperparathyroidism
136.   hypoparathyroidism
137.   vitamin D intoxication
138.   Paget's disease
139.   idiopathic osteoporosis

A. decreased T4
B. decreased T3

140. primary hypothyroidism
141. hyperthyroidism
142. euthyroidism
143. optimal therapy with T3 preparations
144. optimal therapy with T4 preparations

Questions 145-159

Directions. One, some, or all of the responses for each of the following statement.
may be correct. Indicate your response as follows:

A. if items 1 and 3 are correct
B. if items 2 and 4 are correct
C. if three of the items are correct
D. if all of the items are correct
E. if only one of the items is correct

145. In the diagnosis of myocardial infarction, which of the following are increased?

1. total CK activity   3. CK-MB concentration
2. total LD activity   4. LD-5 concentration

146. Which of the following drugs may be found in the sera of patients being treated
for seizures?

1. phenytoin   3. phenobarbital
2. theophylline   4. acetaminophen

147. Which of the following enzymes would be found elevated in obstructive jaundice?

1. amylase   3. lipase
2. alkaline phosphatase   4. gamma-glutamyl transferase

148. Which of the following enzymes are magnesium dependent?

1. hexokinase   3. carboxylases
2. phosphatases   4. transphosphorylases

149. In the enzymatic assay of serum glucose, which of the following enzymes are
utilized?

1. glucose oxidase   3. peroxidase
2. mutarotase   4. amylase

150. Which of the following proteins have a molecular weight of less than 100,000
daltons?

1. pre-albumin   3. hemopexin
2. albumin   4. alpha-1-antitrypsin

151. Which of the following proteins are NOT manufactured in the liver?

    1. fibrinogen   3. pre-albumin
    2. complement fraction Cl   4. immunoglobulin G

152. Which of the following samples may be analyzed for bilirubin content using
      the spectrophotometric assay (bilirubinometer)?

    1. neonatal samples
    2. adult samples
    3. premature neonate samples
    4. neonatal samples after the infant has had an exchange transfusion

153. Which of the following methods may be utilized for the assay of total protein
      in cerebrospinal fluid?

    1. biuret method   3. bromcresol green method
    2. trichloroacetic acid   4. Coomassie Blue method

154. Which of the following methods may be used to determine serum magnesium levels.

    1. atomic absorption   3. calgamite
    2. titan yellow   4. ammonium oxalate

155. In obstructive jaundice, which of the following statements is (are) TRUE?

    1. direct bilirubin is increased
    2. alkaline phosphatase is increased
    3. albumin/globulin ratio is normal
    4. gamma-glutamyltranspeptidase is normal

156. Which of the following disorders will produce decreased levels of serum
      carotene?

    1. diabetes mellitus   3. malabsorption syndromes
    2. myxedema   4. nephritis

157. Which of the following will cause elevations of the serum salicylates?

    1. aspirin   3. tylenol
    2. wintergreen flavoring   4. alka-seltzer

158. Which of the following may result in hypoglycemia?

    1. insulinoma   3. ethanol
    2. hypopituitarism   4. salicylates

159. Which of the following disorders may be adequately diagnosed using only the
      glucose tolerance test?

    1. diabetes mellitus   3. gestational diabetes
    2. hypoglycemia   4. diabetes insipidous

Explanatory Answers

1. (D) In the Jaffe reaction for serum creatinine determination, the active reagent is alkaline picrate which reacts with creatinine to form a yellow-red compound.

2. (B) Uric acid is the end product of purine metabolism in human beings.

3. (B) Ammonium molybdate is used in the chemical determination of serum phosphorus. Ammonium molybdate reacts with the phosphorus to form ammonium phosphomolybdate which is reduced to a molybdenum blue compound.

4. (C) Tetany is associated with decreases in total serum calcium.

5. (C) Meats and sea foods are poor sources of carbohydrates because they contain less than 1% glycogen.

6. (C) Inulin is a polysaccharide which consists mainly of fructose and is classified as a fructosan. Starch and glycogen are principally glucose polysaccharides and are therefore classified as glucosans.

7. (A) Glycogenesis is the term used to indicate the conversion of glucose to glycogen. The breakdown of glycogen to glucose is called glyco-genolysis; the conversion of glucose to lactate or pyruvate is called glycolysis; and the formation of glucose from non-carbohydrate sources is called glucogenesis.

8. (A) Albumin has the fastest electrophoretic mobility because it is the smallest and has the largest number of negative charges.

9. (A) Primary hyperparathyroidism results in elevated serum calcium levels, elevated ionized calcium levels, and decreased serum phosphorus levels.

10. (C) Potassium is the major intra-cellular cation having a concentration of 150 mmoles/L.

11. (D) At the pH of 8.6 all serum proteins are negatively charged, allowing for the separation of these proteins by electrophoretic procedures.

12. (A) Cholesterol is the sterol found most abundantly in man; it is the precursor of the steroid hormones.

13. (C) Two molecules of delta-aminolevulinic acid condense to form porphobilinogen.

14. (B) Most of the "direct" bilirubin is conjugated to the indirect form in the liver.

15. (B) Direct bilirubin is conjugated in the liver with glucuronic acid to form bilirubin deglucuronide.

16. (D) Bilirubin is a product of hemoglobin degradation.

17. (D) The optimal pH for alkaline phosphatase is about 10.0.

18. (C) The peptide bond is the characteristic bond between amino acids in protein chains. The peptide bond is a bond formed by the carboxyl group of one amino acid and the amino group of another amino acid.

19. (D) The optimum pH for acid phosphatase has been found to be between 4.8-5.1. The acid phosphatases are unstable at temperatures above 37°C and pH levels above 7.0.

20. (B) Prostatic acid phosphatase is strongly inhibited by tartrate ions. Since elevated prostatic acid phosphatase levels are important in the diagnosis of prostatic carcinoma, acid phosphatase levels are usually performed with and without tartrate ions present.

21. (C) Glycogen is produced in the liver from glucose and is classified as a polysaccharide.

22. (B) Glucogenesis is the term used to designate the formation of glucose from non carbohydrate sources such as amino acids.

23. (C) Enzymatic procedures for the determination of glucose are specific for β-D-glucose. Since only about 60% of the glucose in serum is in the β-D-glucose form, it is necessary to use a mutarotase to convert all of the glucose to β-D-glucose.

24. (A) β-hydroxybutyric acid is usually formed from acetyl Co A. The acetyl Co A accumulates when there is a decrease or cessation of glucose metabolism resulting in a decrease of oxaloacetic acid.

25. (A) Aldolase belongs to the class known as lyases. The EC designation identifies the class of the enzyme by the first digit in the EC number.

26. (B) Hypernatremia, elevated sodium level, is found in Cushing's syndrome in which there is an increased absorption of sodium by the renal tubules.

27. (A) Magnesium ions are necessary for all kinase reactions.

28. (A) Peptic ulcers usually result in elevated levels of gastric acidity. Pernicious anemia is associated with the absence of hydrochloric acid and most cases of carcinoma of the stomach are associated with achloridia or hypochloridia.

29. (A) In acute pancreatitis, there are significant increases in both serum amylase activity and in serum lipase activity.

30. (A) The end products of amylase activity on starch are glucose and maltose. Amylase splits the starch chain at the alpha-1,4 linkages forming maltose and glucose.

31. (A) Alkaline phosphatase levels are found elevated in any liver disease involving biliary tree obstruction as well as in bone diseases such as Paget's disease.

32. (D) All of the items listed are necessary for immunogenicity. There must be a stable structure, a randomness of structure, a minimal molecular mass of 4,000 to 5,000, and the protein must be foreign to the host.

33. (B) Tripeptides and polypeptides as well as proteins will give a positive reaction with biuret reagent. Amino acids and dipeptides will not give a positive biuret reaction.

34. (C) Alcohol, carbon tetrachloride, and cyanide will all produce respiratory depression. Mercurials will cause nephritis, edema, abdominal pain and a variety of other changes, but will not produce respiratory depression.

35. (D) All of the statements are true of carbon tetrachloride poisoning. Carbon tetrachloride poisoning may lead to cirrhosis of the liver. It is readily absorbed by the respiratory tract, skin, and gastrointestinal tract, and alcohols or dimethyl sulfoxide greatly increases its toxicity.

36. (A) Patients with muscular dystrophy, especially in the early and middle stages of the disease will classically show elevations of serum lactic dehydrogenase. Serum creatine kinase activity is markedly elevated in all types of muscular dystrophy.

37. (A) Bile acts in the small intestine to emulsify dietary fats so that they can be hydrolized by lipase.

38. (B) Vitamins A and D are fat soluble vitamins.

39. (C) The optimum activity of amylase is dependent on the presence of chloride ions or other monovalent anions such as the bromide ions or nitrate ions.

40. (C) Sodium, potassium, and lithium may all be assayed by flame photometry.

41. (B) Cystine and cysteine are classified as aliphatic, neutral, sulfur containing amino acids.

42. (A) Hemolysis and lipemia will result in falsely elevated serum levels of inorganic phosphate. Hemolysis will result in the release of intracellular phosphate ions while lipemia will cause a turbidity in the final reaction.

43. (D) All of the reasons listed will result in non-linearity of results.

44. (A) Phosphotungstic acid and uricase are used in the determination of uric acid levels. Uric acid is oxidized by phosphotungstic

acid producing allantoin, CO_2, and tungsten blue which is measured at 710 nm. Uricase is an enzyme that is specific for uric acid. When uric acid is incubated with uricase the resulting decrease in absorbance is measured at 290 nm.

45. (C) Epinephrine, glucagon, and hydrocortisone will all produce increases in blood sugar levels. Epinephrine stimulates glycogenolysis, glucagon stimulates hepatic glycogenolysis, and hydrocortisone has an antagonistic action to insulin.

46. (B) The pattern of LDH isoenzyme electrophoresis shown indicates an increase or predominance of LD-5, which is found predominantly in liver and skeletal muscle.

47. (C) The fraction that is elevated is LD-4, which is the slowest moving LD fraction. LD-5 is composed of four M units, M_4.

48. (B) Respiratory acidosis is characterized by a decreased pCO_2 and an elevated pH.

49. (B) Respiratory acidosis is characterized by an elevated pCO_2 and a decreased pH.

50. (A) Metabolic acidosis is characterized by a decreased pCO_2 and a decreased pH.

51. (D) Metabolic alkalosis is characterized by an elevated pCO_2 and an elevated pH.

52. (C) Serum LDH levels are found elevated in hemolytic anemias and in patients with progressive muscular dystrophy.

53. (B) Serum CPK levels are elevated in progressive muscular dystrophy, but not in hemolytic anemia.

54. (A) Bilirubin levels are found elevated in hemolytic anemias but not in progressive muscular dystrophy.

55. (A) Serum potassium levels are not usually found elevated in progressive muscular dystrophy, but may be found elevated in hemolytic anemias depending on the degree of hemolysis.

56. (C) The prothrombin time is increased in both acute hepatitis and obstructive jaundice. In acute hepatitis this is due to actual damage to the liver cells while in obstructive jaundice it is due to impaired absorption of vitamin K which is necessary for the formation of prothrombin.

57. (A) Serum aldolase activity is markedly increased in acute hepatitis and normal in obstructive jaundice. This increase is due to liver cell damage in acute hepatitis.

58. (D) Serum globulins are not decreased in either acute hepatitis or obstructive jaundice. In acute hepatitis the serum globulin levels are increased while in obstructive jaundice they are normal.

59. (C) Serum LDH levels are found elevated in both liver disease and myocardial infarctions.

60. (B) Serum CPK levels are found elevated in myocardial infarctions, but are negligible in liver disease.

61. (A) Serum alkaline phosphatase levels are found increased in liver disease and bone disorders, but not in myocardial infarctions.

62. (D) Serum acid phosphatase levels are found elevated in prostatic diseases and bone disorders, but not in liver disease or myocardial infarctions.

63. (A) Triglycerides and chilomicrons are both forms of lipids. Since lipids vary in density and electrical charge, they may be separated by electrophoretic procedures.

64. (C) The biuret method is used for the measurement of protein concentrations, not lipid concentrations.

65. (A) BUN is synthesized in the liver from ammonia produced by deamination of amino acids. It is measured by the diacetyl monoxime method, and is found elevated in renal disease.

66. (C) BUN is not usually found elevated in gout, however, uric acid is found elevated in gout.

67. (A) Glucose is an aldose, which reduces cupric ions and has the basic formula $C_6H_{12}O_6$.

68. (B) Glucose is not a ketose.

69. (B) Haptoglobin, pre-β-lipoprotein, and α_2-macroglobulin all migrate in the α_2-globulin band in protein electrophoresis.

70. (C) β-lipoproteins do not migrate with the α_2-globulins. β-lipoproteins migrate with the β_1-globulins.

71. (B) LDH is found elevated in patients with myocardial infarctions and liver disease, and has 5 distinct isoenzymes.

72. (D) LDH is not found elevated in patients with acute cerebrovascular disease, while CPK is usually found elevated in these patients.

73. (C) Vitamin A is the common name of the chemical retinol.

74. (D) Vitamin B_1 is the common name of the chemical thiamine.

75. (A) Vitamin B_{12} is the common name of the chemical cyanocobalamin.

76. (E) Vitamin B_2 is the common name of the chemical riboflavin.

77. (C) The enzyme found elevated in bone diseases is alkaline phosphatase.

78. (A) The enzyme found elevated in pancreatic disorders is serum amylase.

79. (B) The enzyme found elevated in prostate diseases, particularly cancer of the prostate, is acid phosphatase.

80. (D) One of the enzymes found elevated in heart disorders is lactic dehydrogenase.

81. (E) Alanine aminotransferase has for its standard letter abbreviation ALT. This enzyme was formerly known as SGOT--serum glutamic oxalacetic transaminase.

82. (C) Aspartate transferase has for its standard letter abbreviation AST. This enzyme was formerly known as SGPT--serum glutamic pyruvic transaminase.

83. (D) Lipase has for its standard letter abbreviation LPS.

84. (A) Amylase has for its standard letter abbreviation AMS.

85. (A) Hemoglobin is classified as a chromoprotein. Chromoproteins contain an organic prosthetic group that is linked to a metal ion.

86. (E) Ceruloplasmin, which contains copper, is classified as a metalloprotein. Metalloproteins have a metal ion attached directly to the protein.

87. (C) Orosomucoid is a glycoprotein.

88. (B) Collagens, elastins and keratins are fibrous proteins that are essentially insoluble in most common reagents.

89. (A) Rickets is characterized by decreased serum calcium and serum phosphorus, and elevated alkaline phosphatase levels.

90. (C) Primary hyperparathyroidism is characterized by decreased serum levels of phosphorus, and normal or slightly elevated alkaline phosphatase levels.

91. (B) Paget's disease is characterized by normal serum levels of calcium and phosphorus and elevated alkaline phosphatase levels.

92. (E) Vitamin D intoxication is characterized by elevated serum calcium levels, normal, elevated, or decreased serum phosphorus levels, and normal alkaline phosphatase levels.

93. (B) The determination of the concentration of osmotically active particles utilizes the freezing point depression. This is measured by an analytical instrument known as the osmometer.

94. (C) Cu^{2+} ions in alkaline reacts with the carbonyl (-C=O) and amine (=N-H) groups of peptide bonds to form a colored complex.

95. (B) Addition of lactic acid releases CO_2 from HCO_3^-, CO_3^{2-} and other sources of bound CO_2.

96. (D) Due to the amphoteric property of proteins and depending on the pH of the solution used, different proteins will vary in net positive or negative charge per unit area of surface. Based on these net charges, individual proteins can be separated under the influence of an electrical current and classified accordingly.

97. (C) Standard deviation is equal to the square root of the sum of the squared differences from the mean divided by one less than the number of determination.

98. (D) A normal solution contains one gram equivalent weight of solute in one liter of solution.

99. (B) A 1 N solution contains one gram equivalent weight of solute in 1000 ml of solution or one milligram equivalent weight (milliequivalent) of solute in 1 ml of solution.

100. (C)

$$mEq/l = \frac{mg \ of \ solute/liter \ of \ solution}{equivalent \ weight \ of \ solute}$$

$$\frac{2500}{23} = 108.7 \ mEq/l$$

101. (A) Hyperliporpoteinemias of types II, IV, and V are associated with nephrotic syndrome, while type I is not.

102. (B) Immunoglobulin A, as all of the immunoglobulins, is produced in lymphoid cells, not the liver.

103. (A) Haptoglobin migrates in the alpha-1 region of the electrophoretic pattern. All of the other options for this questions migrate in the beta band.

104. (C) In primary hyperparathyroidism, the serum levels of calcium will be elevated, the serum levels of phosphorous will be decreased, and the urine concentrations of both calcium and phosphorous will be increased.

105. (B) After hemoglobin, the greatest concentration of iron in the normal adult male, will be found in ferritin, (approximately 13% of the total body iron). Myoglobin, transferrin, and enzyme iron are found in concentrations of less than 5% of the total body iron.

106. (B) In primary hypothyroidism, the T4 is decreased, the T3 is normal or slightly decreased and the TSH is increased.

107. (D) In ethanol induced hypoglycemia, as in other drug induced hypoglycemias, the fasting level of glucose will be below normal.

All of the other responses come under the classification of reactive hypoglycemia and usually have normal fasting glucose levels.

108. (D) Pregnancy could cause a type IV secondary hyperlipoproteinemia. None of the other types appear to be affected by pregnancy.

109. (C) Of all the components listed, C3 is formed in the liver. C1 is formed in the intestinal epithelium, C2 is formed in the macrophage, and immunoglobulin G is formed in lymphoid tissue.

110. (D) In neurogenic muscle disorders, neither the total LD nor the total CK will be elevated.

111. (C) In an acute myocardial infarction, both the total LD and total CK will be elevated.

112. (C) In progressive muscular dystrophy, both the total LD and the total CK will be elevated.

113. (A) In megaloblastic anemia, the total LD will be elevated, but, there will not be an elevation of total CK.

114. (A) In pulmonary infarction, there will be an elevation of total LD, but, there will not be an elevation of the total CK.

115. (C) In acute myocardial infarction, there will be an elevation of the total CK as well as an elevation of the CK-MB isoenzyme.

116. (C) In progressive muscular dystrophy, there will be an elevation of the total CK and, though most often associated with heart damage, there may also be an elevation of the CK-MB isoenzyme, particularly in the Duchenne type.

117. (A) In organic brain disease, the total CK will be elevated while

there will be no significant elevation of the CK-MB isoenzyme. The iosenzyme CK-BB will be markedly elevated.

118. (D)   In acute hepatitis, there will be no elevation of the total CK nor of the CK-MB isoenzyme.

119. (D)   In neurogenic muscle disease, there will be no elevation of the total CK nor of the CK-MB isoenzyme.

120. (A)   The total CK activity will be elevated in myocardial infarction, but, will not be elevated in acute hepatitis.

121. (C)   The total LD activity will be increased in both myocardial infarction and in acute hepatitis. Note: Electrophoretic separation of the isoenzymes of LD will disclose the difference in these two disorders.

122. (C)   The total activity of AST (SGOT) will be increased in both myocardial infarction and acute hepatitis.

123. (D)   There will be no increase in total amylase activity in either myocardial infarction or acute hepatitis.

124. (B)   The total activity of ALT (SGPT) will be increased in acute hepatitis with no significant increase in myocardial infarction.

125. (A)   Direct (conjugated) bilirubin is water soluble. Indirect (unconjugated) bilirubin is not water soluble.

126. (C)   Both direct (conjugated) bilirubin and indirect (unconjugated) bilirubin are soluble in alcohol.

127. (B)   Indirect (unconjugated) bilirubin has a high affinity for brain tissue. The deposition of bilirubin in brain tissue (Kernicterus) is associated with high levels of unconjugated bilirubin.

128. (C)   Both direct (conjugated) bilirubin and indirect (unconjugated) bilirubin have a tetrapyrrole structure.

129. (A)   Direct (conjuaged) bilirubin is a polar substance. The conjugated of indirect bilirubin diglucuronide renders it polar and therefore water soluble.

130. (B)   In iron deficiency anemia, the total serum iron is decreased while the total iron binding capacity is increased.

131. (C)   In viral hepatitis, both the total serum iron and the total iron binding capacity will be increased.

132. (A)   In thalassemia, the total serum iron will be markedly increased with a corresponding decrease in the total iron binding capacity.

133. (D)   In nephrosis, the total iron and total iron binding capacity will both be decreased.

134. (A)   The total serum iron will be increased and the total iron binding capacity will be decreased, in iron poisoning.

135. (D)   In primary hyperparathyroidism, both the serum calcium and the urine calcium will be elevated.

136. (C)   The serum calcium and the urine calcium will both be decreased in hypoparathyroidism.

137. (D)   In vitamin D intoxication, both the serum calcium and the urine calcium will be elevated.

138. (D)   In Paget's disease, the serum calcium and the urine calcium will be normal to slightly elevated, neither of them will be decreased.

139. (D) In idiopathic osteoporosis, the serum calcium and the urine calcium will both be normal to slightly increased, neither will be decreased.

140. (C) In primary hypothyroidism, there is a definitive decrease in the T4 concentration and either a normal or decreased T3 concentration.

141. (D) In hyperthyroidism, neither T4 nor T3 will be decreased. They will both be increased.

142. (D) In euthyroidism, neither T4 nor T3 will be decreased. Both will be found in normal concentrations.

143. (A) In optimal therapy with T3 preparations, the T4 concentration will be decreased.

144. (D) In optimal therapy with T4 preparations, neither the T4 nor the T3 concentrations will be decreased. They will both be normal.

145. (C) In acute myocardial infarction, the total CK activity, the total LD activity, and the CK-MB isoenzyme fraction will all be elevated. However, the LD-5 isoenzyme activity will not be increased.

146. (A) Patients treated for seizure disorders, are most frequently treated with phenytoin or phenobarbital. Theophylline is used for asthmatic patients. Acetaminophen is used as an analgesic.

147. (B) In obstructive jaundice, the serum levels of alkaline phosphatase and gammaglutamyl transferase will be elevated, while the lipase and amylase activity will not be affected.

148. (D) All of the enzymes listed are magnesium dependent.

149. (C) In the glucose oxidase method of glucose analysis, the enzymes glucose oxidase, mutarotase, and peroxidase are employed. The glucose oxidase converts glucose to gluconic acid and hydrogen peroxide. The peroxidase converts the hydrogen peroxide to water and oxygen. The glucose oxidase method is specific for beta-D-glucose, therefore, it is necessary to use a mutarotase to convert the alpha-D-glucose to the beta form. Amylase is not utilized.

150. (D) All of the protein fractions listed have molecular weights of less than 100,000 daltons. Prealbumin has a molecular weight of 62,000; albumin has a molecular weight of 66,000; hemopexin has a molecular weight of 60,000; and alpha-1-antitrypsin has a molecular weight of 54,000.

151. (B) Complement fraction Cl is manufactured in the intestinal epithelium. Immunoglobulin G is manufactured in lymphoid cells.

152. (A) The sera from neonates, whether premature or mature, can be assayed on the bilirubinometer. Adult sera contains too many interfering substances for accurate analysis on the bilirubinometer. (Neonates who have had exchange transfusions have been transfused with adult blood.)

153. (C) The measurement of total protein in cerebrospinal fluid may be accomplished using a modification of the biuret method, using the turbidimetric trichloroacetic acid method or by using the Coomassie blue dye binding technique. The bromcresol green dye binding method is used to determine serum albumin.

154. (C) Magnesium levels may be obtained by atomic absorption, the colorimetric titan yellow determination or by the colori-

metric calgamite-magnesium complex
method.

155. (C) In obstructive jaundice, the
direct bilirubin is increased,
alkaline phosphatase is markedly
increased, the albumin/globulin
ratio is normal and the gamma-
glutamyl transpeptidase is
elevated.

156. (E) Carotene levels will be
decreased in malabsorption states.
They will be increased in myxedema,
diabetes mellitus, and chronic
nephritis.

157. (C) Aspirin, wintergreen flavoring
and alka-seltzer all contain salicylates. Since serum determination
of salicylates is not specific for
acetylsalicylic acid, all of these
compounds may cause elevations in
serum salicylate levels. Tylenol,
another analgesic compound, does
not contain salicylates.

158. (D) All of the items listed
may produce hypoglycemia.

159. (A) Only diabetes mellitus and
gestational diabetes may be
diagnosed accurately using only
the glucose tolerance test.
Diabetes insipidous requires
osmolality determinations and
ADH determinations, while accurate
diagnosis of hypoglycemia should
include cortisol determinations
and physical evaluation during
the glucose tolerance test.

Bibliography and Recommended Readings

Annino, J. S. Clinical Chemistry - Principles and Procedures. Fourth Edition. 1976. Little, Brown and Company. Boston.

Bauer, J. D. and P. G. Ackermann. Clinical Laboratory Methods. Ninth Edition. 1982. The C. V. Mosby Company. St. Louis.

Henry, J. B. Todd-Sanford-Davidsohn Clinical Diagnosis and Management by Laboratory Methods. Sixteenth Edition. 1979. W. B. Saunders Company. Philadelphia.

Henry, R. H., Winkelman, J. W. and D. C. Cannon (Editors). Clinical Chemistry Principles and Techniques. Second Edition. 1974. Harper and Row Publishers. Hagerstown, Maryland.

Raphael, S. S. (Senior Author). Lynch's Medical Laboratory Technology. Volume I. Third Edition. 1976. W. B. Saunders Company. Philadelphia.

Richterich, R. and J. P. Colombo (Editors). Clinical Chemistry: Theory, Practice and Interpretation. 1981. John Wiley and Sons., Inc. New York.

Tietz, N. W. (Editor). Fundamentals of Clinical Chemistry. Second Edition. 1976. W. B. Saunders Company. Philadelphia.

CHAPTER 13

Toxicology

Directions. Select the one BEST answer for each of the following statements. Circle the appropriate response on the answer sheet.

1. Which of the following is considered to be a rapidly fatal dose of carbon monoxide?

   A. 0.01% (V/V) in air
   B. 0.04-0.05% (V/V) in air
   C. 0.06-0.07% (V/V) in air
   D. 0.4% (V/V) in air and above

2. Which of the following substances may be detected by its odor on the patient's breath?

   A. arsenic
   B. kerosene
   C. cyanide
   D. lead

3. The Reinsch test is performed on a urine sample and the copper wire is shiny on rubbing. Which of the following substances is most likely responsible?

   A. mercury
   B. arsenic
   C. selenium
   D. antimony

4. Which of the following is used in the determination of bromides in serum?

   A. tumeric paper
   B. hydrochloric acid
   C. benzene
   D. gold trichloride

5. Which of the following reagents is NOT employed in the chemical detection of methanol in blood?

   A. formaldehyde
   B. permanganate
   C. sodium bisulfite
   D. chromotropic acid

6. Upon examination of a patient suspected of being poisoned, the findings reveal a mild anemia and a blue line on the gums. Which of the following substances is most likely responsible?

   A. arsenic
   B. mercury
   C. lead
   D. zinc

7. Both cocaine and chlorpromazine have Rf values of 0.96. Which of the methods of thin-layer chromatography would differentiate between these two drugs?

    A. ultraviolet light
    B. Iodoplatinate
    C. ninhydrin
    D. diphenylcarbazone H_2SO_4

8. Ferric nitrate is the chief ingredient for the detection of:

    A. phenothiazine compounds
    B. salicylates
    C. heavy metals
    D. carbon monoxide

9. Carbon monoxide imparts a bright cherry red color to blood due to the presence of:

    A. carboxyhemoglobin
    B. methemoglobin
    C. cyanmethemoglobin
    D. oxyhemoglobin

10. Which of the following plasma salicylate levels is considered toxic 6 hours after ingestion?

    A. 10 mg/dl
    B. 30 mg/dl
    C. 40 mg/dl
    D. 65 mg/dl

11. Carboxyhemoglobin is best detected spectrophotometrically at which of the following wavelengths?

    A. 535 nm and 572 nm
    B. 630 nm to 634 nm
    C. 618 nm to 620 nm
    D. 550 nm

Questions 12-17

Directions. For each of the numbered items select the appropriate lettered response. Do not use the same letter more than once.

Appearance of Copper in Reinsch test   Heavy metal

12. dull black deposit
13. shiny black deposit
14. dark purple deposit

    A. mercury
    B. arsenic
    C. antimony
    D. bismuth

Substance   Specimen

15. mercury
16. lithium
17. arsenic

    A. hair
    B. urine
    C. whole blood
    D. serum

Questions 18-20

Directions. For each of the numbered words or phrases listed below, select the appropriate response as follows:

A. if the item is associated with A only
B. if the item is associated with B only
C. if the item is associated with both A and B
D. if the item is associated with neither A nor B

A. Long acting
B. Short acting

18. barbital
19. secobarbital
20. pentobarbital

Questions 21-30

Directions. Select the one BEST answer for each of the following statements. Mark the appropriate response on the answer sheet.

21. Which of the following laboratory test(s) is the test of choice for the evaluation of a patient suspected of organophosphate poisoning of greater than one month's duration?

    A. red cell cholinesterase
    B. plasma pseudocholinesterase
    C. fat samples for pesticide
    D. urine samples for pesticide

22. Which of the following reactions occur in phase I metabolism of a drug?

    A. conjugation only
    B. conjugation, oxidation and reducation
    C. reduction only
    D. oxidation, reducation and hydrolysis

23. Drugs with low elimination rates are:

    A. only soluble in lipids
    B. only water soluble and bound to plasma proteins
    C. only water soluble and inhibit enzymes in the liver cells
    D. only inhibit enzymes in the liver cells

24. Which of the following may affect the concentration of procainamide in a drug assay?

    A. specimen drawn from an arm with a running IV and the patient having missed the 12 noon dose
    B. specimen drawn from an arm with a running IV, hemolysis and the patient having missed the 12 noon dose
    C. specimen drawn from an arm with a running IV, drawing the specimen immediately after a dose and the patient having missed the 12 noon dose
    D. specimen drawn from the arm with a running IV, hemolysis, drawing the specimen immediately after a dose and the patient having missed the 12 noon dose

25. Which of the following is the best indicator of the amount of drug at the site of action?

    A. urine concentration
    B. urine/serum ratio of less than 1.0
    C. serum concentration
    D. urine/serum ratio of greater than 1.0

26. Specimens should be allowed to clot for 30 minutes at room temperature, prior to centrifugation, because:

    A. glycolysis is inhibited by waiting
    B. there is decreased fibrin formation and a minimum of hemolysis
    C. there is decreased fibrin formation and increased yield of serum
    D. there is decreased fibrin formation, a minimum of hemolysis and increased yield of serum

27. Breath specimens for alcohol are best because:

    A. simple, rapid, noninvasive, reflects the content in arterial circulation, and reflects the content at brain tissue
    B. simple, rapid, noninvasive, reflects the content in venous circulation, and reflects the content at brain tissue
    C. simple, rapid, noninvasive reflects the content in venous circulation
    D. simple, rapid, noninvasive, reflects the content at brain tissue

28. In the serum alcohol procedure utilizing the alcohol dehydrogenase, a positive response can be seen with which of the following?

    A. ethanol only
    B. ethanol and methanol
    C. ethanol, methanol and isopropanol
    D. ethanol, methanol, isopropanol and acetone

29. Effective theophylline concentrations in serum are generally:

    A. 20 - 30 micrograms/ml   C. 20 - 30 mg/ml
    B. 10 - 20 micrograms/ml   D. 10 - 20 mg/ml

30. Which of the following toxicologic overdoses are generally associated with children?

    A. lead only   C. lead, iron and salicylate
    B. lead and salicylate   D. lead, digoxin, iron and salicylate

Questions 31-34

Directions. The following statement contains numbered blanks. For each numbered blank there is a corresponding set of lettered responses. Select the BEST answer from each lettered set.

In a substrate labeled fluorescent immunoassay (SLFIA), the order of occurence of the following events is 31, 32, 33, and 34.

31. A. free substrate-labeled drug produces fluorescence
    B. drug and substrate-labeled drug compete for binding sites on an anti-drug antibody
    C. beta-galactosidase is added to the reaction mixture
    D. the substrate-labeled drug is inactive as a substrate for beta-galactosidase

32. A. free substrate-labeled drug produces fluorescence
    B. drug and substrate-labeled drug compete for binding sites on an anti-drug antibody
    C. beta-galactosidase is added to the reaction mexture
    D. the substrate-labeled drug is inactive as a substrate for beta-galactosidase

33. A. free substrate-labeled drug produces fluorescence
    B. drug and substrate-labeled drug compete for binding sites on an anti-drug antibody
    C. beta-galactosidase is added to the reaction mexture
    D. the substrate-labeled drug is inactive as a substrate for beta-galactosidase

34. A. free substrate-labeled drug produces fluorescence
    B. drug and substrate-labeled drug compete for binding sites on an anti-drug antibody
    C. beta-galactosidase is added to the reaction mixture
    D. the substrate-labeled drug is inactive as a substrate for beta-galactosidase

Questions 35-51

Directions. For each of the numbered words or phrases listed below, select the appropriate response as follows:

A. if the item is associated with A only
B. if the item is associated with B only
C. if the item is associated with both A and B
D. if the item is associated with neither A nor B

A. nephelometry
B. turbidimetry

35. yields poor results at low concentrations
36. measures light scattered at an angle of incidence
37. affected by turbid samples

A. heterogeneous assay
B. homogeneous assay

38. turbidimetry
39. radioimmunoassay (RIA)
40. nephelometry

A. enzyme-linked immunsorbent assay (ELISA)
B. enzyme-multiplied immunoassay (EMIT)

41. similar to radioimmunoassay (RIA)
42. uses enzyme, not radioisotopic label
43. binding of enzyme alters the substrate, thereby inactivating it as a substrate for the enzyme

44. degree of enzyme activity expressed by bound and free forms of conjugate must be substantially different

      A. fluorescent polarization immunoassay (FPIA)
      B. substrate-labeled fluorescent immunoassay (SFLIA)

45. uses a fluorophore
46. produces a by-product which requires strict disposal and bookkeeping policies
47. based on the degree of rotational Brownian movement of molecules

      A. increases renal excretion of lithium
      B. decreases renal excretion of lithium

48. thiazide diuretics
49. water restriction
50. osmotic diuretics
51. dehydration

Questions 52-63

Directions. For each of the numbered items select the appropriate lettered response. Do not use the same letter more than once.

52. carbamazepine	A.	mysoline
53. primidone	B.	zarontin
54. valproate sodium	C.	dilantin
55. phenytoin	D.	tegretol
	E.	depakene

56. amitriptyline	A.	tofranil
57. doxepin	B.	aventyl
58. imimpramine	C.	elavil
59. nortriptyline	D.	sinequam
	E.	tylenol

60. tylenol	A.	propoxyphene
61. darvocet	B.	lysergic acid diethylamide
62. valium	C.	acetominophen
63. thorazine	D.	chlorpromazine
	E.	diazepam

Explanatory Answers

1. (D) 0.4% and greater levels of carbon monoxide in air is considered to be fatal in less than an hour.

2. (B) Very often the odor of kerosene on the breath is an indication of the ingestion of that substance.

3. (A) In the presence of mercury, the copper wire will have a film of light gray to black which will become shiny on rubbing.

4. (D) The chloride of gold trichloride ($AuCl_3$) is replaced by the bromide in an acid solution.

5. (A) Formaldehyde is not used in the chemical detection of methanol because in the chemical method, methanol is converted by oxidation to formaldehyde.

6. (C) Lead poisoning is usually responsible for a mild anemia and in anywhere from 2-50% of lead poisoning cases, a blue gum line is present.

7. (B) Cocaine, when reacted with iodoplatinate, will produce an orange-violet color, while chlorpromazine will produce a blue-violet color.

8. (B) Ferric sulfate, at a concentration of 1%, in 0.07 N nitric acid, forming ferric nitrate, is used for the qualitative determination of salicylates.

9. (A) The bright cherry red color of blood is due to the presence of carboxyhemoglobin.

10. (D) At six hours, the level of serum salicylates that is associated with toxicity is above 45 mg/dl for mild toxicity, above 65 mg/dl for moderate toxicity, and above 90 mg/dl for severe toxicity.

11. (A) The optimum wavelength for carboxyhemoglobin is 535 nm and 572 nm; methemoglobin is best detected at 630-634 nm, sulfhemoglobin at 618-620 nm and cyanmethemoglobin at 550 nm.

12. (B) The copper plate or copper spiral on the Reinsch test will produce a dull black deposit in the presence of arsenic.

13. (D) The copper plate or spiral in the Reinsch test will produce a shiny black deposit in the presence of bismuth.

14. (C) The copper plate or spiral in the Reinsch test will produce a dark purple sheen in the presence of antimony.

15. (B) The Reinsch test for heavy metal poisoning is performed on urine or gastric secretions.

16. (D) Lithium levels are determined by flame photometry which is performed on blood serum.

17. (A) Hair has been shown to contain arsenic for periods of up to 30 hours after ingestion.

18. (A) Barbital is considered to be a long acting barbiturate, having a hypnotic action of 6 or more hours of duration.

19. (B) Secobarbital is considered to be a short acting barbiturate, having a hypnotic action of less than 3 hours.

20. (B) Pentobarbital is considered to be a short acting barbiturate, having a hypnotic action of less than 3 hours.

21. (A) Red cell cholinesterase is the test of choice. Plasma psuedocholine-sterase alterations may be reflec-tive of a genetic variation and cholinesterase inhibition is longer lasting in red blood cells.

22. (D) Phase I metabolism of a drug consists of oxidation, reduction or hydrolysis reactions. Phase II consists of conjugation reactions.

23. (A) The more lipid soluble the drug the greater the amount retained in the body. Lipid soluble drugs require oxidation to polar sub-stances before being eliminated.

24. (D) IV fluid will dilute the sample; hemolysis interferes with the reaction; specimens drawn too soon will affect the distribution and equilibration of the drug, and missed doses affect the distribu-tion, equilibration and elimina-tion of the drug.

25. (C) The serum concentration of a drug is a direct consequence of the interaction of the absorption, metabolism and excretion processes of the drug and is therefore the best indicator of the amount of drug at the site of action.

26. (D) Allowing one-half hour for complete clot formation increases the yield of serum, minimizes hemolysis, and insures that fibrin will not appear in the sera later. Glycolysis occurs when the sample is drawn, but, measurable effects do not begin until 1 hour after the specimen is collected.

27. (A) Breath samples for alcohol are best because they are simple to obtain, rapid, noninvasive, they reflect the arterial content of the alcohol and they reflect the concentration of alcohol at the brain tissue site.

28. (C) The major disadvantage to the alcohol dehydrogenase method is that it measures methanol, isopro-panol and other alcohols as well as the desired alcohol, ethanol.

29. (B) The effective therapeutic range for theophylline is 10 - 20 micrograms/ml. The bronchodilator effect of theophylline is in direct proportion to the logarithm of the drug concentration.

30. (C) Though lead and salicylates are often associated with child-hood overdoses, iron is also toxicologically dangerous for children. Small amounts of iron can cause death in children, ingestion of lead based paints can result in anemia and neurologic damage and salicylates, which are often easily obtained by children, may cause severe acido-sis. Children can tolerate higher doses of digoxin than adults.

31. (B) The first step in the sequence of events in a labeled fluorescent immunoassay is the competition for binding sites on the anti-drug antibody.

32. (D) Once the substrate-labeled drug is bound to the antibody, the substrate-labeled drug is inactive as a substrate for the

enzyme beta-galactosidase.

33. (C) The substrate-labeled drug will fluoresce only after it reacts with the beta-galactosidase.

34. (A) Only the substrate-labeled drug that is NOT attached to the antibody will fluoresce.

35. (B) Turbidimetry yields poor results at low concentrations because of its difficulty in detecting small changes from full illumination.

36. (A) Nephelometry measures the amount of light scattered by particles at an angle of incidence from a light source.

37. (C) Nephelometric assays cannot be performed on turbid samples because of the particle interference. Turbidimetric assays are also affected by turbid samples, however, this can be corrected by the use of a serum blank in the testing process.

38. (B) Turbidimetry does not require preparatory steps prior to measuring the light absorbed and therefore is considered to be a homogeneous assay.

39. (A) Bound and free forms of an analyte must be separated prior to measurement by radioimmunoassay and therefore is considered to be a heterogeneous assay.

40. (B) As is true of turbidimetry, nephelometry does not require special handling procedures prior to performance of the assay and is therefore considered to be a homogeneous assay.

41. (A) The drug specific antibody has no impact on enzyme activity and the bound and free phases must be separated before substrate is converted to measurable product, as is done in an RIA procedure.

42. (C) Both the EMIT and ELISA assays utilize enzymes instead of radioisotopic labels.

43. (B) The enzyme-drug conjugate of EMIT assays has its enzyme activity modulated when it is bound to a specific antibody to the measured drug.

44. (B) This is a necessary requirement that allows quantitation in EMIT assays. It is also a quality that precludes separation techniques in the EMIT assays.

45. (C) All fluorescent assays utilize fluorophores. The major fluorophores are fluorescein, rhodamine and umbelliferone.

46. (D) The major advantage to fluorescent immunoassays is that they are fast, have a long shelf life and lack the problems associated with radioisotopic assays which require special handling of byproducts and detailed bookkeeping.

47. (A) The fluorophore-drug conjugate has a very rapid Brownian movement and produces fluorescence that is depolarized; when the drug is bound to antibody the Brownian rotation movement is decreased which results in an increase in the polarization of fluorescence.

48. (B) Thiazide diuretics decrease the renal excretion of lithium.

49. (B) Water restriction decreases the renal excretion of lithium.

50. (A) Osmotic diuretics increase the renal excretion of lithium.

51. (B) Dehydration decreases the renal excretion of lithium.

52. (D) The trade name for carbamazepine is tegretol.

53. (A) The trade name for primidone is mysoline.

54. (E) The trade name for valproate sodium is depakene.

55. (C) The trade name for phentoin is dilantin.

56. (C) The trade name for amitriptyline is elavil.

57. (D) The trade name for doxepin is sinequam.

58. (A) The trade name for imimpramine is tofranil.

59. (B) The trade name for nortriptyline is aventyl.

60. (C) The generic name for tylenol is acetominophen.

61. (A) The generic name for darvocet is propoxyphene.

62. (E) The generic name for valium is diazepam.

63. (D) The generic name for thorazine is chlorpromazine.

Bibliography and Recommended Readings

Bauer, J. D. and P. G. Ackermann. <u>Clinical Laboratory Methods</u>. Ninth Edition. 1982. The C. V. Mosby Company. St. Louis.

Doull, J. et.al. <u>Casarett and Doull's Toxicology</u>. Second Edition. 1980. Macmillan Publishing Company, Inc. New York.

Hanenson, I. B. <u>Quick Reference to Clinical Toxicology</u>. 1980. J. B. Lippincott. Philadelphia.

Henry, R. J. (Editor). <u>Todd-Sanford-Davidsohn Clinical Diagnosis and Management by Laboratory Methods</u>. Sixteenth Edition. 1979. W. B. Saunders Company. Philadelphia.

Thienes, C. H. and T. J. Haley. <u>Clinical Toxicology</u>. Fifth Edition. 1972. Lea and Febiger. Philadelphia.

CHAPTER 14

Endocrinology

Directions. For each of the numbered items select the appropriate lettered response. Do not use the same letter more than once.

Gland	Hormone
1. Pituitary gland	A. Gastrin
2. Parathyroid gland	B. Epinephrine
3. Adrenal gland	C. Adrenocorticotropin
4. Ovary	D. Parathormone
	E. Relaxin

Hormone	Site of Action
5. Antidiuretic hormone	A. Liver
6. Glucagon	B. Renal tubules
7. Oxytocin	C. Male sex organs
8. Testosterone	D. Smooth muscle
	E. Female sex organs

Questions 9-18

Directions. Select the one BEST answer for each of the following statements. Circle the appropriate response on the answer sheet.

9. Which of the following is responsible for the regulation of calcium metabolism?

   A. Thyroxin   C. Parathormone
   B. Leutinizing hormone D. Insulin

10. Stimulation of, and secretion of the thyroid hormones is the principle action of:

    A. Triiodothyronine   C. Thyrocalcitonin
    B. Thyrotrophin   D. Thyroxin

11. The Zimmerman reaction is used to detect which of the following hormones?

    A. Thyroid hormones   C. 17-Ketosteroids
    B. Adrenocortical hormones   D. Catecholamines

275

12. Which of the following hormones is NOT secreted by the anterior pituitary gland?

    A. Thyroid stimulating hormone (TSH)
    B. Adrenocorticotrophic hormone (ACTH)
    C. Antidiuretic hormone (ADH)
    D. Growth hormone (GH)

13. Which of the following disease states will exhibit a decrease in the ketogenic steroids?

    A. Addison's disease   C. adrenal hyperplasia
    B. Cushing's syndrome   D. precocious puberty

14. Which of the following is the normal range for plasma levels of growth hormone in males?

    A. 0-8 ng/ml   C. 15-24 ng/ml
    B. 10-15 ng/ml   D. 18-30 ng/ml

15. Which of the following would NOT be considered an abnormal level for VMA (Vanilmandelic acid), in a 24 hour urine sample, for an infant?

    A. 75 µg/kg/day   C. 125 µg/kg/day
    B. 100 µg/kg/day   D. 150 µg/kg/day

16. Which of the following methods is used for the determination of urinary corticosteroids?

    A. Zimmerman reaction   C. both A and B
    B. Porter-Silber method   D. neither A nor B

17. The use of Estriol determinations as a measure of fetal viability is best accomplished during:

    A. 1st and 2nd trimesters   C. 2nd and 3rd trimesters
    B. 1st and 3rd trimesters   D. all stages of pregnancy

18. Which of the following hormones is a protein hormone?

    A. Estriol   C. Luteinizing hormone
    B. Progesterone   D. Aldosterone

Questions 19-25

Directions.   For each of the numbered words or phrases listed below, select the appropriate response as follows:

A.   if the item is associated with A only
B.   if the item is associated with B only
C.   if the item is associated with both A and B
D.   if the item is associated with neither A nor B

A.   Increased Thyroid Binding Globulin
B.   Increased Serum Thyroxin

19.   Graves' disease (active)
20.   Thyrotoxicosis (T_3)
21.   Primary hypothyroidism

A.   Negative feedback mechanism of control
B.   Control by production of neurohumors

22.   Thyroid gland
23.   Adrenals
24.   Posterior pituitary
25.   Anterior pituitary

Explanatory Answers

1. (C) Adrenocorticotrophic hormone is secreted by the anterior pituitary gland.

2. (D) Parathormone is the hormone that is excreted by the parathyroid glands.

3. (B) Epinephrine and norepinephrine, or adrenalin and noradrenalin, are secreted by the adrenal medulla.

4. (E) Relaxin, a polypeptide hormone, is secreted by the ovaries.

5. (B) Antidiuretic hormone, or vasopressin, acts on the renal tubules for the reabsorption of water by the tubules.

6. (A) Glucagon, which is secreted by the pancreas, has its site of action in the liver where it stimulates glycogenolysis.

7. (D) Oxytocin, which is secreted by the posterior pituitary, has its site of action on the smooth muscles of the uterus and mammary glands.

8. (C) Testosterone, which is secreted by the testis, has its site of action on the male accessory sex organs for the development of secondary sex characteristics.

9. (C) Parathormone, which is secreted by the parathyroid glands, controls the metabolism of calcium.

10. (B) Thyrotrophin (TSH) stimulates the formation of the thyroid hormones and regulates the secretion of those hormones.

11. (C) The Zimmerman reaction is used for the detection of 17-ketosteroids. The reaction is based on the formation of a reddish purple complex that has a maximum absorption at 520 nm.

12. (C) Antidiuretic hormone (ADH) is secreted by the posterior pituitary gland. Thyroid stimulating hormone, growth hormone, and adrenocorticotrophic hormone are all secreted by the anterior pituitary gland.

13. (A) There is a decrease in the excretion of ketogenic steroids in Addison's disease. All of the other conditions listed will characteristically show increases in the ketogenic steroids.

14. (A) The normal range for plasma levels of growth hormone in males is 0-8 ng/ml, while in females it is 0-30 ng/ml.

15. (A) The normal levels of VMA for infants is less than 83 μg/kg/day. Therefore, the value of 75 μg/kg/day would not be considered abnormal.

16. (B) The Porter-Silber method produces a yellow pigment when corticosteroids react with phenylhydrazine.

17. (C) Estriol levels for the determination of fetal viability is most useful during the 2nd and 3rd trimesters of pregnancy because during the 1st trimester Estriol levels are relatively low.

18. (C) Luteinizing hormone is a pituitary hormone, all of which are protein hormones. Estriol, Progesterone, and Aldosterone are all steroid hormones.

19. (B) In Graves' disease the serum thyroxin levels will be increased or elevated, while the TBG levels will be normal or decreased.

20. (D) Neither TBG nor thyroxin will be increased in T₃ thyrotoxicosis; their levels will be normal. The T_3 levels will be increased.

21. (D) Neither TBG nor thyroxin will be elevated or increased in primary hypothyroidism. The thyroxin levels will be decreased, while the TBG levels will be normal or decreased.

22. (A) The control of the thyroid gland is by negative feedback mechanism. Thyrotrophic hormone secreted by anterior pituitary, stimulates the thyroid to secrete thyroxin. When the thyroxin levels reach normal, the thyroxin inhibits the secretion of thyrotrophic hormone.

23. (A) The control of the adrenals is by negative feedback mechanism. ACTH secreted by the anterior pituitary stimulates the production of hormones of the adrenal cortex. When normal levels are reached, the hormones of the adrenal cortex inhibit the secretion of ACTH.

24. (D) The posterior pituitary and the adrenal medulla are not controlled by negative feedback mechanism nor by production of neurohumors. They are controlled by stimulation of nerves.

25. (B) The anterior pituitary is controlled by neurohumors which are chemicals produced by nerve cells to control secretion of the hormones. The anterior pituitary is controlled in this manner by the hypothalamus.

Bibliography and Recommended Readings

Davidsohn, I., and J. B. Henry (Editors). <u>Todd-Sanford Clinical Diagnosis by Laboratory Methods</u>. Fifteenth Edition. 1974. W. B. Saunders Company. Philadelphia.

Hall, R., Anderson, J., Smart, G., and G. M. Besser. <u>Clinical Endocrinology</u>. Second Edition. 1974. J. B. Lippincott Company. Philadelphia.

Henry, R. J., Winkelman, J. W., and D. C. Cannon (Editors). <u>Clinical Chemistry Principles and Technics</u>. Second Edition. 1974. Harper and Row Publishers. Hagerstown, Maryland.

Tietz, N. W. (Editor). <u>Fundamentals of Clinical Chemistry</u>. Second Edition. 1976. W. B. Saunders Company. Philadelphia.

Weiss, L. and R. O. Greep. <u>Histology</u>. Fourth Edition. 1977. McGraw-Hill, Inc. New York.

CHAPTER 15

Urinalysis

Directions. Select the one BEST answer for each of the following statements. Circle the appropriate response on the answer sheet.

1. In what part of the kidney are the nephrons located?

   A. medulla   C. calyces
   B. cortex   D. hilum

2. At which point in the nephron is glucose reabsorbed from the glomerular filtrate?

   A. Proximal convoluted tubule   C. Distal convoluted tubule
   B. Loop of Henle   D. Collecting tubule

3. Which of the following is considered to be a familial kidney disorder?

   A. Nephrosis   C. Polycystic kidney
   B. Pyelitis   D. Pyelonephritis

4. Which of the following urine pigments will usually precipitate with amorphous urate crystals?

   A. Urochrome   C. Urobilin
   B. Uroerythrin   D. Urobilinogen

5. The production of ammonia by the renal tubular cells prevents the urine pH from going below which of the following pH levels?

   A. 3.5   C. 4.0
   B. 4.5   D. 5.0

6. While examining a urine sediment, a technologist observes flat, hexagonal, colorless crystals. The next step to be taken is:

   A. Report the number of cystine crystals per low power field
   B. Examine another sample of the urine before reporting anything
   C. Perform a chemical confirmation for cystine
   D. Perform a chemical confirmation for leucine

7. Which of the following sugars will NOT react with the tests for reducing substances?

    A. Glucose   C. Lactose
    B. Fructose   D. Sucrose

8. A urine sample from a patient with a hemolytic transfusion reaction is sent to the laboratory. Which of the following would you expect to find?

    A. elevated levels of both bile and urobilinogen
    B. elevated level of bile, but no urobilinogen
    C. elevated level of urobilinogen, but no bile
    D. no bile or urobilinogen

9. Which of the following tests is NOT a test for urine bilirubin?

    A. Harrison test   C. Obermayers test
    B. Franklin test   D. Ictotest

10. A test for occult blood on a urine sample was performed, and a positive result was obtained. The test was a STIX test. Microscopic examination revealed no red blood cells. The urine sample was then tested with 80% ammonium sulfate, and there was no precipitate formed. The substance giving the positive result was most likely:

    A. Hemoglobin   C. Casts
    B. Myoglobin   D. Pus

11. Urinary casts are found in a microscopic examination under which of the following conditions?

    A. Low power with dim illumination
    B. Low power with bright illumination
    C. High power with dim illumination
    D. High power with bright illumination

12. Porphyrins will show a red fluoresence when irradiated with an ultraviolet light, but normal urine will fluoresce an intense blue-green which may mask the porphyrin unless there is a large amount. Which of the following reagents will also demonstrate the presence of porphyrins?

    A. Guaiacol   C. Erhlich's reagent
    B. 10% ferric chloride   D. Sodium nitroprusside reagent

13. Active reabsorption of protein by the brush border of the renal tubules is accompanied by a process known as:

    A. Athrocytosis   C. Osmosis
    B. Diffusion   D. Filtration

14. In the heat and acetic acid method, sodium chloride is added to the acetic acid to prevent interference by which of the following substances?

    A. Glucose   C. Proteoses
    B. Mucin   D. Bence-Jones protein

15. If a normal person were to be severely restricted from consuming water, he/she should be able to concentrate his/her urine to a specific gravity of at least:

    A. 1.020   C. 1.040
    B. 1.030   D. 1.025

16. Each gram of protein per dl of urine raises the specific gravity by:

    A. 0.001   C. 0.003
    B. 0.002   D. 0.004

17. Which of the following methods for determining the concentration of dissolved solids in urine relies upon the principle of freezing point depression?

    A. Refractometry   C. Measurement of surface tension
    B. Specific gravity   D. Osmolality

18. How much urine does the average adult excrete in a 24 hour period?

    A. 800 - 1000 ml   C. 1800 - 2000 ml
    B. 1200 - 1500 ml   D. 2000 - 2400 ml

19. The dipstick method for protein determination is based upon which of the following principles?

    A. Protein precipitation in heat
    B. Protein precipitation in acids
    C. Protein precipitation in alkali
    D. Protein error of indicators

20. A technologist was performing a microscopic examination of a urine sample and saw what he believed to be red blood cells. Because he was unsure that they were in fact red blood cells and not simply yeast cells, he decided to confirm his findings. Which of the following would he use to differentiate between red blood cells and yeasts?

    A. Ascorbic acid   C. Acetic acid
    B. Hydrochloric acid   D. Ferric chloride

21. Which of the following would NOT give false positive results with Benedict's test?

    A. Ascorbic acid   C. Homogentisic acid
    B. Elevated levels of uric acid D. Peroxide

22. The protein seen in approximately 50% of the patients with multiple myeloma is unique in that it will precipitate at temperatures between 40 and 60°C and redissolve at 100°C. This protein is known as:

    A. Bence-Jones protein   C. Glycoprotein
    B. Tamm-Horsfall protein   D. Lipoprotein

23. The term used to denote decreased urine output is:

    A. Polyuria   C. Nocturia
    B. Pyuria   D. Oliguria

24. Which of the following is NOT one of the primary functions of the kidney?

    A. Acid-base balance
    B. Detoxification of harmful substances
    C. Water balance
    D. Excretion of waste products

25. Which of the following porphyrins is usually elevated in lead poisoning?

    A. Uroporphyrin I   C. Coproporphyrin I
    B. Coproporphyrin III   D. Protoporphyrin III

26. Which of the following amino acids is NOT found in the urine of patients with Maple Syrup Urine Disease?

    A. Leucine   C. Isoleucine
    B. Valine   D. Phenylalanine

27. A mother who has been breast feeding her newborn infant noticed that the infant was having gastrointestinal problems. She notified her pediatrician who ordered a urinalysis and specifically requested a test for reducing sugars. When he received the report he found that the dipstick (glucose specific) test for sugar was negative, but that the Clinitest was positive. Which sugar most likely causes these results?

    A. Glucose   C. Galactose
    B. Fructose   D. Pentose

Questions 28-37

Directions. For each of the numbered items select the appropriate lettered response. Do not use the same letter more than once.

28. Phenylketonuria   A. Faintly aromatic

29. Bacterial decomposition of urea B. Thymol odor

30. Normal urine   C. Maple syrup odor

                                     D. Mousy odor

                                     E. Ammonia odor

31. Rhubarb

32. Azure A

33. Melanin

34. Phenol poisoning

A. Blue color

B. Reddish orange

C. Olive green

D. Black

E. Yellow

10% ferric chloride is utilized in several testing procedures in the urinalysis laboratory. Match each of the following results with the appropriate testing procedure.

35. Deep blue color that lasts for a split second

36. Precipitation of ferric phosphate that turns black in about 30 minutes

37. Red wine color that disappears after boiling

A. Acetoacetic acid

B. Homogentisic acid

C. Salicylates

D. Melanin

E. Acetone

Questions 38-41

Directions. One, some, or all of the responses for each of the following statements may be correct. Indicate your response as follows:

A. if items 1 and 3 are correct
B. if items 2 and 4 are correct
C. if three of the items are correct
D. if all of the items are correct
E. if only one of the items is correct

38. The formation of casts is dependent on which of the following conditions?

1. High solute concentration
2. Low pH
3. High protein concentration
4. High pH

39. Gerhardt's test will give purple to red wine colors in urine samples containing which of the following?

1. Acetoacetic acid
2. Acetone
3. Salicylates
4. Beta-hydroxybutyric acid

40. Which of the following substances will yield false positive results for protein when tested by the sulfosalicylic acid procedure?

1. Highly buffered alkaline urines
2. Tolbutamid
3. High creatine levels
4. Myoglobin

41. Which of the following, if present in the urine, will result in falsely elevated
     readings when using the glucose oxidase, peroxidase, chromagen system for
     glucose determination?

     1. Penicillin   3. Salicylates
     2. Hydrogen peroxide   4. Bilirubin

                    Questions 42-44

Directions. Select and circle the one BEST answer for each of the following statements utilizing the information presented in either the following graph, tracing,
table or laboratory data.

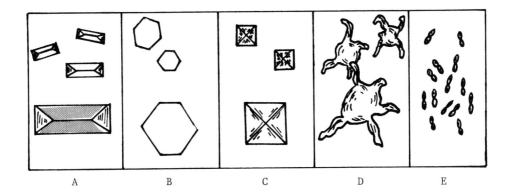

        A   B   C   D   E

42. Which of the crystals above are found in alkaline urine, and effervesce when
     acetic acid is added to the sample?

     A.   B.   C.   D.   E.

43. Which of the above crystals are found in acid, neutral, or alkaline samples?

     A.   B.   C.   D.   E.

44. Which of the above crystals would require a chemical confirmation test before
     being reported?

     A.   B.   C.   D.   E.

Questions 45-46

Directions. The column on the left contains 3 scientifically related categories while
the column on the right contains 4 items which may illustrate scientific phenomena or
processes. Three of the items in the column on the right relate to only one of the
categories in the column on the left. FIRST, indicate the category in which the 3
processes or phenomena belong. SECOND, indicate the one process or phenomenon which
is not related to that category.

Category	Phenomenon

45. A. Multiple myeloma   46. A. Tamm-Horsfall mucoprotein
    B. Urinary casts   B. Dissolve in alkaline urine
    C. Cystine crystals   C. Accompanied by proteinuria
                                                  D. Require chemical confirmation

Questions 47-63

Directions. Select the one BEST answer for each of the following statements. Circle
the appropriate response on the answer sheet.

47. The mucopolysaccharide that is found in Sanfilippo syndrome, as well as in
Hurler's syndrome is:

    A. Dermatan sulfate   C. Keratan sulfate
    B. Heparin sulfate   D. Hyaluronic acid

48. While performing a microscopic examination of a urinary sediment, a technologist
sees what he believes are oval fat bodies. Which of the following tests would
confirm his finding?

    A. Sudan III stain   D. A and B, but not C
    B. polarized light microscopy   E. A, B and C
    C. Sudan IV stain

49. The first morning specimen is considered the best specimen for routine
urinalysis because:

    A. it is the most concentrated specimen
    B. it is the most dilute specimen
    C. orthostatic proteinuria is best detected
    D. A and C, but not B

50. The Rothera test for ketones will measure:

    A. acetone only   D. A and B, but not C
    B. acetoacetic acid only   E. B and C, but not A
    C. beta-hydroxybutric acid only

51. Which of the following would you select to preserve the organized sediment in a urine sample, particularly the casts?

    A. sodium carbonate
    B. chloroform
    C. formalin (40% V/V)
    D. thymol

52. Postural proteinuria or orthostatic proteinuria is usually detected by examining which of the following specimens?

    A. first morning specimen collected while the patient is still lying down
    B. a urine sample collected after the patient has been erect or walking for at least 2 hours
    C. a urine sample collected at bedtime
    D. a urine sample collected at any time

53. Which of the following is the correct order of the aging process of casts?

    A. cellular, fine granular, coarse granular, waxy
    B. cellular, coarse granular, fine granular, waxy
    C. hyaline, coarse granular, fine granular, waxy
    D. hyaline, fine granular, coarse granular, waxy

54. Which of the following is the recommended specimen to be used when searching for urobilinogen?

    A. first morning specimen
    B. any randomly voided specimen
    C. a specimen collected during the hours of 2-4 P.M.
    D. a 24 hour urine collection

55. What time period is recommended for collection of a urine sample that is to have an Addis count performed?

    A. any random specimen
    B. a two hour collection
    C. a 12 hour collection
    D. a 24 hour collection

56. White blood cells in hypotonic solution swell, and the granules exhibit Brownian movement. These cells are known as:

    A. glitter cells
    B. oval fat bodies
    C. siderocytes
    D. lymphocytes

57. What does the term cylinduria indicate?

    A. increase in the number of cylindroids
    B. increase in the number of casts
    C. increase in the number of leucine spheres
    D. increase in the number of pseudocasts

58. Acute glomerulonephritis usually follows an untreated infection with which of the following organisms?

    A. Group A, beta-hemolytic streptococcus
    B. Staphylococcus aureus
    C. Staphylococcus epidermidis
    D. Group D, streptococcus

59. A build-up of nitrogenous waste products in the blood due to renal disease or failure is called:

    A. proteinemia   C. anemia
    B. uremia   D. bilirubinemia

60. Which of the following foods is most likely to produce an acid urine?

    A. citrus fruits   D. A and B, but not C
    B. meats   E. B and C, but not A
    C. cranberries

61. Which of the following conditions is associated with a defect in renal tubular reabsorption?

    A. Phenylketonuria   C. Maple Syrup Urine Disease
    B. Alkaptonuria   D. Cystinuria

62. The resorcinol test is used to confirm the presence of which of the following sugars?

    A. glucose   C. fructose
    B. galactose   D. lactose

63. The active ingredient in Ehrlich's reagent is:

    A. paradimethylaminobenzaldehyde
    B. p-nitrobenzene diazonium p-toluene
    C. delta-amino-levulinic acid
    D. barium chloride and 10% ferric chloride

Questions 64-67

Directions. One, some, or all of the responses for each of the following statements may be correct. Indicate your response as follows:

A. if items 1 and 3 are correct
B. it items 2 and 4 are correct
C. if three of the items are correct
D. if all of the items are correct
E. if only one of the items is correct

64. The ICTOTEST procedure for bilirubinuria is performed and the results show an orange-red reaction. This result is most likely due to which of the following:

    1. bilirubin   3. chlorpromazine
    2. salicylates   4. pyridium

65. A physician suspects that a child has alkaptinuria and sends a urine sample to the laboratory for analysis. Which of the following testing procedures could you use to determine the prescence of homogentisic acid?

    1. add 10% NaOH drop by drop
    2. add 10% ferric chloride drop by drop
    3. add alkalinized urine to photographic paper
    4. perform a Benedict's test on the sample

66. Excessively high levels of urine calcium would be expected in which of the following diseases?

    1. Hyperparathyroidism
    2. Renal tubular acidosis
    3. Increased absorption of Vitamin D
    4. Vitamin D deficiency

67. Increased urine glucose levels can be found in which of the following disease states?

    1. Pheochromocytoma
    2. Pancreatitis
    3. Hyperthyroidism
    4. Fanconi syndrome

Questions 68-85

Directions. Select the one BEST answer for each of the following statements. Circle the appropriate response on the answer sheet.

68. Water reabsorption due to antidiuretic hormone takes place in which of the following protions of the nephron?

    A. glomerulus
    B. proximal convoluted tubule
    C. loop of Henle
    D. distal convoluted tubule

69. Which of the following substances is excreted in adult men, in muscle-wasting diseases only?

    A. urea
    B. creatine
    C. creatinine
    D. uric acid

70. 5-Hydroxyindole Acetic Acid (5-HIAA) is usually found elevated in carcinoid tumors of the argentaffin cells of the intestinal tract. 5-HIAA is the metabolite of which of the following substances?

    A. serotonin
    B. fumaric acid
    C. homogentisic acid
    D. tyrosine

71. When the final color of a urine glucose determination, utilizing the ortho-toluidine reagent, is brown instead of green, which of the following substances is likely to be responsible?

    A. fructose
    B. xylose
    C. galactose
    D. lactose

72. Which of the following is NOT usually included in a "routine" urinalysis?

A. pH
B. glucose
C. phenylketones
D. protein

73. When trying to distinguish between neutrophilic leukocytes and small renal epithelial cells in a urine microscopic exam, which of the following would be most useful?

A. glacial acetic acid
B. hydrochloric acid
C. sulfuric acid
D. picric acid

74. Which of the following substances is the most commonly found constituent of renal calculi?

A. calcium oxalate
B. uric acid
C. cystine
D. magnesium ammonium phosphate

75. A urine sepcimen was examined at a temperature of 23°C. The specific gravity was found to be 1.021. This specific gravity was measured with a urinometer calibrated at 20°C, and should be corrected to which of the following?

A. 1.014
B. 1.020
C. 1.021
D. 1.022

76. Which of the following is most common in diabetes mellitus?

A. polyuria
B. dysuria
C. oliguria
D. anuria

77. The osmometer is an instrument used for the determination of urine osmolality on the basis of freezing point depression. Which of the following best illustrates the principle behind the test?

A. the lower the freezing point, the higher the osmotic pressure
B. the lower the freezing point, the lower the osmotic pressure
C. the lower the freezing point, the higher the water content
D. A and C, but not B

78. Homocystinuria can be distinguished from cystinuria by which of the following?

A. high voltage electrophoresis
B. thin layer chromatography
C. paper chromatography
D. A and B, but not C

79. Which of the following tests is designed to detect the presence of beta-hydroxybutyric acid?

A. Rothera test
B. Gerhardt test
C. Hart test
D. Gmelin test

80. Which of the following is the qualitative test for urine calcium?

    A. Fantus test   C. Sulkowitch test
    B. Gmelin test   D. Guthrie test

81. Of the following tests for protein in urine, which is NOT a quantitative test?

    A. Kingsbury-Clark test   C. Roberts test
    B. Esbach's test   D. Tsuchiya test

82. Antidiuretic hormone (ADH) is excreted by:

    A. posterior pituitary gland   C. thyroid gland
    B. anterior pituitary gland   D. adrenal cortex

83. The presence of large numbers of leukocytes and clumps of leukocytes is usually indicative of:

    A. polycystic kidney   C. renal calculi
    B. urinary tract infection   D. cystic fibrosis

84. Which urinary cast displays the following characteristics: homogenous, refractile, irregular in shape, blunt ends, cracks or clefts?

    A. hyaline cast   C. waxy cast
    B. blood cast   D. fine granular cast

85. Trichomonads, yeast cells, or Enterobius vermicularis in a urine microscopic is usually indicative of which of the following?

    A. contamination   C. diabetes
    B. massive infection   D. glomerular membrane defect

                        Questions 86-94

Directions. One, some, or all of the responses for each of the following statements may be correct. Indicate your response as follows:

A. if items 1 and 3 are correct
B. if items 2 and 4 are correct
C. if three of the items are correct
D. if all of the items are correct
E. if only one of the items is correct

86. The polysaccharide inulin is more appropriate for renal clearance tests than urea because:

    1. approximately 40% of urea is reabsorbed by the renal tubules
    2. approximately 75% of the inulin is excreted
    3. inulin is not reabsorbed by the renal tubules
    4. urea is not reabsorbed by the renal tubules

87. Which of the following substances should be avoided prior to performing a quantitative test for 5-HIAA (5-hydroxyindole acetic acid)?

1. phenothiazine drugs
2. bananas
3. pineapple
4. sulfa drugs

88. A 14 year old boy is admitted to the hospital with swollen ankles after having a streptococcal infection. The following results were obtained upon analysis of his blood: Glucose - 90 mg/dl
BUN - 75 mg/dl
Creatinine - 5.2 mg/dl

Which of the following would you most likely find in his urine sediment?

1. red blood cells
2. white blood cells
3. casts
4. renal epithelial cells

89. Pathologic conditions in which cholesterol crystals may be found in the urine include:

1. chyluria
2. pyelitis
3. cystitis
4. nephritis

90. Which of the following would not normally appear in the urine?

1. albumin
2. immunoglobulin M
3. immunoglobulin G
4. Bence-Jones protein

91. Which of the following is usually found in the urine sediment?

1. red blood cells
2. squamous epithelial cells
3. tubular epithelial cells
4. transitional epithelial cells

92. Which of the following kidney disorders will frequently result in oliguria?

1. dehydration
2. renal ischemia
3. acute glomerulonephritis
4. obstruction

93. The Watson-Schwartz test is used for which of the following?

1. urobilinogen
2. phenylketones
3. porphyrins
4. alkaptonuria

94. Which of the following generally favor the formation of urinary calculi?

1. hyperparathyroidism
2. hyperthyroidism
3. cystinuria
4. homocystinuria

Questions 95-100

Directions. The column on the left contains 3 scientifically related categories while the column on the right contains 4 items which may illustrate scientific phenomena or processes. Three of the items in the column on the right relate to only one of the categories in the column on the left. FIRST, indicate the category in which the 3 processes or phenomenon belong. SECOND, indicate the one process or phenomenon which is not related to that category.

Category

Phenomenon

95. A. normal pH
     B. alkaline pH
     C. acid pH

96. A. diet high in meat protein
     B. metabolic acidosis
     C. respiratory acidosis
     D. hyperaldosteronism

97. A. tyrosinuria
     B. cystinuria
     C. alkaptonuria

98. A. renal calculi
     B. hexagonal crystals
     C. inborn error of metabolism
     D. aminoaciduria

99. A. renal plasma flow
     B. glomerular filtration rate
     C. tubular function

100. A. inulin clearance
      B. PAH clearance
      C. creatinine clearance
      D. urea clearance

Questions 101-110

Directions. Select the one BEST answer for each of the following statements. Circle the appropriate response on the answer sheet.

101. Which of the following is the active ingredient in the dipstick method for protein in the urine?

     A. 10% ferric chloride
     B. azure A
     C. tetrabromphenol blue
     D. sodium nitroprusside

102. A daily urine output which is over 2000 ml/24 hours is referred to as:

     A. anuria
     B. oliguria
     C. polyuria
     D. pyuria

103. Which of the following crystals will not normally be found in a urine specimen with a pH of 8.0?

     A. ammonium biurates
     B. triple phosphates
     C. calcium carbonates
     D. uric acid

104. When the organized sediment of a urine is obscured by innumerable red blood cells, the organized sediment can be evaluated by:

     A. adding acetic acid
     B. heating
     C. adding hydrochloric acid
     D. adding sodium hydroxide

105. Which of the following are considered to be abnormal crystals when found in urine sediment?

    A. cystine crystals   C. tyrosine crystals
    B. cholesterol crystals   D. all of the above

106. When performing concentration tests, which of the following measurements is performed?

    A. specific gravity   C. ketones
    B. glucose   D. albumin

107. The presence of renal disease, as opposed to lower urinary tract disease, is most strongly suggested by:

    A. squamous epithelial cells   C. pyuria
    B. proteinuria   D. calcium carbonate crystals

108. The Guthrie test and the ferric chloride test are useful in the screening for:

    A. glycosuria   C. amino aciduria
    B. proteinuria   D. cylinduria

109. Which of the following specimens is the specimen of choice for the performance of a routine urinalysis?

    A. random specimen   C. first early morning specimen
    B. 12 hour timed specimen   D. 24 hour timed specimen

110. Which of the following specimens is the specimen of choice for a quantitative protein determination?

    A. random specimen   C. first early morning specimen
    B. 12 hour timed specimen   D. 24 hour timed specimen

Explanatory Answers

1. (B) The nephrons, or functional units of the kidney, are located in the renal cortex.

2. (A) Glucose along with large amounts of water, involved with the enzymatic coupling and uncoupling actions for glucose reabsorption, takes place in the proximal convoluted tubule.

3. (C) Polycystic kidney is familial in nature, whereas the other disorders listed are caused by poisons and bacterial infection.

4. (B) Uroerythrin normally co-precipitates with the amorphous urate crystals giving them their characteristic pink color.

5. (B) Production of ammonia by the renal tubular cells prevents the urine pH from going below 4.5.

6. (C) The crystals described suggest the presence of cystine. Because cystine is an abnormal finding, the next step to be taken is to chemically confirm this with sodium nitroprusside in an alkaline solution.

7. (D) Sucrose will not react with the reducing substance tests because it is not a reducing sugar. Even though sucrose is composed of the two reducing sugars glucose and fructose, it will not react because both the aldehyde group of the glucose and the ketone group of the fructose are involved in the coupling to make sucrose, and therefore are not free to react with the reducing substance tests.

8. (C) Hemolytic anemias and transfusion reactions usually show elevated levels of urobilinogen and stercobilinogen but no bile.

9. (C) Obermayers test is a test for indican.

10. (B) Myoglobin is the most likely substance. Myoglobin will give positive results on tests for occult blood as will hemoglobin and red cells. Since no red cells were found, the positive reaction is most likely due to either hemoglobin or myoglobin. Myoglobin is soluble in 75-80% ammonium sulfate, hemoglobin will precipitate at that concentration.

11. (A) Because the protein matrix of casts is made principally of Tamm-Horsfall protein, the refractive index of the casts is very close to that of glass, so casts are found most easily under low power with dim or reduced illumination.

12. (C) Ehrlich's reagent will demonstrate the presence of porphyrins yielding a red color. This color reaction will have to be differentiated from the same type of color reaction observed between Ehrlich's reagent and urobilinogen.

13. (A) Athrocytosis is the mechanism by which the brush border of the renal tubular cells actively re-

absorb protein. This is accomplished in the proximal tubule and is an energy producing process.

14. (B) Mucin will precipitate in acetic acid and heat yielding false positive tests for protein. The addition of the sodium chloride prevents the mucin from precipitating.

15. (B) The normal person whose water intake has been severely restricted should be able to concentrate his/her urine to a specific gravity of at least 1.030.

16. (C) The specific gravity of urine will be raised 0.003 for each gram of protein per dl. .004 gm 1

17. (D) The measurement of total dissolved solids in urine by the osmolality method employs the freezing point depression principle.

18. (B) The average adult excretes 1200 - 1500 ml of urine per day.

19. (D) The dipstick method of protein determination is based on the principle of protein error of indicators. Protein error of indicators involves the use of tetrabromphenol blue indicator which at a pH of 3.0 is yellow in the absence of protein and blue in the presence of protein.

20. (C) The addition of acetic acid under the cover slip would dissolve the red blood cells but not the yeast cells.

21. (D) Peroxide is an oxidizing agent. Benedict's test is a test for reducing substances, therefore peroxide would not produce a false positive result.

22. (A) Bence-Jones protein is found in the urine of approximately 50% of the patients with multiple myeloma. It will precipitate at 40-60°C, redissolve at 100°C, and reprecipitate at 40-60°C.

23. (D) Oliguria is the term commonly used to denote a decreased urinary output.

24. (B) The kidney has three primary functions: acid-base balance, water balance, and excretion of waste products. The liver is primarily responsible for the detoxification of harmful substances.

25. (B) Porphyrinuria in heavy metal poisoning is usually due to increased amounts of coproporphyrin III.

26. (D) Phenylalanine is not found in elevated amounts in the urine of patients with Maple Syrup Urine Disease. This disease is characterized by its maple syrup odor and the presence of abnormally high levels of methionine, leucine, isoleucine, and valine.

27. (C) Galactose intolerance, a rare inherited disorder, is characterized by gastrointestinal disorders in breast feeding infants a few days after they have started breast feeding. The disease is caused by a deficiency of galactose-1-phosphate-uridyl-transferase and leads to mental retardation and cirrhosis.

28. (D) A mousy odor is characteristic of the presence of phenylpyruvic acid, a metabolite of phenylalanine, which is found in patients with phenylketonuria.

29. (E) The strong ammoniacal odor sometimes present in some urine specimens comes from the bacterial decomposition of urea.

30. (A) Normal urine, devoid of long standing infection, has a faintly aromatic odor.

31. (B) Rhubarb, produces a reddish-orange color in urine specimens, particularly alkaline urines.

32. (A) Azure A, a constituent of the Diagnex Blue Test, will produce a blue colored urine.

33. (D)   Melanin in urine will cause the urine specimen to turn black when left standing.

34. (C)   Phenol poisoning will produce an olive green urine.

35. (B)   Homogentisic acid in a urine sample will react with 10% ferric chloride by producing a deep blue color that lasts for only a split second.

36. (D)   Melanin in a urine sample will react with 10% ferric chloride by precipitating ferric phosphate which, left standing, will turn black in approximately 30 minutes.

37. (A)   Acetoacetic acid will react with 10% ferric chloride by producing a red wine color. Salicylates will also do this, which is why it is necessary to boil the tube. After boiling, if the color persists it is due to salicylates.

38. (C)   The formation of casts is dependent on three conditions: high solute concentration, high protein concentration, and low pH. Casts very easily and readily dissolve in alkaline solutions.

39. (A)   Gerhardt's test will give positive results in the presence of acetoacetic acid and salicylates, but will not detect the presence of acetone or betahydroxybutyric acid.

40. (E)   Tolbutamid, the oral hypoglycemic, will give false positive results if it is present in a urine sample being tested for protein by the sulfosalicylic acid method.

41. (E)   False positive results on the glucose oxidase, peroxidase, chromagen system for glucose are obtained when the urine specimen is contaminated by strong oxidizing agents such as hydrogen peroxide. The peroxidase will react with the hydrogen peroxide, allowing the chromagen to accept the released oxygen and change colors.

42. (E)   Calcium carbonate crystals are found in alkaline urine and will effervesce, releasing carbon dioxide, when acetic acid is added.

43. (C)   Calcium oxalate crystals are the only crystals found in acid, neutral, and alkaline urine samples. Cystine crystals will dissolve in alkaline urines, while triple phosphate, calcium carbonate, and ammonium biurate crystals are found only in alkaline urines.

44. (B)   Cystine crystals are abnormal crystals in the urine and therefore require chemical confirmation prior to reporting.

45. (B)   The category that is associated with three of the phenomena is (B). Tamm-Horsfall mucoprotein is found in urinary casts; it is the protein that makes up the matrix of the cast. Casts rapidly dissolve in alkaline urines. Since casts require a high protein concentration for their formation there is usually an accompanying proteinuria.

46. (D)   The phenomenon that does not belong in this group is (D): casts do not require chemical confirmation.

47. (B)   Heparin sulfate is the predominant mucopolysaccharide found in Sanfilippo syndrome. Heparin sulfate is also found in Hurler's syndrome, as well as dermatan sulfate.

48. (E)   Sudan III or Sudan IV stains are both good stains for lipids. Polarized light microscopy will also confirm the presence of oval fat bodies by displaying the characteristic "maltese cross" pattern.

49. (A)   The first morning specimen is best for routine urinalysis because it is the most concentrated.

50. (D) Rothera's nitroprusside test will detect both acetone and acetonacetic acid, but not beta-hydroxybutyric acid.

51. (C) Formalin (40% V/V) is a useful preservative for the formed elements in a urine sample. Sodium carbonate and chloroform are not good preservatives of formed elements.

52. (B) A urine sample collected after the patient has been standing or walking at least 2 hours is the best sample to use for the detection of postural or orthostatic proteinuria. Protein is excreted in these patients when they have been standing or walking, and usually disappears when the individual lies down.

53. (B) Cellular casts, particularly epithelial casts upon aging and degeneration will become coarsely granular, then with further degeneration, finely granular and ultimately waxy.

54. (C) A specimen collected over the 2 hour period between 2 and 4 P.M. is the specimen of choice because this is when urobilinogen excretion is thought to be at its peak.

55. (C) The Addis count is a quantitative procedure for the determination of formed elements excreted in the urine. This procedure is performed on a 12 hour urine specimen.

56. (A) In hypotonic urines, when the specific gravity is low, white blood cells will swell and the granules exhibit Brownian movement, causing a "glittering" effect. These cells are known as "glitter cells."

57. (B) The term cylinduria indicates an increase in the number of casts which usually indicates renal disease.

58. (A) Acute glomerulonephritis is usually the result of an untreated infection with a Group A, beta hemolytic streptococcus.

59. (B) Uremia is the term used to indicate a build-up of nitrogenous waste products in the blood due to renal disease or failure.

60. (E) Acid urines may be produced by ingestion of fruits such as cranberries and when diets are high in meats and meat proteins. Citrus fruits will often produce an alkaline urine.

61. (D) Cystinuria is the result of a defect in renal tubular reabsorption whereas each of the other options are in-born errors of metabolism.

62. (C) The resorcinol test is used to test for the presence of fructose.

63. (A) p-dimethylaminobenzaldehyde in concentrated hydrochloric acid reacts with urobilinogen to produce a red color.

64. (B) Salicylates and pyridium will give a red to orange-red reaction with the ICTOTEST procedure. Bilirubin will result in a blue-purple color reaction as will chlorpromazine (Thorazine).

65. (D) All four of the testing procedures could be used. Adding 10% NaOH will cause the urine to darken; adding 10% ferric chloride will cause a rapidly disappearing blue color; adding alkalinized urine to photographic paper will cause the paper to turn black; and performing a Benedict's test will produce a yellow-orange precipitate which darkens to a muddy orange.

66. (C) Increased urine calcium levels are found in hyperparathyroidism, increased intestinal absorption of Vitamin D, and in renal tubular acidosis where there is excessive loss of base.

67. (D) Increased urine glucose levels can be found in all of the disease states listed: pheochromocytoma due to epinephrine excretion; pancreatitis

due to disturbance in the function of cells of the islets of Langerhans; hyperthyroidism due to increased rate of intestinal absorption of glucose; and Fanconi syndrome due to lowered renal absorption of glucose.

68.   (D)   Antidiuretic hormone (ADH) acts on the distal convoluted tubule and the collecting tubule.

69.   (B)   Creatine is normally excreted in small amounts in adult women, pregnant and lactating women and children of both sexes.   However, in adult men it is usually excreted as its anhydride creatinine. Creatine found in the urine of an adult male is usually due to muscle-wasting diseases.

70.   (A)   5-hydroxyindole acetic acid is the metabolite of serotonin, 5-hydroxytryptamine.

71.   (B)   Xylose, a pentose, will produce a brown color instead of a green color in the orthotoluidine reaction.

72.   (C)   Phenylketones are usually NOT tested for in a routine urinalysis. Phenylketones are usually screened for when there is a possibility of PKU (phenylketonuria).

73.   (A)   A small amount of glacial acetic acid run under the cover glass will aid in the differentiation of white blood cells from renal epithelial cells by bringing the nucleus more clearly into view.

74.   (A)   Calcium oxalate is the most commonly found constituent of renal calculi.   The mechanism and origin of this phenomenon is not entirely understood.

75.   (D)   Specific gravity is influenced by temperature and this urinometer was calibrated at 20°C.   For each 3°C above or below 20°C the specific gravity should be corrected by 0.001.

76.   (A)   Polyuria, or increased urine output, is a common characteristic of diabetes mellitus.

77.   (A)   The measurement of urine osmolality is based on the principle of freezing point depression which states that the lower the freezing point, the higher the osmotic pressure.

78.   (A)   Homocystinuria may be distinguished from cystinuria by means of high voltage electrophoresis.

79.   (C)   Hart test is designed for the detection of beta-hydroxybutyric acid.   It utilizes hydrogen peroxide to change the beta-hydroxybutyric acid to acetone and the Lange nitroprusside test to detect acetone and acetoacetic acid.

80.   (C)   The Sulkowitch test is used for rapid rough qualitative determination of the presence of urine calcium.

81.   (C)   Roberts test is a qualitative test for protein whereas the Kingsbury-Clark, Esbach's, and Tsuchiya tests are all quantitative tests.

82.   (A)   Antidiuretic hormone, or ADH, is excreted almost entirely by the posterior pituitary gland.

83.   (B)   Large numbers of leukocytes and clumps of leukocytes usually indicate the presence of a bacterial urinary tract infection.

84.   (C)   Waxy casts characteristically display a homogenous appearance with irregular shape, blunt ends, cracks or clefts, and is highly refractile and brittle looking.

85.   (A)   Trichomonads and yeast cells, when found in the urine, are usually the result of vaginal contamination, while the presence of Enterobius vermicularis is usually the result of fecal contamination.

86. (A) Approximately 40% of urea is reabsorbed by the tubules, while insulin is completely excreted by the kidney.

87. (C) Phenothiazine drugs result in false negatives, while banana or pineapple ingestion results in a false positive test in the quantitative test for 5-HIAA.

88. (D) This child has indications of acute glomerular nephritis, and the finding of red blood cells, white blood cells, casts, and renal epithelial cells would be consistent with acute glomerular nephritis.

89. (D) All of the listed conditions may result in the presence of cholesterol crystals in the urine.

90. (B) Albumin and immunoglobulin G are normally found in urine. Bence-Jones protein is only found in multiple myeloma and immunoglobulin M is not usually found in urine due to its pentameric structure.

91. (A) Red blood cells and tubular epithelial cells are common findings in renal disease.

92. (D) All of the disease entities listed can result in oliguria and often anuria.

93. (A) The Watson-Schwartz test is a chemical test for the presence of urobilinogen and porphobilinogen.

94. (A) Both hyperparathyroidism and cystinuria will often result in the formation of renal calculi.

95. (C) An acid pH is found in a diet high in meat protein, metabolic acidosis, and respiratory acidosis.

96. (D) Hyperaldosteronism produces an alkaline urine.

97. (B) Cystinuria often results in the formation of renal calculi; cystine crystals are hexagonal flat plates; and since cystine is an amino acid found in above normal limits, it is classified as an aminoaciduria.

98. (C) Cystinuria is not an inborn error of metabolism, rather it is a congenital defect of the kidney's ability to reabsorb cystine, lysine, ornithine, and arginine.

99. (B) The inulin clearance test, creatinine clearance test and the urea clearance tests are all tests for GFR, glomerular filtration rate.

100. (B) The PAH or para-aminohippurate clearance is essentially for renal plasma flow, since the PAH clearance is almost equal to the renal plasma flow.

101. (C) Tetrabromphenol blue is the active ingredient in the dipstick method for protein. The dipstick method is based on the principle of protein error of indicators, the indicator used is tetrabromphenol blue.

102. (C) Since the normal daily output of urine is generally below 2000 ml, an output of over 2000 ml would be considered polyuria, meaning increased urine output.

103. (D) Uric acid crystals are only found in acid urines. At alkaline pH's uric acid crystals will go back into solution.

104. (A) The addition of acetic acid to the urine sediment will dissolve the red blood cells allowing the other elements of the organized sediment to be evaluated.

105. (D) All of the crystals listed as choices are considered to be abnormal crystals when found in the urine sediment.

106. (A) Concentration, as well as dilution, tests are monitored by performing specific gravity measurements.

107. (B) Proteinuria is the most likely sign of renal disease. Squamous epithelial cells are found routinely in the urine sediment of individuals with or without urinary tract disease. dysuria could be the result of a bladder or urethral infection. Calcium carbonate crystals may normally be found in alkaline urines.

108. (C) The Guthrie test and the ferric chloride test are both utilized for the determination of the presence of phenylpyruvic acid. Phenylpyruvic acid is a metabolite of phenylalanine which is increased in pheylketonuria.

109. (C) The first morning specimen is the best specimen for routine urinalysis because it is the most concentrated specimen.

110. (D) All quantitative chemical analysis should be performed using 24 hour timed specimens due to circadian variation in the output of chemical constituents.

Bibliography and Recommended Readings

Bauer, J. D. and P. G. Ackermann. Clinical Laboratory Methods. Ninth Edition. 1982. The C. V. Mosby Company. St. Louis.

Freeman, J. A. and M. F. Beeler (Editors). Laboratory Medicine - Urine Analysis and Medical Microscopy. Second Edition. 1982. Lea and Febiger. Philadelphia.

Graff, Sr. L. Handbook of Routine Urinalysis. 1982. J. B. Lippincott Company. Philadelphia.

Henry, J. B. Todd-Sanford-Davidsohn Clinical Diagnosis and Management by Laboratory Methods. Sixteenth Edition. 1979. W. B. Saunders Company. Philadelphia.

Henry, R. J., Winkelman, J. W. and D. C. Cannon (Editors). Clinical Chemistry Principles and Techniques. Second Edition. 1974. Harper and Row Publishers. Hagerstown, Maryland.

Race, G. J. and M. G. White. Basic Urinalysis. 1979. J. B. Lippincott Company. Philadelphia.

Raphael, S. S. (Senior Author). Lynch's Medical Laboratory Technology. Volume I. Third Edition. 1976. W. B. Saunders Company. Philadelphia.

Ross, D. and A. E. Neely. Textbook of Urinalysis and Body Fluids. 1982. Appleton-Centry-Crofts. Englewood Cliffs, New Jersey.

Tietz, N. W. (Editor). Fundamentals of Clinical Chemistry. Second Edition. 1976. W. B. Saunders Company. Philadelphia.

CHAPTER 16

Body Fluid Analysis

Directions. Select the one BEST answer for each of the following statements. Circle the appropriate response on the answer sheet.

1. Which of the following amounts of gastric juice would be considered abnormal when a patient is in a fasting state?

   A. 20 ml
   B. 40 ml

   C. 60 ml
   D. 100 ml

2. Normal semen will show motility in a fresh specimen to be:

   A. at least 60%
   B. at least 70%

   C. at least 80%
   D. at least 90%

3. Which of the following is used as a stimulant in the tubeless gastric analysis Diagnex Blue test?

   A. caffeine
   B. histolog

   C. histamine
   D. ethanol

4. The normal pH range for a semen specimen is:

   A. 6.8 - 7.0
   B. 7.0 - 7.2

   C. 7.2 - 7.6
   D. 7.6 - 8.0

5. Which of the following enzymes is found in seminal fluid?

   A. alkaline phosphatase
   B. acid phosphatase

   C. amylase
   D. lactic dehydrogenase

6. In which of the following disease states would the assay of hexoseaminidase A and B, on amniotic fluid, be useful?

   A. erythroblastosis fetalis
   B. Down's syndrome

   C. Cooley's anemia
   D. Tay-Sachs disease

7. Which of the following would be considered an abnormal cerebrospinal fluid glucose?

   A. 30 mg/dl
   B. 45 mg/dl

   C. 60 mg/dl
   D. 70 mg/dl

8. A yellow discoloration of spinal fluid is referred to as:

   A. jaundice   C. hyperlipidemia
   B. xanthochromia   D. hemoglobinemia

9. The Pandy test is a test used for the determination of which of the following substances?

   A. fibrinogen   C. glucose
   B. globulin   D. chlorides

10. The color of normal synovial fluid is:

   A. colorless   C. straw
   B. red   D. dark yellow

11. The normal liquefaction of semen takes place in:

   A. 1 – 10 minutes   C. 30 – 60 minutes
   B. 10 – 30 minutes   D. 60 – 120 minutes

12. Charcot-Leyden crystals are often found in sputum specimens of patients with asthma. Charcot-Leyden crystals are formed from:

   A. eosinophils   C. fatty acids
   B. hematoidin   D. myelin

13. Synovial fluid glucose is usually decreased in which of the following?

   A. gout   C. disarticulations
   B. inflammatory arthritis   D. xanthochromia

14. Increased amounts of pericardial fluid may produce symptoms which depend on:

   A. the rate of fluid build up
   B. the volume of fluid accumulated
   C. both A and B
   D. neither A nor B

15. Which of the enzymes listed below is most commonly found elevated, in CSF, in infectious processes of the central nervous system?

   A. Lactic dehydrogenase (LD)
   B. Phosphohexose isomerase (PHI)
   C. Glutamic oxalacetic transaminase (GOT)
   D. Cholinesterase

16. An India ink preparation is performed on cerebrospinal fluid in an attempt to detect which of the following?

   A. bacteria   C. fungus
   B. protein   D. glucose

17. Normally, how much fluid is contained in the pericardial sac?

    A. 1 - 10 ml   C. 50 - 100 ml
    B. 20 - 50 ml   D. 100 - 150 ml

18. The chemical examination for glucose, in a pleural fluid, was found to be 65 mg/dl, while the blood glucose was 105 mg/dl. Which of the following is the most likely reason for these results?

    A. it is normal   C. bacterial infection
    B. Lupus erythematosus   D. adenocarcinoma

19. The normal color of peritoneal fluid is:

    A. red   C. colorless
    B. yellow   D. brown

20. Which of the following sperm counts is usually considered to be distinctly abnormal?

    A. less than 100 million   C. less than 20 million
    B. less than 200 million   D. less than 60 million

21. Which of the following is used in the Ropes' test on synovial fluid?

    A. 5% acetic acid   C. 10% acetic acid
    B. 5% hydrochloric acid   D. 10% hydrochloric acid

22. The process of tapping the peritoneal cavity to withdraw fluid is called:

    A. amniocentesis   C. lumbar puncture
    B. paracentesis   D. catheterization

23. What is the normal cerebrospinal fluid glucose concentration?

    A. 20 - 50 mg/dl   C. 80 - 110 mg/dl
    B. 50 - 80 mg/dl   D. 110 - 130 mg/dl

24. The measurement of sweat chloride is useful in the diagnosis of a disorder of which of the following organs?

    A. heart   C. kidney
    B. liver   D. pancreas

25. Upon microscopic examination of a synovial fluid specimen a technologist finds the following: White blood cell count = 150

                                            74% lymphocytes
                                            5% monocytes
                                            21% neutrophils
    This would indicate which of the following?

    A. a normal finding   C. viral infection
    B. bacterial infection   D. Lupus erythematosus

26. Which of the following would you expect to find in synovial fluid in "pseudogout"?

    A. monosodium urate crystals   C. A and B
    B. calcium pyrophosphate crystals   D. neither A nor B

27. Which of the following will typically form a transudate effusion in pleural fluid?

    A. congestive heart failure   C. metastatic carcinoma
    B. malignant lymphoma   D. pleural infections

Questions 28-36

Directions. One, some or all of the responses for each of the following statements may be correct. Indicate your response as follows:

A. if items 1 and 3 are correct
B. if items 2 and 4 are correct
C. if three of the items are correct
D. if all of the items are correct
E. if only one of the items is correct

28. Which of the following may be responsible for a turbid peritoneal fluid?

    1. appendicitis   3. ruptured bowel
    2. pancreatitis   4. primary bacterial infection

29. Which of the following are normal ways in which synovial fluid is produced?

    1. osteoarthritis
    2. active secretion
    3. mild rheumatoid arthritis
    4. dialysis of plasma across the synovial membrane

30. Which of the following can be used to stimulate the secretion of gastric acid?

    1. histamine   3. ethanol
    2. caffeine   4. histolog

31. Which of the following conditions will produce a firm clot in the Ropes' test?

    1. normal fluid   3. lupus erythematosus
    2. rheumatoid arthritis   4. acute rheumatic fever

32. Which of the following substances will produce a black stool specimen?

    1. blackberries   3. bismuth
    2. huckleberries   4. rhubarb

33. Pleural surfaces are normally lubricated by 1 - 10 ml of fluid. Abnormal amounts of fluid may be caused by which of the following?

    1. inflammation   3. congestive heart failure
    2. decreased osmotic pressure   4. decreased lymphatic drainage

34. Which of the following are tests for occult blood in stool specimens?

    1. guaiac test
    2. benzidine test
    3. ortho-tolidine test
    4. ortho-toluidine test

35. Traumatic taps for synovial fluid typically show which of the following?

    1. blood initially decreasing as you aspirate
    2. streaking of blood in the syringe
    3. clotting of blood streaks within 15 minutes
    4. xanthochromia

36. Hemothorax may be distinguished from a hemorrhagic effusion by performing which of the following?

    1. hematocrit of the pleural fluid
    2. turbidity of the pleural fluid
    3. hematocrit of the capillary blood
    4. red blood cell count of the pleural fluid

Questions 37-38

Directions. The column on the left contains 3 scientifically related categories while the column on the right contains 4 items which may illustrate scientific phenomena or processes. Three of the items in the column on the right relate to only one of the categories in the column on the left. FIRST, indicate the category in which the 3 processes or phenomena belong. SECOND, indicate the one process or phenomenon which is not related to that category.

Category

37. A. pleural fluid
     B. synovial fluid
     C. amniotic fluid

Phenomenon

38. A. ragocytes
     B. Reiter cells
     C. monosodium urate crystals
     D. elevated amylase levels

Questions 39-50

Directions. For each of the numbered items select the appropriate lettered response. Do not use the same letter more than once.

Synovial Fluid

39. Turbid, yellow
40. Milky fluid
41. Xanthochromia
42. Grossly bloody

Cause

A. Previous hemorrhage
B. WBC's present
C. Mucin present
D. Lymphatic obstruction
E. Hemophilia

Disorder

43. Pancreatitis
44. Intestinal necrosis
45. Congestive heart failure
46. Tuberculosis peritonitis

Finding

A. Elevated ammonia levels
B. Transudate
C. Lymphocytosis
D. Elevated peritoneal amylase
E. Erythrocyte count of 50,000

Feces Color

47. Clay colored
48. Black
49. Red streaked
50. Very dark brown

Cause

A. Iron ingestion
B. Excretion of urobilin
C. Obstructive jaundice
D. Bleeding in lower colon
E. Steatorrhea

Questions 51-65

Directions. For each of the numbered words or phrases listed below, select the appropriate response as follows:

A. if the item is associated with A only
B. if the item is associated with B only
C. if the item is associated with both A and B
D. if the item is associated with neither A nor B

A. normal synovial fluid viscosity
B. good mucin clot test

51. gouty arthritis
52. traumatic arthritis
53. systemic lupus erythematosus
54. osteoarthritis
55. rheumatoid arthritis

A. transudative effusion
B. exudative effusion

56. clear fluid
57. total proteins greater than 50% of serum levels
58. clot formation
59. fibrinogen level of less than 4%
60. turbid fluid

A. increased spinal fluid protein
B. decreased spinal fluid chloride

61. encephalitis
62. subdural hemorrhage
63. tuberculosis meningitis
64. submeningeal abscess
65. spinal cord tumor

Questions 66-70

Directions. One, some, or all of the responses for each of the following statements may be correct. Indicate your response as follows:

A. if items 1 and 3 are correct
B. if items 2 and 4 are correct
C. if three of the items are correct
D. if all of the items are correct
E. if only one of the items is correct

66. Infertility is associated with which of the following seminal fluid analyses?

1. volume of less than 0.5 ml
2. sperm count of less than 60 million
3. motility of 30% in the first hour
4. pH of 7.6

67. Which of the following findings would be suggestive of pseudogout?

1. many sodium urate crystals
2. many calcium pyrophosphate crystals
3. poor mucin clot test
4. good mucin clot test

68. Which of the following values obtained during the analysis of an amniotic fluid sample would indicate fetal immaturity?

1. L/S ratio of less than 1.2
2. optical density at 650 nm of less than 0.15
3. Creatinine value of 1.0 mg/dl or less
4. AFP level of less than 4,000 ng/ml

69. Which of the following substances are associated with pneumoconiosis?

1. silica (sand)   3. coal
2. lime or marble   4. asbestos

70. Which of the following tests are utilized in the assessment of erythroblastosis fetalis?

1. amniotic fluid bilirubin   3. alpha-feto protein
2. alpha-1-antitrypsin assay   4. mucin clot test

Explanatory Answers

1. (D) The stomach in a fasting state usually will not excrete more than 60 ml; amounts of 100 ml or more are considered abnormal.

2. (A) Motility below 60% in a fresh semen specimen is generally considered to be abnormal.

3. (A) Caffeine in the form of caffeine sodium benzoate is taken one hour before the ingestion of the azure resin.

4. (C) The normal pH of semen is between 7.2 and 7.6.

5. (B) Since seminal fluid is composed of some excretions from the prostate gland which is rich in acid phosphatase, there is a considerable amount of acid phosphatase in semen.

6. (D) In Tay-Sachs disease, assay of an amniotic fluid for levels of hexoseaminidase A and B would show a low activity of hexoseaminidase A and a normal or elevated level of activity of hexoseaminidase B.

7. (A) The normal glucose range for cerebrospinal fluid is 40-70 mg/dl.

8. (B) Xanthochromia is the term applied to a yellow discoloration of spinal fluid which may be due to bilirubin, hemoglobin derivatives or substances from brain destruction.

9. (B) The Pandy test is used for the determination of the presence of globulins in cerebrospinal fluid.

10. (C) Normal synovial fluid is straw colored or lighter.

11. (B) The normal liquefaction of semen, which is dependent on the fibrinolysin present, should take place within 10 to 30 minutes.

12. (A) Charcot-Leyden crystals arise from the disintegration of eosinophils which are usually abundant in patients with asthma.

13. (B) Synovial fluid normally reflects the plasma glucose levels; in inflammatory arthritis glucose levels are decreased.

14. (C) Symptoms from pericardial fluid build up depend on the rate of fluid build up and the volume accumulated.

15. (B) Phosphohexose isomerase (PHI) elevations are found in infectious processes of the CNS caused by fungi, bacteria or viruses.

16. (C) The India ink preparation is designed for the detection of the fungus Cryptococcus neoformans.

17. (B) The pericardial sac normally contains about 20 - 50 ml of clear, straw colored transudate.

18. (C) Glucose in pleural fluid is usually about equal to that of whole

blood. Pleural fluid glucose of 30 - 40 mg/dl lower than the blood glucose strongly suggests bacterial infection.

19. (B) Peritoneal fluid is typically clear, and pale yellow to amber.

20. (C) The normal sperm count usually falls between the range of 60 - 150 million, and counts of less than 20 million are usually considered abnormal.

21. (A) 5% acetic acid is the acid used in the Ropes' test. One ml of synovial fluid is added to the 20 ml of 5% acetic acid and the clot formation is observed.

22. (B) Paracentesis is the term applied to the tapping of the peritoneal cavity for obtaining fluid for either relieving pressure or for the purposes of testing.

23. (B) Normal cerebrospinal fluid contains 50 - 80 mg/dl of glucose. Decreased levels are often found in infections and malignancies, whereas normal levels are often found in virus infections.

24. (D) The sweat chloride test is performed for the detection of cystic fibrosis, a congenital pancreatic disease.

25. (A) Normal synovial fluid will contain less than 200 wbc's and most of these will be lymphocytes and monocytes; less than 25% of the cells will be neutrophils.

26. (B) Pseudogout is characterized by the finding of calcium pyrophosphate crystals in the synovial fluid.

27. (A) Congestive heart failure typically produces a transudative pleural effusion, while malignant lymphomas, metastatic carcinoma, and pleural infections typically produce an exudative effusion.

28. (D) All of the choices may produce a turbid peritoneal fluid.

29. (B) Normally, synovial fluid is produced in one of two ways; by active secretion or by dialysis of plasma across the synovial membrane.

30. (D) All of the items listed will stimulate gastric acid secretion.

31. (C) The Ropes' test is performed to observe the ropy clot of mucoproteins that forms. It is a firm clot in normal fluid, lupus erythematosus and acute rheumatic fever. In rheumatoid arthritis the clot is friable and the surrounding fluid is turbid.

32. (C) Blackberries, huckleberries, and bismuth all produce a black stool specimen.

33. (D) All of the choices may produce abnormal amounts of pleural fluid. Inflammation may result in increased capillary permeability; decrease in plasma colloid osmotic pressure, increased hydrostatic pressure due to congestive heart failure, and, decreased lymphatic drainage due to tumor, inflammation, or fibrosis of the mediastinal lymph nodes may all result in increased fluid build up.

34. (C) The guaiac test, benzidine test, and ortho-tolidine test are all tests for occult blood. The ortho-toluidine test is one used for glucose determinations.

35. (C) Traumatic synovial fluid taps characteristically show one or more of the following: blood initially decreasing as aspiration continues, streaking of blood, and clotting of these streaks. In hemorrhagic fluids, the blood would be prevalent throughout the aspiration, would be uniform, and, unless fibrinogen were present, would not show any clotting.

36. (A) Performance of the simultaneous measurement of the hematocrit of the pleural fluid and the capillary blood will distinguish between hemothorax and a hemorrhagic effusion. With a hemothorax, the hematocrit of the pleural fluid is similar to that of the capillary blood.

37. (B) Synovial fluid may contain ragocytes, or so-called RA cells, Reiter cells, which are large phagocytic cells containing ingested neutrophils, or, in acute gouty arthritis, monosodium urate crystals.

38. (D) Elevated amylase levels are not frequently encountered in synovial fluid.

39. (B) Turbid yellow fluid usually indicates the presence of white blood cells, whether due to septic or non-septic inflammation.

40. (D) Grossly milky synovial fluid may occur in effusions due to rheumatoid arthritis, acute gout, and lymphatic obstruction.

41. (A) Although xanthochromia may be difficult to evaluate, a deep yellow color or brown color may suggest previous hemorrhage.

42. (E) Grossly bloody synovial fluid occurs with effusions due to trauma, hemophilia, or acute synovitis.

43. (D) 90% of the cases of pancreatitis have amylase levels of the peritoneal fluid higher than the serum amylase levels.

44. (A) Increased levels of peritoneal ammonia suggests intestinal necrosis or perforation.

45. (B) Transudates rather than exudates are found in conditions such as congestive heart failure, cirrhosis, or nephrotic syndrome.

46. (C) Lymphocytosis may be due to tuberculosis peritonitis or chylosis ascites.

47. (C) Clay colored stool specimens are characteristic of obstructive jaundice.

48. (A) Iron ingestion, ingestion of bismuth preparations, and bleeding high in the digestive tract will all result in the passage of black stools.

49. (D) Bleeding in the lower colon, the recturm, or the anus, may result in red streaked stool specimens.

50. (B) The excretion of urobilin, as occurs in hemolytic anemias may result in the passage of very dark brown stool specimens.

51. (D) Gouty arthritis is associated with a low synovial fluid viscosity and a poor mucin clot test.

52. (C) Traumatic arthritis is associated with a normal synovial fluid viscosity and a good mucin clot test.

53. (C) Systemic lupus erythematosus is associated with a normal synovial fluid viscosity and a good mucin clot test.

54. (C) Osteoarthritis is associated with a normal synovial fluid viscosity and a good mucin clot test.

55. (D) Rheumatoid arthritis is associated with a low synovial fluid viscosity and a fair mucin clot test.

56. (C) Both transudative and exudative fluids may be clear in appearance. Normally, all transudative effusions are clear and straw colored, while exudative effusions may be clear, turbid, bloody or purulent.

57. (B) Exudative effusions characteristically have total protein concentrations that are greater than

50% of the serum total protein concentration.

58. (B) Clot formation is associated with exudative effusions since there is an increased amount of fibrinogen present.

59. (A) Fibrinogen levels of less than 4% in an effusion is generally associated with a transudative type of effusion.

60. (B) Turbid fluids are generally exudative since transudative fluids are always clear.

61. (D) Encephalitis is usually characterized by a slightly decreased spinal fluid protein and a normal spinal fluid chloride.

62. (D) Subdural hemorrhage is characterized by a normal spinal fluid protein and a normal spinal fluid chloride.

63. (C) Tuberculosis meningitis is associated with a moderate increase in spinal fluid protein and a decrease in the spinal fluid chloride.

64. (A) Submeningeal abscesses are associated with moderate elevations of the spinal fluid protein and normal spinal fluid chloride.

65. (A) Spinal cord tumors are associated with a marked elevation of the spinal fluid protein and a normal spinal fluid chloride.

66. (A) The lower limits of normal for seminal fluid volume is 0.5 ml and the motility is 50% or more. Therefore, levels of both volume and motility being below normal would be suggestive of infertility.

67. (B) Pseudogout is characterized by the presence of calcium pyrophosphate crystals and a good mucin clot test. Many sodium urate crystals and a poor mucin clot test would be suggestive of gouty arthritis.

68. (C) An L/S ratio of less than 1.2, an optical density of 650 nm of less than 0.15 and a creatinine value of 1.0 mg/dl or less are all indicative of fetal immaturity. The AFP (alpha-feto protein) level of less than 4,000 is not directly associated with fetal maturity though it would be consistent with a normal pregnancy in the third trimester.

69. (D) All of the items listed are associated with pneumoconiosis. Silica or sand causes silocosis, lime or marble dust causes calicosis, coal dust causes anthracosis and asbestos causes asbestosis.

70. (E) Only the amniotic bilirubin assay, from the choices offered, is a measurement that would assess erythroblastosis fetalis. The alpha-feto protein assay is normally used to detect neural tube defects, the alpha-1-antitrypsin test is not performed on amniotic fluid, and the mucin clot test is used to measure the hyaluronic acid content of synovial fluid.

Bibliography and Recommended Readings

Bauer, J. D. and P. G. Ackermann. <u>Clinical</u> <u>Laboratory</u> <u>Methods</u>. Ninth Edition. 1982. The C. V. Mosby Company. St. Louis.

Burke, S. R. <u>The</u> <u>Composition</u> <u>and</u> <u>Function</u> <u>of</u> <u>Body</u> <u>Fluids</u>. Third Edition. 1980. The C. V. Mosby Company. St. Louis.

Freeman, J. A. and M. F. Beeler (Editors). <u>Laboratory</u> <u>Medicine</u> - <u>Urine</u> <u>Analysis</u> <u>and</u> Medical Microscopy. Second Edition. 1982. Lea and Febiger. Philadelphia.

Henry, J. B. <u>Todd-Sanford-Davidsohn</u> <u>Clinical</u> <u>Diagnosis</u> <u>and</u> <u>Management</u> <u>by</u> <u>Laboratory</u> <u>Methods</u>. Sixteenth Edition. 1979. W. B. Saunders Company. Philadelphia.

Henry, R. J., Winkelman, J. W. and D. C. Cannon (Editors). <u>Clinical</u> <u>Chemistry</u> <u>Principles</u> <u>and</u> <u>Techniques</u>. Second Edition. 1974. Harper and Row Publishers. Hagerstown, Maryland.

Raphael, S. S. (Senior Author). <u>Lynch's</u> <u>Medical</u> <u>Laboratory</u> <u>Technology</u>. Volumes I and II. Third Edition. 1976. W. B. Saunders Company. Philadelphia.

Ross, D. and A. E. Neely. <u>Textbook</u> <u>of</u> <u>Urinalysis</u> <u>and</u> <u>Body</u> <u>Fluids</u>. 1982. Appleton-Century-Crofts. Englewood Cliffs, New Jersey.

Tietz, N. W. (Editor). <u>Fundamentals</u> <u>of</u> <u>Clinical</u> <u>Chemistry</u>. Second Edition. 1976. W. B. Saunders Company. Philadelphia.

CHAPTER 17

Cytogenetics/Cytology

Directions. Select the one BEST answer for each of the following statements. Circle the appropriate response on the answer sheet.

1. A child's karyotype displayed three number 21 chromosomes instead of the normal two. Trisomy-21 is compatible with life; however, the child will demonstrate:

   A. Tay Sachs disease
   B. cat cry syndrome
   C. Down's syndrome
   D. Klinefelter's syndrome
   E. Turner's syndrome

2. A karyotype showed that a section of chromosome 22 was missing. Which of the following disorders is associated with the deletion of a portion of chromosome 22?

   A. Cooley's anemia
   B. chronic myelogenous leukemia
   C. Tay Sachs disease
   D. Turner's syndrome
   E. systemic lupus erythematosus

3. A karyotype displayed normal and abnormal cells. This mosaic is the result of nondisjunction in the:

   A. zygote
   B. mother
   C. father
   D. maternal grandmother
   E. paternal grandmother

4. Certain chromosomal deletions are not lethal but they produce deleterious effects. People who have one normal chromosome 5 and a partially deleted homologue so that part of the short arm of the homologous chromosome 5 is deleted illustrate body abnormalities and severe mental retardation. These patients have a condition referred to as:

   A. Turner's syndrome
   B. Down's syndrome
   C. Guillain-Barre syndrome
   D. cat cry syndrome
   E. Klinefelter's syndrome

5. The chromosomal aberration most frequently observed cytologically is due to:

   A. inversions
   B. terminal deletions
   C. translocations
   D. interstitial deletions
   E. duplications

6. When the inverted region of the chromosome includes the centromere it is referred to as:

    A. paracentric
    B. pericentric
    C. intrachromosomal

    D. interstitial
    E. bivalent

7. In man, the Y chromosome is male determining. Male gonads are found in individuals with the following chromosomal arrangement:

    A. XY
    B. XXY
    C. XXXY

    D. all of the above
    E. A and B but not C

8. In humans the XO karyotype is associated with:

    A. Down's syndrome
    B. Klinefelter's syndrome
    C. Turner's syndrome

    D. Guillain-Barre syndrome
    E. cri-du-chat syndrome

9. Individuals with an XXY karyotype usually demonstrate:

    A. Sjogren's syndrome
    B. cat cry syndrome
    C. Klinefelter's syndrome

    D. Ellis van Creveld syndrome
    E. Down's syndrome

10. Dwarfism is a rare recessive condition. This condition is generally referred to as:

    A. Ellis van Creveld syndrome
    B. Sjogren's syndrome
    C. Aldrich's syndrome

    D. Hoffman's disease
    E. Hunter's disease

11. With many cytological stains and staining techniques the Y chromosome cannot be differentiated from chromosomes 21 and 22 so that there are:

    A. five such chromosomes in males and only four in females
    B. six such chromosomes in males and only five in females
    C. four such chromosomes in males and four in females
    D. five such chromosomes in males and females
    E. three such chromosomes in males and two in females

12. If a woman's somatic cell nuclei contain two sex chromatin body masses, her sex chromosome configuration is:

    A. XX
    B. XXY
    C. XYY

    D. XXX
    E. none of the above

13. If a female has Turner's syndrome, how many Barr bodies would her somatic cells contain?

    A. three
    B. two

    C. one
    D. none

14. Megakaryocytes are bone marrow cells which demonstrate a large nucleus and a great deal of cytoplasm. Megakaryocytes form:

    A. basophils   D. platelets
    B. eosinophils   E. osteoclasts
    C. red blood cells

15. Conventional staining techniques and E/M have demonstrated the presence of Hassal's corpuscles in the medulla of this gland. This gland is the:

    A. thyroid   D. adrenal
    B. thymus   E. pituitary
    C. parathyroid

16. An H and E preparation of this tissue showed a dark blue section which was identified as Peyer's patches. This slide bears a section of the:

    A. small intestine   D. liver
    B. large intestine   E. spleen
    C. kidney

17. Chief cells are hormone producing cells found in the:

    A. pituitary   D. thyroid
    B. pancreas   E. adrenal
    C. parathyroid

18. The arms of chromosomes vary somewhat in length depending upon the location of the primary constriction. When the centromere is median in location an equal armed chromosome results. This equal armed chromosome is called:

    A. metacentric   D. concentric
    B. telocentric   E. pericentric
    C. acrocentric

19. Deletion of part of the long arm of chromosome 22, called the "Philadelphia" chromosome, is indicative of:

    A. chronic myelogenous leukemia   D. Down's syndrome
    B. sickle cell anemia   E. dwarfism
    C. Guillain-Barre syndrome

20. Generally, chromosome replication occurs simultaneously with cell division so that the two sets of daughter chromosomes segregate into separate cells. However, in certain cell types cell division does not accompany chromosome replication and consequently the replicated chromosomes accumulate in the same nucleus rather than in separate nuclei. This process whereby cell division does not accompany chromosome replication is called:

    A. puffing   C. chromosome folding
    B. Balbiani ring   D. endoduplication

21. Huntington's chorea is a disease of the nervous system. This disease is rare but fatal and the symptoms are not exhibited until middle age. This disease is inherited as an autosomal dominant trait. If an apparently normal man in his late twenties is informed that his father has been diagnosed as having Huntington's chorea, what are the chances of the son developing the disease himself?

    A. 100%
    B. 75%
    C. 50%
    D. 25%
    E. none at all

22. A person is a sexual mosaic with sex chromosome constituents of XX/XXXY. How many Barr bodies would be found in that person's cells?

    A. one or two
    B. two or three
    C. only one
    D. only two
    E. only three

23. Down's syndrome is the result of trisomy 21. Consequently the somatic cells of individuals with Down's syndrome have 47 chromosomes instead of 46. Down's syndrome is then the result of:

    A. crossing over
    B. chromosome deletion
    C. chromosome inversion
    D. translocation
    E. nondisjunction

24. Mucus secreting cells of the intestine protect the absorptive cells of the intestine. These protective mucus secreting cells when stained with H and E appear membrane bound. These intestinal mucus secreting cells are:

    A. chief cells
    B. parietal cells
    C. basket cells
    D. goblet cells
    E. lacunae

25. Color blindness and hemophilia are said to be "sex linked" disorders. Which of the following best explains why they are classified in this manner?

    A. because males have XY chromosomes
    B. because males have two YY chromosomes
    C. because females never acquire these disorders
    D. because males never acquire these disorders
    E. none of the above

Explanatory Answers

1. (C) Trisomy-21 causes Mongolism or Down's syndrome.

2. (B) Chronic myelogenous leukemia is associated with the deletion of a portion of chromosome 22.

3. (A) Mosaics are the result of non-disjunction of chromosomes in the developing zygote.

4. (D) Individuals who have a partially deleted chromosome 5 suffer from cri-du-chat (cat cry) syndrome which is characterized with several body abnormalities and severe mental retardation. Although the body abnormalities are less severe in adulthood, mental retardation is severe and persists throughout the life span of the individual.

5. (A) Inversions are most frequently observed primarily because they are easily identified and also they rarely produce lethal effects in either the homozygous or hetero-zygous form.

6. (B) When the inverted region of the aberrant chromosome contains the centromere, it is said to be pericentric.

7. (D) Males demonstrating an XY, XXY and XXXY chromosomal constitution will have developed testes although they may be nonfunctional in XXY and XXXY individuals. The normal male sex-chromosome configuration is XY.

8. (C) Individuals with an XO karyotype demonstrate Turner's syndrome which is characterized by a short stature, infantilism, underdeveloped gonads, multiple birthmarks and a severe webbing of the neck.

9. (C) The most frequent chromosome constitution demonstrating Kline-felter's syndrome is XXY. Individuals with this syndrome have male internal and external genitalia but the testes are small and non-functional. Mental retardation may or may not occur. Individuals with 48 XXXY, 49 XXXXY may also demonstrate Klinefelter syndrome traits but more severely than a 47 XXY chromosome constitution.

10. (A) Dwarfism is a condition referred to as Ellis van Creveld syndrome.

11. (A) The Y chromosome resembles chromosomes 21 and 22. Chromosomes 21 and 22 are in pairs while the Y chromosome is not. Consequently 5 similar chromosomes would be found in male karyotypes and 4 in females who lack the Y chromosome.

12. (D) Because of the relationship between sex chromatin and X chromosomes, a triple X female would have two sex chromatin bodies in the nuclei of her body cells.

13. (D) If a woman has Turner's syndrome her sex chromosome constitution is XO. The one X chromosome becomes extended and cannot be seen cytologically. The only reason a Barr body is seen in female body cells is that the female contains two XX chromosomes, one of which may extend and be non-visible and the other which may remain contracted and visible under light microscopy. No Barr bodies are visualized in the nuclei of male cells because males have an XY sex chromosome configuration and the one X chromosome is extended and non-visible under the light microscope.

14. (D) The function of megakaryocytes is to form platelets.

15. (B) Hassal's corpuscles are found only in the medulla of the thymus.

16. (A) Peyer's patches which are made up of lymphatic nodules are characteristically found in the lower part of the small intestine.

17. (C) The chief cells produce the hormones of the parathyroid gland.

18. (A) Equal armed chromosomes are referred to as being metacentric. Submetacentric chromosomes have arms which differ slightly in length while the arms of acrocentric chromosomes differ markedly in length. Chromosomes which have only one arm are termed telocentric.

19. (A) The "Philadelphia" chromosome is found in the bone marrow of individuals suffering from chronic myelogenous leukemia.

20. (D) Endoduplication occurs when cell division is not synchronized with chromosome replication.

21. (C) Since the disease is rare, the father is most likely heterozygous for Huntington's chorea (Hh). All of the father's children would then have a 50% chance of inheriting the dominant allele.

22. (A) Depending upon which cells are examined, one or two Barr bodies could be found. Some of this person's cells are XX and have one Barr body, but other cells are XXXY and have two Barr bodies.

23. (E) Nondisjunction occurs when chromosomes fail to separate properly during meiosis. Consequently some cells receive two chromosomes-21 and Down's syndrome results.

24. (D) The goblet cells of the small intestine secrete mucus. The mucus appears magenta when stained with the PA-Schiff technique and the membrane bound goblet cell may be seen also with H and E.

25. (A) They are classified as "sex-linked" because the Y chromosome, found in males is lacking the genetic information found on upper arms of the X chromosome.

Bibliography and Recommended Readings

Avers, Charlotte J. Cell Biology. 1976. D. Van Nostrand Company. New York.

Crispens, Charles G. Essentials of Medical Genetics. 1971. Harper and Row Publishers, Inc. Hagerstown, Maryland.

DeRobertis, E. D. P., Saez, Francisco A. and E. M. F. De Robertis, Jr. Cell Biology. 1975. W. B. Saunders Company. Philadelphia.

Gompel, Claude. Atlas of Diagnostic Cytology. 1978. John Wiley and Sons, Inc. New York.

Ham, Arthur W. Histology. Seventh Edition. 1974. J. B. Lippincott Company. Philadelphia.

Koss, Leopold G. Diagnostic Cytology. Second Edition. 1968. J. B. Lippincott Company. Philadelphia.

Purtilo, David T. A Survey of Human Diseases. 1978. Addison-Wesley Publishing Company, Inc. Reading, Massachusetts.

Singer, Sam. Human Genetics. 1978. W. H. Freeman and Company. San Francisco.

CHAPTER 18

Quality Control/Laboratory Safety/ Laboratory Management

Directions. Select the one BEST answer for each of the following statements. Circle the appropriate response on the answer sheet.

1. Care should be taken in properly and carefully grinding tissue with a mortar and pestle, opening a lyophilized culture, shaking cultures in high-speed mixers and withdrawing culture samples from vaccine bottles because:

   A. the cultures may be old
   B. mutations may occur
   C. aerosols may be produced

   D. no cultures may grow
   E. none of the above

2. The accepted standard for steam sterilization is assumed to be "15 pounds of pressure for 15 minutes." However, quality control measures for steam sterilization should emphasize:

   A. pressure and time
   B. temperature and time
   C. the type of steam sterilizer used

   D. pressure only
   E. temperature only

3. Good bacteriological techniques in sample collections:

   A. prevent specimen contamination only
   B. facilitate things for the patient
   C. prevent specimen contamination and protect the worker against infections
   D. prevent the worker from having to collect a second specimen
   E. ensure good culture plate results

4. Biological indications are used to monitor sterilizers. The bacteriological genus most commonly used as a biological indicator is:

   A. Clostridium
   B. Bacillus
   C. Corynebacterium

   D. Mycobacterium
   E. A and B but not C or D

5. To obtain reproducible results in a diagnostic laboratory it is essential to have:

   A. detailed procedures for diagnostic tests
   B. the best instrumentation available
   C. no change in personnel
   D. a limited number of diagnostic tests

6. Although manufacturers of bacteriological media do quality control studies on their products, users should monitor these products prior to use to:

   A. comply with regulations
   B. assure that the product is still good at the time of use
   C. check the storage conditions
   D. check the pH and color of the medium in question
   E. check the environmental influence on the media

7. Which of the following cultures should be maintained to check for the V and X growth factors?

   A. Staphylococcus aureus
   B. Streptococcus pyogenes
   C. Haemophilus influenzae
   D. Pseudomonas aeruginosa
   E. Citrobacter freundii

8. Which of the following should be maintained in a laboratory to check bacitracin disks, group A antiserum quality and the production of beta hemolysis on blood agar plates?

   A. Streptococcus salivarus
   B. Streptococcus mitis
   C. Streptococcus pneumoniae
   D. Streptococcus fecalis
   E. Streptococcus pyogenes

9. Which of the following is necessary for checking optochin disks and an organism's ability to produce alpha hemolysis on blood agar plates?

   A. Streptococcus salivarus
   B. Streptococcus mitis
   C. Streptococcus pneumoniae
   D. Streptococcus fecalis
   E. Streptococcus pyogenes

10. Which culture should be maintained in the laboratory to check for chlamydospore production?

    A. Aspergillus flavus
    B. Aspergillus niger
    C. Penicillium notatum
    D. Penicillium roqueforti
    E. Candida albicans

11. The medium recommended for the Bauer-Kirby disk susceptibility test is:

    A. trypticase soy agar
    B. Mueller-Hinton agar
    C. blood agar
    D. Thayer-Martin medium
    E. Fletcher's medium

12. Quality control records should be kept in every laboratory. A record should be kept on test results, equipment performance and the age and quality of laboratory reagents. The best place for these records is:

    A. in a locked cabinet so no one can use or lose them
    B. at each bench so as to be available for everyone to use
    C. in the business office
    D. in the laboratory director's possession only

13. Bacterial stock cultures may be maintained longest when:

    A. kept in broth
    B. streaked on slants
    C. lyophilized
    D. streaked on slants and covered with mineral oil
    E. grown on blood agar plates

14. Which of the following should be maintained as a stock culture to test for coagulase activity?

    A. Staphylococcus epidermidis   D. Streptococcus pyogenes
    B. Staphylococcus aureus   E. Citrobacter sp.
    C. Staphylococcus citreus

15. Which of the following should be maintained as stock cultures to demonstrate deaminase activity?

    A. Proteus vulgaris   D. Shigella dysenteriae
    B. Escherichia coli   E. Staphylococcus aureus
    C. Salmonella typhi

16. Which of the following should be maintained to check for oxidase production?

    A. Neisseria gonococci   D. Haemophilus influenzae
    B. Treponema pallidum   E. Salmonella typhimurium
    C. Streptococcus pyogenes

17. Which of the following is the best method to sterilize materials which denature readily?

    A. soak in alcohol   C. tyndallization
    B. soak in ethanol   D. all of the above

18. Kovac's reagent should be used to determine the presence of:

    A. indole   D. lecithin
    B. esculin   E. hydrogen sulfide
    C. starch

19. Which of the following should be maintained to check for typhus fever?

    A. Pseudomonas OX 19   D. Both A and B
    B. Proteus OX 19   E. Both B and C
    C. Providencia OX 19

20. If typhoid fever is suspected, the patient's serum should be set up against the following Salmonella typhi and antigen(s):

    A. the H antigen only   C. both the H and O antigens
    B. the O antigen only   D. none of the above

Questions 21-36

Directions. For each of the numbered items select the appropriate lettered response. Do not use the same letter more than once.

21. accuracy
22. precision
23. sensitivity
24. standard

A. degree of discrimination
B. closeness to the true mean
C. composition closely resembling the test specimen
D. reproducibility
E. highly purified material

25. standard deviation
26. 95% confidence limit
27. systematic shift
28. systematic trend

A. percentage of variance from the mean
B. the measure of scatter around the mean
C. change in values caused by sudden failure or bias
D. gradual increase or decrease
E. encompasses 95.45% of the results in a normal curve

Term

29. mean
30. median
31. mode
32. C. V.

Definition

A. the middle value in a set
B. percent of the mean value
C. the average value
D. difference between the smallest and largest values
E. the value in a set occuring most frequently

Chemical agent

33. Sulfur dioxide
34. Carbon tetrachloride
35. Benzidine
36. Phenol

Effect

A. carcinogenic
B. contact dermatitis
C. severe burns to the lungs
D. liver damage
E. prevents oxygenation of blood

Questions 37-42

Directions. One, some, or all of the responses for each of the following statements may be correct. Indicate your response as follows:

A. if items 1 and 3 are correct
B. if items 2 and 4 are correct
C. if three of the items are correct
D. if all of the items are correct
E. if only one of the items is correct

37. In which of the following situations is the median a better measure of the center than the mean?

1. positively skewed curve
2. standard Gaussian curve
3. negatively skewed curve
4. a relatively flat curve

38. In which of the following areas can a properly prepared and stained blood smear be of value in quality control?

1. platelet count
2. RBC indices
3. white blood cell count
4. hematocrit

39. Reagent red cells for ABO reverse grouping should be tested for their ability to react with weak antisera. Which of the following dilutions of commerical anti-A and anti-B should be used for this purpose?

1. 1:50
2. 1:100
3. 1:75
4. 1:200

40. Coomb's sera should be tested for their reactivity to which of the following?

1. IgG
2. IgM
3. C3
4. C4

41. Which of the following should have separate serum pools established for quality control purposes?

1. enzymes
2. glucose
3. thyroid tests
4. bilirubin

42. Which of the following will demonstrate the reactivity of antisera used in blood banking?

1. avidity testing
2. titration of the antisera
3. dilution of the antisera
4. ionic strength

Questions 43-57

Directions. Select the one BEST answer for each of the following statements. Circle the approrpiate response on the answer sheet.

43. How often should the temperature of Rh view boxes be recorded?

    A. every day
    B. every other day
    C. once a week
    D. once a month

44. Which of the following time periods is recommended for the use of a pooled serum control?

    A. one month
    B. three months
    C. six months
    D. one year

45. Quality control programs are used to determine or check which of the following?

    A. precision and accuracy of results
    B. technical performance of laboratory personnel
    C. performance of laboratory equipment
    D. performance of reagents
    E. all of the above

46. A pooled serum has been thawed, mixed, filtered, and assayed. The assay value for glucose is 75 mg/ml. The desired value for glucose is 100 mg/dl. How much glucose would have to be added to 2 liters of this sera to reach the desired value?

    A. 25 mg
    B. 250 mg
    C. 50 mg
    D. 500 mg

47. Which of the following levels of sodium would NOT be acceptable in distilled or deionized water?

    A. 0.05 mg/1
    B. 0.1 mg/1
    C. 0.05 mg/ml
    D. 0.0001 mg/ml

48. Which of the following is the maximum allowable concentration of carbon dioxide in distilled or deionized water?

    A. 0.1 mg/1
    B. 0.5 mg/1
    C. 1 mg/1
    D. 3 mg/1

49. Which of the following chemical reagent grades for the analysis of trace metals?

    A. Analytical Reagent Grade (AR)
    B. Chemically Pure Grade (CP)
    C. Technical grade
    D. Practical grade

50. In the SI system of units of measure and weights, which of the following is the unit used for the "amount of substance"?

    A. kilogram
    B. candela
    C. mole
    D. radian

51. All of the following statements concerning borosilicate glass are TRUE except:

   A. if has a high stress point
   B. it can withstand all temperatures encountered in the routine laboratory
   C. it is resistant to attack by alkaline solutions
   D. it has a very low change in volume with change in temperature

52. Which of the following chemical "grades" is acceptable for making reagents?

   A. NF grade   C. AR grade
   B. technical grade   D. practical grade

53. Organic chemicals, in a dry crystalline form, (unless otherwise stated), are stable for:

   A. 1 year   C. 3 years
   B. 2 years   D. 5 years

54. Lyophilized materials, when stored unopen and frozen, are stable for:

   A. 1 month   C. 9 months
   B. 6 months   D. 12 months

55. According to CAP specifications, water of reagent grade Type I must have a specific conductivity of not more than:

   A. 0.1 micromhos/cm   C. 2.0 micromhos/cm
   B. 1.0 micromhos/cm   D. 5.0 micromhos/cm

56. According to the CAP specifications for Type I reagent grade water, the water must have a specific resistance of no less than:

   A. 0.2 megohms/cm   C. 5.0 megohms/cm
   B. 0.5 megohms/cm   D. 10.0 megohms/cm

57. One of the tests for purity of water is the test for substances that reduce permanganate. This test measures:

   A. silicates   C. dissolved organic compounds
   B. heavy metals   D. hardness

Questions 58-60

Directions. Select and circle the one BEST answer for each of the following statements utilizing the information presented in either the following graph, tracing, table or laboratory data.

A technologist, during the process of testing a new lot number of glucose reagent, performs a reproducibility study on a single sample and obtains the following results:

100, 101, 101, 100, 99, 102, 99, 100, 100, 98 mg/dl

58. Assuming that the actual value for this sample was, in fact, 120 mg/dl, this person's results are an example of:

    A. accuracy
    B. precision

    C. reliability
    D. both A & B

59. Assuming that the actual value for this sample was 100 mg/dl, then, these results are an example of:

    A. accuracy
    B. precision

    C. reliability
    D. both A & B

60. Assuming that the actual value for this sample is 120 mg/dl, the coefficient of variation for this series would be:

    A. 0.1%
    B. 1.0%

    C. 10%
    D. 20%

Questions 61-80

Directions. Select the one BEST answer for each of the following statements. Mark the appropriate response on the answer sheet.

61. As laboratory productivity increases, it is essential to:

    A. increase the number of qualified technologists
    B. buy more reagents
    C. enlarge the laboratory facility
    D. lower the cost of laboratory tests

62. A test result will be as good as:

    A. the Standard Operational Procedure Manual
    B. the supervisor
    C. the pathologist
    D. the manner in which the sample was obtained

63. The Standard Operational Procedure Manual should be used:

    A. periodically
    B. weekly

    C. daily
    D. monthly

64. Each instrument:

    A. need not have a separate function sheet
    B. should have a separate function sheet
    C. should be checked monthly
    D. should be checked weekly

65. The Occupational Safety and Health Administration (OSHA) is a regulatory agency which is:

    A. governmental in nature
    B. an ASCP agency

    C. an AMA agency
    D. a CDC agency

66. A laboratory has the following organizational structure: pathologist→ chief technologist→ supervisor→bench technologist. You are a bench technologist in bacteriology and feel a test result may be incorrect. You should immediately seek assistance from:

    A. the pathologist
    B. the chief technologist
    C. your immediate supervisor
    D. no one for you would appear incompetent

67. In order to make the best decision, a laboratory manager should:

    A. consult only with laboratory supervisors
    B. consult only with the bench technologists
    C. consult only with the pathologist
    D. be certain he/she has all the facts

68. Internal quality control refers to a laboratory's method of assuring the quality of routine test results on a:

    A. weekly basis
    B. daily basis
    C. monthly basis
    D. yearly basis

69. An internal quality control system can be established and maintained using several methods including the:

    A. Shewhart chart
    B. OSHA regulations
    C. J C A H regulations
    D. C A P regulations

70. The person responsible for purchasing laboratory reagents:

    A. need not know anything about the laboratory
    B. should know about the laboratory and testing
    C. should try to save money
    D. should buy substitute reagents

71. Laboratory glassware has been found to:

    A. never interfere with test results
    B. rarely interfere with test results
    C. frequently interfere with test results
    D. none of the above

72. According to the Gaussian normal distribution curve, $\pm$ 1 standard deviation equals:

    A. 67% of the group of values
    B. 95% of the group of values
    C. 99.7% of the group of values
    D. none of the above

73. External survey programs:

    A. are a nuisance and should be avoided
    B. are not essential if a laboratory is efficiently managed
    C. are not essential if the technologists are competent
    D. should be used by laboratories

74. Continuing education:

    A. is not necessary for technologists
    B. is a personal choice and should not be imposed
    C. should be the responsibility of the hospital solely
    D. is essential and should be encouraged

75. Two examples of quality control charts are:

    A. Shewhart and Tonk
    B. Shewhart and Gaussian

    C. Levy-Jennings and Tonk
    D. Levy-Jennings and Shewhart

76. Accuracy is:

    A. how close a test result comes to the true value
    B. merely reproducibility
    C. reliability
    D. repeated measurements of the same specimen

77. In laboratory medicine, the term quality control refers to:

    A. how close the test result comes to the true value
    B. merely reproducibility
    C. reproducibility and how close the result comes to the true value
    D. repeated reliable measurements of the same specimen

78. Precision is:

    A. how close a test result comes to the true value
    B. reproducibility
    C. reliability
    D. repeated measurements of the same specimen

79. Control samples are used to monitor a technique's:

    A. accuracy only
    B. precision and accuracy

    C. precision only
    D. primary calibration

80. A standard calibration is used as a:

    A. reference value only
    B. quality control value

    C. both A and B
    D. neither A nor B

Explanatory Answers

1. (C) Appreciable amounts of aerosols may be produced when the designated procedures are employed; therefore, these should be performed with caution.

2. (B) When steam sterilizing, one should not only consider 15 lbs. pressure for 15 minutes as the sole criterion for complete sterilization. Air pressure gauges are often inaccurate, therefore the time and temperature factors should be significant for proper sterilization. Sterilization for 15 minutes at 250°F (121°C) would ensure more reliable results. This is also further supported by the fact that at a high altitude a 15 lb. pressure reading will not correspond to 250°F (121°C). Clinics and laboratories in high altitudes would have to adjust the pressure gauge to correspond to a 250°F reading.

3. (C) Safety measures must be taken collecting bacteriological specimen. Good bacteriological techniques prevent specimen contamination and protect the worker against infectious agents.

4. (B) Members of the genus Bacillus are most frequently used as biological indicators for monitoring sterilizers.

5. (A) Detailed procedures would minimize variables and aid in obtaining reproducible results in laboratory work.

6. (B) A routine checking of commercially prepared media will assure the worker that the quality of the product has not been diminished during storage.

7. (C) Cultures of Haemophilus influenzae should be maintained to check for the X and V growth factors.

8. (E) Streptococcus pyogenes can be employed for checking bacitracin disks, group A antiserum quality and beta hemolysis on blood agar plates.

9. (C) A culture of Streptococcus pneumoniae would be necessary to check optochin disks and an organism's ability to produce alpha hemolysis on blood agar plates.

10. (E) Candida albicans cultures should be maintained to determine Chlamydospore production. Chlamydospore agar or Wolin and Bevis agar are recommended media for Chlamydospore production.

11. (B) Mueller-Hinton agar is recommended for the Bauer-Kirby disk susceptibility test.

12. (B) Quality control records should be kept where everyone can see and use them. All entries should be initialed and dated. It is recommended that one person be in charge of quality control in each laboratory.

13. (C) Lyophilization maintains stock cultures for a long time period. Certain cultures have been recorded as remaining viable twenty years after lyophilization.

14. (B) The Staphylococcus aureus strains are the producers of coagulase and should be maintained as stock cultures to demonstrate coagulase activity.

15. (A) Proteus species are able to deaminate several amino acids. The deaminase activity of Proteus serves as a means of differentiating Proteus from other Enterobacteriaceae.

16. (A) It is recommended that strains of Neisseria gonococci be kept to check for oxidase production.

17. (C) Tyndallization, also called fractional sterilization, may be employed to sterilize materials which would denature if sterilized by conventional methods.

18. (A) Several reagents can be used to determine the production of indole by bacteria. Kovac's reagent is such a reagent and it is widely used to this purpose.

19. (B) When diagnosing typhus fever, antigens prepared from Proteus OX 19 should be used.

20. (C) When typhoid fever is suspected, the patient's serum should be set up against both the O and H antigens of Salmonella typhi.

21. (B) Accuracy is defined as the closeness to the true mean.

22. (D) Precision is the degree of reproducibility in a method. Precision is the spread between replicates.

23. (A) Sensitivity is the degree to which an analytical system can discriminate between two values that are significantly different.

24. (E) A standard is a highly purified material of known standard composition.

25. (B) Standard deviation is the measure of the scatter of values around the mean value in a Gaussian distribution.

26. (E) 95% Confidence Limit encompasses 95.45% of the results in a normal Gaussian distribution, if the number of samples is large enough the results fall into a symmetrical distribution.

27. (C) A systematic shift is the result of a sudden failure or bias of the test system. The systematic shift is characterized by results that are consistently high or low.

28. (D) A systematic trend is a gradual increase or decrease of the test system. The systematic trend is characterized by a lack of random scatter.

29. (C) The mean is defined as the average value, or the arithmetic mean.

30. (A) The median is defined as the value that is the middle value in a set.

31. (E) The mode is defined as the value in a set that occurs most frequently.

32. (B) The C. V., or coefficient of variation, is the percent of the mean value, and is determined by dividing the standard deviation by the mean and multiplying by 100.

33. (C) Sulfur dioxide is extremely toxic and produces severe burns to the lungs.

34. (D) Carbon tetrachloride causes liver damage. This substance is toxic at levels that are not detectable by odor, and has a cumulative effect.

35. (A) Benzidine and its salts are considered carconogenic.

36. (B) Phenol is corrosive to the skin and may produce a contact dermatitis even in dilute solution.

37. (A) Positively or negatively skewed curves are asymetrical curves in which the median is a better measure of the center than the mean because it will not be affected by the extremes of the distribution.

38. (C) A properly prepared and stained blood smear can be of value in quality control in verifying the platelet count, the white blood cell count, and the red blood cell indices.

39. (B) Dilutions of 1:100 or 1:200 should be used to check the reactivity of reagent red cells used for reverse blood grouping.

40. (C) Coomb's sera should be tested for their reactivity to IgG, C3, and C4. Anti human globulin must contain anti IgG, anti C3, especially anti C3d, and anti C4.

41. (A) Separate pools of sera should be collected for enzymes and thyroid tests. A separate pool of sera for enzymes is desirable because elevated levels of enzymes are desired, and a separate pool of sera for thyroid tests is desirable because the sera should not be frozen.

42. (C) Reactivity of antisera is demonstrated by avidity, titration of the antisera, and dilution of the antisera.

43. (A) The temperature of the Rh viewbox surface should be 45-50°C in order to achieve the 37°C temperature for the Rh slide test. The temperature of the view box surface should be checked every day that it is used.

44. (B) Serum collected for a pooled serum control should be collected in an amount sufficient to last three months; shorter periods just provide a greater amount of work, while sera frozen for longer periods tend to deteriorate.

45. (E) The goals of quality control programs are to assure the precision and accuracy of test results, to check the technical performance of laboratory personnel, to check the performance of laboratory equipment, and to check the performance of reagents.

46. (D) In order to get the desired value, 25 mg of glucose would have to be added for each 100 ml of sera, so 25 x 20 = 500 mg.

47. (C) Distilled or deionized water to be used for analytical purposes should not contain more than 0.1 mg/1 of sodium.

48. (D) The maximum allowable carbon dioxide concentration in distilled or deionized water is 3 mg/l.

49. (A) Analytical reagent grade chemicals are recommended for trace metal analysis because of high level of purity.

50. (C) The basic unit in the International System of Units (SI system) for the amount of substance is the mole. Kilogram is the unit of mass, candella is the unit of luminous intensity, and radian is the unit of plane angle.

51. (C) While borosilicate glass does have a high stress point, can withstand all temperatures encountered in the routine laboratory and has a very low change in volume for change in temperature, it cannot resist attack by alkaline solutions.

52. (C) AR, or Analytical Reagent grade, is the only grade of chemical listed that is suitable for making reagents

for analytical purposes. All of the other grades listed may contain impurities that render them unsuitable for use in the preparation of reagents.

53. (C) Unless otherwise stated on the container, organic chemicals in a dry crystalline form, are stable up to 3 years.

54. (D) Lyophilized materials, when sotred unopened and frozen, are considered to be stable for 1 year.

55. (A) The CAP specifications for Type I reagent grade water require that the water have a specific conductivity of not more than 0.1 micromhos/cm.

56. (D) The CAP specifications for Type I reagent grade water require that the water have a specific resistance of no less than 10.0 megohms/cm.

57. (C) The test for substances that reduce permanganate is a test for dissolved organic substances.

58. (B) The results presented are all very close to one another, however, if we consider the normal or actual value to be 120 mg/dl, the results are an example of precision in that they are all very close to one another. They are not accurate in this case.

59. (D) If, we assume that the normal or actual value for this sample is 100 mg/dl, then the results obtained are an example of both accuracy and precision in that they are not only very close to one another, but, they are also very close to the actual value.

60. (A) Regardless of the actual value, the coefficient of variation is a determination derived from a particular set of values. The coefficient of variation is a means of expressing standard deviation in unitless terms.

61. (A) As laboratory productivity increases, the number of qualified technologists should increase to maintain quality.

62. (D) A test result will be as good as the manner in which the specimen was collected.

63. (C) The Standard Operational Procedure Manual is one of the most important items at the bench. It should be updated yearly, but used frequently, if not daily.

64. (B) Each instrument should have a separate function sheet and should be checked on a daily basis.

65. (A) OSHA is a governmental agency.

66. (C) If a bench worker doubts a result, he/she should consult the immediate supervisor. The supervisor should consult on other levels, if necessary. One should always seek assistance when results are doubtful.

67. (D) In order to make the best decision or to resolve a problem, a laboratory manager should try to obtain all the facts in the situation.

68. (B) Quality control in a laboratory assures the quality of routine test results on a daily basis.

69. (A) The Shewhart chart is one method of establishing an internal quality control system.

70. (B) Laboratory quality begins with reagent quality. The purchasing agent should know how the laboratory functions and should avoid substitute reagents unless these have been proven to be as good and as reliable as those reagents recommended by the vendor.

71. (C) Dirty glassware and/or water are probably the two greatest sources responsible for poor laboratory test results. A quality control

program should include glassware and water checks.

72. (A) According to the Gaussian normal standard deviation curve, ± 1 standard deviation equals 67% of the group of values.

73. (D) Hospital laboratories should participate in external survey evaluation programs. These will allow a laboratory to compare methodologies with other laboratories. It is also a licensing requirement that hospitals show active files on external surveys.

74. (D) Continuing education is essential. During this time of rapid technological advances it is vital for the technologists to remain informed. Ideally, hospitals should encourage and support internal and external continuing education for technologists.

75. (D) Levy-Jennings and Shewhart charts are two charts used in quality control programs.

76. (A) Accuracy is how close a test result comes to the true value.

77. (D) In laboratory medicine, the term quality control mostly refers to repeated measurement of the same specimen. From these measurements laboratory personnel can determine the mean, standard deviation and coefficient of variation and by using a Levy-Jennings chart plot these determinations daily to show upper and lower levels of "control".

78. (B) Precision is reproducibility of a result.

79. (B) Control samples are used to check on a laboratory's performance. Control samples will monitor the precision (reproducibility) and accuracy of a technique.

80. (C) A calibrator is used as a reference value against which other samples are measured and may also be used as a quality control value measuring accuracy.

Bibliography and Recommended Readings

Becan-McBride, Kathleen. Editor. Textbook of Clinical Laboratory Supervision. 1981. Appleton-Crofts. New York.

Doucet, Lorraine. Editor. Medical Technology Review. 1981. Chapter 11. Quality Control/Management in the Clinical Laboratory. Shirley Brien, Contributor. J. B. Lippincott Company. Philadelphia.

Snyder, John R. and Arthur Lilarsen. Administration and Supervision in Laboratory Medicine. 1983. Harper and Row Publishers. Philadelphia.

Todd, J. C. Clinical Diagnosis and Management by Laboratory Methods. 1979. W. B. Saunders Company. Philadelphia.

CHAPTER 19

Tips From a High Scoring Registry Applicant

Registry, certification or proficiency examinations are like any other tests in that they seek to measure knowledge and ability in a specific area - in your case the clinical field.

Several successful registry applicants, who have achieved high scores, have been asked to explain the "key" to their success. The following recommendations were most frequently mentioned as being helpful:

1. Review previously taken quizzes and examinations from the clinical rotations.

2. Utilize Examination Review books to find your "strong" and "weak" areas.

3. Once the "weak" areas are established, brush up on these using your clinical notes and pertinent texts in the particular area or areas.

4. Pace yourself using Examination Review book practice tests so as to establish a work pace for the actual examination.

5. Repeat the Examination Review book diagnostic and practice tests to determine your improvement.

6. Be consistent! Do not prepare for the examination sporadically. Do not answer a few practice questions or read a few notes then "shelf" the preparation material for a few months.

7. Prepare long enough in advance so as to assimilate the material. DO NOT CRAM!

8. Meet with other examinees and test each other - serious group study is frequently beneficial.

9. Attend review courses if they are offered.

10. Frequently, examination boards send applicants examination information, such as question formats and sample questions. Read these carefully and answer the sample questions.

11. The night before the actual examination - get plenty of sleep to be alert and refreshed for the examination.

12. Arrive at the testing center early.

13. When taking the examination read the instructions carefully and thoroughly.

14. Do not read into the questions.

15. Answer the question asked, not the question <u>you</u> <u>think</u> is asked.

16. Be certain that the answer you mark on the answer sheet corresponds with the question number in the examination.

17. Answer the questions you are certain of first, and keep the difficult questions for last.

18. Think! Do not answer questions without sufficient thought.

19. Bring sharpened number 2 lead pencils in case needed.

N.B. Students frequently feel that it is not essential to review for the certification examination, since they recently completed the "rotations". We cannot urge students enough to review prior to the examination. Some rotations could have been made months before the registry, hence the recall ability is limited. The <u>key</u> to success is <u>proper</u> and <u>in-depth</u> preparation.

L.D.
A.P.

Illustrative Chapter
Answer Forms

Procedures in Microbiology

1 A B C D E	12 A B C D E	23 A B C D E	34 A B C D E	45 A B C D E
2 A B C D E	13 A B C D E	24 A B C D E	35 A B C D E	46 A B C D E
3 A B C D E	14 A B C D E	25 A B C D E	36 A B C D E	47 A B C D E
4 A B C D E	15 A B C D E	26 A B C D E	37 A B C D E	48 A B C D E
5 A B C D E	16 A B C D E	27 A B C D E	38 A B C D E	49 A B C D E
6 A B C D E	17 A B C D E	28 A B C D E	39 A B C D E	50 A B C D E
7 A B C D E	18 A B C D E	29 A B C D E	40 A B C D E	51 A B C D E
8 A B C D E	19 A B C D E	30 A B C D E	41 A B C D E	52 A B C D E
9 A B C D E	20 A B C D E	31 A B C D E	42 A B C D E	53 A B C D E
10 A B C D E	21 A B C D E	32 A B C D E	43 A B C D E	54 A B C D E
11 A B C D E	22 A B C D E	33 A B C D E	44 A B C D E	

Bacteriology

1 A B C D E	14 A B C D E	27 A B C D E	40 A B C D E	53 A B C D E
2 A B C D E	15 A B C D E	28 A B C D E	41 A B C D E	54 A B C D E
3 A B C D E	16 A B C D E	29 A B C D E	42 A B C D E	55 A B C D E
4 A B C D E	17 A B C D E	30 A B C D E	43 A B C D E	56 A B C D E
5 A B C D E	18 A B C D E	31 A B C D E	44 A B C D E	57 A B C D E
6 A B C D E	19 A B C D E	32 A B C D E	45 A B C D E	58 A B C D E
7 A B C D E	20 A B C D E	33 A B C D E	46 A B C D E	59 A B C D E
8 A B C D E	21 A B C D E	34 A B C D E	47 A B C D E	60 A B C D E
9 A B C D E	22 A B C D E	35 A B C D E	48 A B C D E	61 A B C D E
10 A B C D E	23 A B C D E	36 A B C D E	49 A B C D E	62 A B C D E
11 A B C D E	24 A B C D E	37 A B C D E	50 A B C D E	63 A B C D E
12 A B C D E	25 A B C D E	38 A B C D E	51 A B C D E	64 A B C D E
13 A B C D E	26 A B C D E	39 A B C D E	52 A B C D E	65 A B C D E

66 A B C D E	79 A B C D E	92 A B C D E	105 A B C D E	118 A B C D E
67 A B C D E	80 A B C D E	93 A B C D E	106 A B C D E	119 A B C D E
68 A B C D E	81 A B C D E	94 A B C D E	107 A B C D E	120 A B C D E
69 A B C D E	82 A B C D E	95 A B C D E	108 A B C D E	121 A B C D E
70 A B C D E	83 A B C D E	96 A B C D E	109 A B C D E	122 A B C D E
71 A B C D E	84 A B C D E	97 A B C D E	110 A B C D E	123 A B C D E
72 A B C D E	85 A B C D E	98 A B C D E	111 A B C D E	124 A B C D E
73 A B C D E	86 A B C D E	99 A B C D E	112 A B C D E	125 A B C D E
74 A B C D E	87 A B C D E	100 A B C D E	113 A B C D E	126 A B C D E
75 A B C D E	88 A B C D E	101 A B C D E	114 A B C D E	127 A B C D E
76 A B C D E	89 A B C D E	102 A B C D E	115 A B C D E	128 A B C D E
77 A B C D E	90 A B C D E	103 A B C D E	116 A B C D E	129 A B C D E
78 A B C D E	91 A B C D E	104 A B C D E	117 A B C D E	130 A B C D E

Bacteriology continued

131 A B C D E	143 A B C D E	155 A B C D E	167 A B C D E	179 A B C D E
132 A B C D E	144 A B C D E	156 A B C D E	168 A B C D E	180 A B C D E
133 A B C D E	145 A B C D E	157 A B C D E	169 A B C D E	181 A B C D E
134 A B C D E	146 A B C D E	158 A B C D E	170 A B C D E	182 A B C D E
135 A B C D E	147 A B C D E	159 A B C D E	171 A B C D E	183 A B C D E
136 A B C D E	148 A B C D E	160 A B C D E	172 A B C D E	184 A B C D E
137 A B C D E	149 A B C D E	161 A B C D E	173 A B C D E	185 A B C D E
138 A B C D E	150 A B C D E	162 A B C D E	174 A B C D E	186 A B C D E
139 A B C D E	151 A B C D E	163 A B C D E	175 A B C D E	187 A B C D E
140 A B C D E	152 A B C D E	164 A B C D E	176 A B C D E	188 A B C D E
141 A B C D E	153 A B C D E	165 A B C D E	177 A B C D E	189 A B C D E
142 A B C D E	154 A B C D E	166 A B C D E	178 A B C D E	

Mycology

1 A B C D E	16 A B C D E	31 A B C D E	46 A B C D E	61 A B C D E
2 A B C D E	17 A B C D E	32 A B C D E	47 A B C D E	62 A B C D E
3 A B C D E	18 A B C D E	33 A B C D E	48 A B C D E	63 A B C D E
4 A B C D E	19 A B C D E	34 A B C D E	49 A B C D E	64 A B C D E
5 A B C D E	20 A B C D E	35 A B C D E	50 A B C D E	65 A B C D E
6 A B C D E	21 A B C D E	36 A B C D E	51 A B C D E	66 A B C D E
7 A B C D E	22 A B C D E	37 A P C D E	52 A B C D E	67 A B C D E
8 A B C D E	23 A B C D E	38 A B C D E	53 A B C D E	68 A B C D E
9 A B C D E	24 A B C D E	39 A B C D E	54 A B C D E	69 A B C D E
10 A B C D E	25 A B C D E	40 A B C D E	55 A B C D E	70 A B C D E
11 A B C D E	26 A B C D E	41 A B C D E	56 A B C D E	71 A B C D E
12 A B C D E	27 A B C D E	42 A B C D E	57 A B C D E	72 A B C D E
13 A B C D E	28 A B C D E	43 A B C D E	58 A B C D E	73 A B C D E
14 A B C D E	29 A B C D E	44 A B C D E	59 A B C D E	74 A B C D E
15 A B C D E	30 A B C D E	45 A B C D E	60 A B C D E	75 A B C D E

Parasitology

1 A B C D E	18 A B C D E	35 A B C D E	52 A B C D E	69 A B C D E
2 A B C D E	19 A B C D E	36 A B C D E	53 A B C D E	70 A B C D E
3 A B C D E	20 A B C D E	37 A B C D E	54 A B C D E	71 A B C D E
4 A B C D E	21 A B C D E	38 A B C D E	55 A B C D E	72 A B C D E
5 A B C D E	22 A B C D E	39 A B C D E	56 A B C D E	73 A B C D E
6 A B C D E	23 A B C D E	40 A B C D E	57 A B C D E	74 A B C D E
7 A B C D E	24 A B C D E	41 A B C D E	58 A B C D E	75 A B C D E
8 A B C D E	25 A B C D E	42 A B C D E	59 A B C D E	76 A B C D E
9 A B C D E	26 A B C D E	43 A B C D E	60 A B C D E	77 A B C D E
10 A B C D E	27 A B C D E	44 A B C D E	61 A B C D E	78 A B C D E
11 A B C D E	28 A B C D E	45 A B C D E	62 A B C D E	79 A B C D E
12 A B C D E	29 A B C D E	46 A B C D E	63 A B C D E	80 A B C D E
13 A B C D E	30 A B C D E	47 A B C D E	64 A B C D E	81 A B C D E
14 A B C D E	31 A B C D E	48 A B C D E	65 A B C D E	82 A B C D E
15 A B C D E	32 A B C D E	49 A B C D E	66 A B C D E	83 A B C D E
16 A B C D E	33 A B C D E	50 A B C D E	67 A B C D E	84 A B C D E
17 A B C D E	34 A B C D E	51 A B C D E	68 A B C D E	85 A B C D E

Virology

1 A B C D E	15 A B C D E	29 A B C D E	43 A B C D E	57 A B C D E
2 A B C D E	16 A B C D E	30 A B C D E	44 A B C D E	58 A B C D E
3 A B C D E	17 A B C D E	31 A B C D E	45 A B C D E	59 A B C D E
4 A B C D E	18 A B C D E	32 A B C D E	46 A B C D E	60 A B C D E
5 A B C D E	19 A B C D E	33 A B C D E	47 A B C D E	61 A B C D E
6 A B C D E	20 A B C D E	34 A B C D E	48 A B C D E	62 A B C D E
7 A B C D E	21 A B C D E	35 A B C D E	49 A B C D E	63 A B C D E
8 A B C D E	22 A B C D E	36 A B C D E	50 A B C D E	64 A B C D E
9 A B C D E	23 A B C D E	37 A B C D E	51 A B C D E	65 A B C D E
10 A B C D E	24 A B C D E	38 A B C D E	52 A B C D E	66 A B C D E
11 A B C D E	25 A B C D E	39 A B C D E	53 A B C D E	67 A B C D E
12 A B C D E	26 A B C D E	40 A B C D E	54 A B C D E	68 A B C D E
13 A B C D E	27 A B C D E	41 A B C D E	55 A B C D E	69 A B C D E
14 A B C D E	28 A B C D E	42 A B C D E	56 A B C D E	70 A B C D E

Immunology/Serology

1 A B C D E	11 A B C D E	21 A B C D E	31 A B C D E	41 A B C D E
2 A B C D E	12 A B C D E	22 A B C D E	32 A B C D E	42 A B C D E
3 A B C D E	13 A B C D E	23 A B C D E	33 A B C D E	43 A B C D E
4 A B C D E	14 A B C D E	24 A B C D E	34 A B C D E	44 A B C D E
5 A B C D E	15 A B C D E	25 A B C D E	35 A B C D E	45 A B C D E
6 A B C D E	16 A B C D E	26 A B C D E	36 A B C D E	46 A B C D E
7 A B C D E	17 A B C D E	27 A B C D E	37 A B C D E	47 A B C D E
8 A B C D E	18 A B C D E	28 A B C D E	38 A B C D E	48 A B C D E
9 A B C D E	19 A B C D E	29 A B C D E	39 A B C D E	49 A B C D E
10 A B C D E	20 A B C D E	30 A B C D E	40 A B C D E	50 A B C D E
51 A B C D E	61 A B C D E	71 A B C D E	81 A B C D E	91 A B C D E
52 A B C D E	62 A B C D E	72 A B C D E	82 A B C D E	92 A B C D E
53 A B C D E	63 A B C D E	73 A B C D E	83 A B C D E	93 A B C D E
54 A B C D E	64 A B C D E	74 A B C D E	84 A B C D E	94 A B C D E
55 A B C D E	65 A B C D E	75 A B C D E	85 A B C D E	95 A B C D E
56 A B C D E	66 A B C D E	76 A B C D E	86 A B C D E	96 A B C D E
57 A B C D E	67 A B C D E	77 A B C D E	87 A B C D E	97 A B C D E
58 A B C D E	68 A B C D E	78 A B C D E	88 A B C D E	98 A B C D E
59 A B C D E	69 A B C D E	79 A B C D E	89 A B C D E	99 A B C D E
60 A B C D E	70 A B C D E	80 A B C D E	90 A B C D E	100 A B C D E
101 A B C D E	111 A B C D E	121 A B C D E	131 A B C D E	141 A B C D E
102 A B C D E	112 A B C D E	122 A B C D E	132 A B C D E	142 A B C D E
103 A B C D E	113 A B C D E	123 A B C D E	133 A B C D E	143 A B C D E
104 A B C D E	114 A B C D E	124 A B C D E	134 A B C D E	144 A B C D E
105 A B C D E	115 A B C D E	125 A B C D E	135 A B C D E	145 A B C D E
106 A B C D E	116 A B C D E	126 A B C D E	136 A B C D E	146 A B C D E
107 A B C D E	117 A B C D E	127 A B C D E	137 A B C D E	147 A B C D E
108 A B C D E	118 A B C D E	128 A B C D E	138 A B C D E	148 A B C D E
109 A B C D E	119 A B C D E	129 A B C D E	139 A B C D E	149 A B C D E
110 A B C D E	120 A B C D E	130 A B C D E	140 A B C D E	150 A B C D E

Immunohematology

1	A B C D E	13	A B C D E	25	A B C D E	37	A B C D E	49	A B C D E
2	A B C D E	14	A B C D E	26	A B C D E	38	A B C D E	50	A B C D E
3	A B C D E	15	A B C D E	27	A B C D E	39	A B C D E	51	A B C D E
4	A B C D E	16	A B C D E	28	A B C D E	40	A B C D E	52	A B C D E
5	A B C D E	17	A B C D E	29	A B C D E	41	A B C D E	53	A B C D E
6	A B C D E	18	A B C D E	30	A B C D E	42	A B C D E	54	A B C D E
7	A B C D E	19	A B C D E	31	A B C D E	43	A B C D E	55	A B C D E
8	A B C D E	20	A B C D E	32	A B C D E	44	A B C D E	56	A B C D E
9	A B C D E	21	A B C D E	33	A B C D E	45	A B C D E	57	A B C D E
10	A B C D E	22	A B C D E	34	A B C D E	46	A B C D E	58	A B C D E
11	A B C D E	23	A B C D E	35	A B C D E	47	A B C D E	59	A B C D E
12	A B C D E	24	A B C D E	36	A B C D E	48	A B C D E	60	A B C D E

61	A B C D E	73	A B C D E	85	A B C D E	97	A B C D E	109	A B C D E
62	A B C D E	74	A B C D E	86	A B C D E	98	A B C D E	110	A B C D E
63	A B C D E	75	A B C D E	87	A B C D E	99	A B C D E	111	A B C D E
64	A B C D E	76	A B C D E	88	A B C D E	100	A B C D E	112	A B C D E
65	A B C D E	77	A B C D E	89	A B C D E	101	A B C D E	113	A B C D E
66	A B C D E	78	A B C D E	90	A B C D E	102	A B C D E	114	A B C D E
67	A B C D E	79	A B C D E	91	A B C D E	103	A B C D E	115	A B C D E
68	A B C D E	80	A B C D E	92	A B C D E	104	A B C D E	116	A B C D E
69	A B C D E	81	A B C D E	93	A B C D E	105	A B C D E	117	A B C D E
70	A B C D E	82	A B C D E	94	A B C D E	106	A B C D E	118	A B C D E
71	A B C D E	83	A B C D E	95	A B C D E	107	A B C D E	119	A B C D E
72	A B C D E	84	A B C D E	96	A B C D E	108	A B C D E	120	A B C D E

Hematology

1	A B C D E	11	A B C D E	21	A B C D E	31	A B C D E	41	A B C D E
2	A B C D E	12	A B C D E	22	A B C D E	32	A B C D E	42	A B C D E
3	A B C D E	13	A B C D E	23	A B C D E	33	A B C D E	43	A B C D E
4	A B C D E	14	A B C D E	24	A B C D E	34	A B C D E	44	A B C D E
5	A B C D E	15	A B C D E	25	A B C D E	35	A B C D E	45	A B C D E
6	A B C D E	16	A B C D E	26	A B C D E	36	A B C D E	46	A B C D E
7	A B C D E	17	A B C D E	27	A B C D E	37	A B C D E	47	A B C D E
8	A B C D E	18	A B C D E	28	A B C D E	38	A B C D E	48	A B C D E
9	A B C D E	19	A B C D E	29	A B C D E	39	A B C D E	49	A B C D E
10	A B C D E	20	A B C D E	30	A B C D E	40	A B C D E	50	A B C D E

51	A B C D E	61	A B C D E	71	A B C D E	81	A B C D E	91	A B C D E
52	A B C D E	62	A B C D E	72	A B C D E	82	A B C D E	92	A B C D E
53	A B C D E	63	A B C D E	73	A B C D E	83	A B C D E	93	A B C D E
54	A B C D E	64	A B C D E	74	A B C D E	84	A B C D E	94	A B C D E
55	A B C D E	65	A B C D E	75	A B C D E	85	A B C D E	95	A B C D E
56	A B C D E	66	A B C D E	76	A B C D E	86	A B C D E	96	A B C D E
57	A B C D E	67	A B C D E	77	A B C D E	87	A B C D E	97	A B C D E
58	A B C D E	68	A B C D E	78	A B C D E	88	A B C D E	98	A B C D E
59	A B C D E	69	A B C D E	79	A B C D E	89	A B C D E	99	A B C D E
60	A B C D E	70	A B C D E	80	A B C D E	90	A B C D E	100	A B C D E

Hematology continued

101	A B C D E	111	A B C D E	121	A B C D E	131	A B C D E	141	A B C D E
102	A B C D E	112	A B C D E	122	A B C D E	132	A B C D E	142	A B C D E
103	A B C D E	113	A B C D E	123	A B C D E	133	A B C D E	143	A B C D E
104	A B C D E	114	A B C D E	124	A B C D E	134	A B C D E	144	A B C D E
105	A B C D E	115	A B C D E	125	A B C D E	135	A B C D E	145	A B C D E
106	A B C D E	116	A B C D E	126	A B C D E	136	A B C D E	146	A B C D E
107	A B C D E	117	A B C D E	127	A B C D E	137	A B C D E	147	A B C D E
108	A B C D E	118	A B C D E	128	A B C D E	138	A B C D E	148	A B C D E
109	A B C D E	119	A B C D E	129	A B C D E	139	A B C D E	149	A B C D E
110	A B C D E	120	A B C D E	130	A B C D E	140	A B C D E	150	A B C D E
151	A B C D E	161	A B C D E	171	A B C D E	181	A B C D E	191	A B C D E
152	A B C D E	162	A B C D E	172	A B C D E	182	A B C D E	192	A B C D E
153	A B C D E	163	A B C D E	173	A B C D E	183	A B C D E	193	A B C D E
154	A B C D E	164	A B C D E	174	A B C D E	184	A B C D E	194	A B C D E
155	A B C D E	165	A B C D E	175	A B C D E	185	A B C D E	195	A B C D E
156	A B C D E	166	A B C D E	176	A B C D E	186	A B C D E	196	A B C D E
157	A B C D E	167	A B C D E	177	A B C D E	187	A B C D E	197	A B C D E
158	A B C D E	168	A B C D E	178	A B C D E	188	A B C D E		
159	A B C D E	169	A B C D E	179	A B C D E	189	A B C D E		
160	A B C D E	170	A B C D E	180	A B C D E	190	A B C D E		

Nuclear Medicine

1	A B C D E	11	A B C D E	21	A B C D E	31	A B C D E	41	A B C D E
2	A B C D E	12	A B C D E	22	A B C D E	32	A B C D E	42	A B C D E
3	A B C D E	13	A B C D E	23	A B C D E	33	A B C D E	43	A B C D E
4	A B C D E	14	A B C D E	24	A B C D E	34	A B C D E	44	A B C D E
5	A B C D E	15	A B C D E	25	A B C D E	35	A B C D E	45	A B C D E
6	A B C D E	16	A B C D E	26	A B C D E	36	A B C D E	46	A B C D E
7	A B C D E	17	A B C D E	27	A B C D E	37	A B C D E	47	A B C D E
8	A B C D E	18	A B C D E	28	A B C D E	38	A B C D E	48	A B C D E
9	A B C D E	19	A B C D E	29	A B C D E	39	A B C D E	49	A B C D E
10	A B C D E	20	A B C D E	30	A B C D E	40	A B C D E	50	A B C D E
51	A B C D E	56	A B C D E						
52	A B C D E	57	A B C D E						
53	A B C D E	58	A B C D E						
54	A B C D E	59	A B C D E						
55	A B C D E	60	A B C D E						

Clinical Chemistry

1 A B C D E	17 A B C D E	33 A B C D E	49 A B C D E	65 A B C D E
2 A B C D E	18 A B C D E	34 A B C D E	50 A B C D E	66 A B C D E
3 A B C D E	19 A B C D E	35 A B C D E	51 A B C D E	67 A B C D E
4 A B C D E	20 A B C D E	36 A B C D E	52 A B C D E	68 A B C D E
5 A B C D E	21 A B C D E	37 A B C D E	53 A B C D E	69 A B C D E
6 A B C D E	22 A B C D E	38 A B C D E	54 A B C D E	70 A B C D E
7 A B C D E	23 A B C D E	39 A B C D E	55 A B C D E	71 A B C D E
8 A B C D E	24 A B C D E	40 A B C D E	56 A B C D E	72 A B C D E
9 A B C D E	25 A B C D E	41 A B C D E	57 A B C D E	73 A B C D E
10 A B C D E	26 A B C D E	42 A B C D E	58 A B C D E	74 A B C D E
11 A B C D E	27 A B C D E	43 A B C D E	59 A B C D E	75 A B C D E
12 A B C D E	28 A B C D E	44 A B C D E	60 A B C D E	76 A B C D E
13 A B C D E	29 A B C D E	45 A B C D E	61 A B C D E	77 A B C D E
14 A B C D E	30 A B C D E	46 A B C D E	62 A B C D E	78 A B C D E
15 A B C D E	31 A B C D E	47 A B C D E	63 A B C D E	79 A B C D E
16 A B C D E	32 A B C D E	48 A B C D E	64 A B C D E	80 A B C D E

81 A B C D E	97 A B C D E	113 A B C D E	129 A B C D E	145 A B C D E
82 A B C D E	98 A B C D E	114 A B C D E	130 A B C D E	146 A B C D E
83 A B C D E	99 A B C D E	115 A B C D E	131 A B C D E	147 A B C D E
84 A B C D E	100 A B C D E	116 A B C D E	132 A B C D E	148 A B C D E
85 A B C D E	101 A B C D E	117 A B C D E	133 A B C D E	149 A B C D E
86 A B C D E	102 A B C D E	118 A B C D E	134 A B C D E	150 A B C D E
87 A B C D E	103 A B C D E	119 A B C D E	135 A B C D E	151 A B C D E
88 A B C D E	104 A B C D E	120 A B C D E	136 A B C D E	152 A B C D E
89 A B C D E	105 A B C D E	121 A B C D E	137 A B C D E	153 A B C D E
90 A B C D E	106 A B C D E	122 A B C D E	138 A B C D E	154 A B C D E
91 A B C D E	107 A B C D E	123 A B C D E	139 A B C D E	155 A B C D E
92 A B C D E	108 A B C D E	124 A B C D E	140 A B C D E	156 A B C D E
93 A B C D E	109 A B C D E	125 A B C D E	141 A B C D E	157 A B C D E
94 A B C D E	110 A B C D E	126 A B C D E	142 A B C D E	158 A B C D E
95 A B C D E	111 A B C D E	127 A B C D E	143 A B C D E	159 A B C D E
96 A B C DE	112 A B C D E	128 A B C D E	144 A B C D E	

Toxicology

1 A B C D E	14 A B C D E	27 A B C D E	40 A B C D E	53 A B C D E
2 A B C D E	15 A B C D E	28 A B C D E	41 A B C D E	54 A B C D E
3 A B C D E	16 A B C D E	29 A B C D E	42 A B C D E	55 A B C D E
4 A B C D E	17 A B C D E	30 A B C D E	43 A B C D E	56 A B C D E
5 A B C D E	18 A B C D E	31 A B C D E	44 A B C D E	57 A B C D E
6 A B C D E	19 A B C D E	32 A B C D E	45 A B C D E	58 A B C D E
7 A B C D E	20 A B C D E	33 A B C D E	46 A B C D E	59 A B C D E
8 A B C D E	21 A B C D E	34 A B C D E	47 A B C D E	60 A B C D E
9 A B C D E	22 A B C D E	35 A B C D E	48 A B C D E	61 A B C D E
10 A B C D E	23 A B C D E	36 A B C D E	49 A B C D E	62 A B C D E
11 A B C D E	24 A B C D E	37 A B C D E	50 A B C D E	63 A B C D E
12 A B C D E	25 A B C D E	38 A B C D E	51 A B C D E	
13 A B C D E	26 A B C D E	39 A B C D E	52 A B C D E	

Endocrinology

1 A B C D E	6 A B C D E	11 A B C D E	16 A B C D E	21 A B C D E
2 A B C D E	7 A B C D E	12 A B C D E	17 A B C D E	22 A B C D E
3 A B C D E	8 A B C D E	13 A B C D E	18 A B C D E	23 A B C D E
4 A B C D E	9 A B C D E	14 A B C D E	19 A B C D E	24 A B C D E
5 A B C D E	10 A B C D E	15 A B C D E	20 A B C D E	25 A B C D E

Urinalysis

1 A B C D E	12 A B C D E	23 A B C D E	34 A B C D E	45 A B C D E
2 A B C D E	13 A B C D E	24 A B C D E	35 A B C D E	46 A B C D E
3 A B C D E	14 A B C D E	25 A B C D E	36 A B C D E	47 A B C D E
4 A B C D E	15 A B C D E	26 A B C D E	37 A B C D E	48 A B C D E
5 A B C D E	16 A B C D E	27 A B C D E	38 A B C D E	49 A B C D E
6 A B C D E	17 A B C D E	28 A B C D E	39 A B C D E	50 A B C D E
7 A B C D E	18 A B C D E	29 A B C D E	40 A B C D E	51 A B C D E
8 A B C D E	19 A B C D E	30 A B C D E	41 A B C D E	52 A B C D E
9 A B C D E	20 A B C D E	31 A B C D E	42 A B C D E	53 A B C D E
10 A B C D E	21 A B C D E	32 A B C D E	43 A B C D E	54 A B C D E
11 A B C D E	22 A B C D E	33 A B C D E	44 A B C D E	55 A B C D E

56 A B C D E	67 A B C D E	78 A B C D E	89 A B C D E	100 A B C D E
57 A B C D E	68 A B C D E	79 A B C D E	90 A B C D E	101 A B C D E
58 A B C D E	69 A B C D E	80 A B C D E	91 A B C D E	102 A B C D E
59 A B C D E	70 A B C D E	81 A B C D E	92 A B C D E	103 A B C D E
60 A B C D E	71 A B C D E	82 A B C D E	93 A B C D E	104 A B C D E
61 A B C D E	72 A B C D E	83 A B C D E	94 A B C D E	105 A B C D E
62 A B C D E	73 A B C D E	84 A B C D E	95 A B C D E	106 A B C D E
63 A B C D E	74 A B C D E	85 A B C D E	96 A B C D E	107 A B C D E
64 A B C D E	75 A B C D E	86 A B C D E	97 A B C D E	108 A B C D E
65 A B C D E	76 A B C D E	87 A B C D E	98 A B C D E	109 A B C D E
66 A B C D E	77 A B C D E	88 A B C D E	99 A B C D E	110 A B C D E

Body Fluid Analysis

1 A B C D E	15 A B C D E	29 A B C D E	43 A B C D E	57 A B C D E
2 A B C D E	16 A B C D E	30 A B C D E	44 A B C D E	58 A B C D E
3 A B C D E	17 A B C D E	31 A B C D E	45 A B C D E	59 A B C D E
4 A B C D E	18 A B C D E	32 A B C D E	46 A B C D E	60 A B C D E
5 A B C D E	19 A B C D E	33 A B C D E	47 A B C D E	61 A B C D E
6 A B C D E	20 A B C D E	34 A B C D E	48 A B C D E	62 A B C D E
7 A B C D E	21 A B C D E	35 A B C D E	49 A B C D E	63 A B C D E
8 A B C D E	22 A B C D E	36 A B C D E	50 A B C D E	64 A B C D E
9 A B C D E	23 A B C D E	37 A B C D E	51 A B C D E	65 A B C D E
10 A B C D E	24 A B C D E	38 A B C D E	52 A B C D E	66 A B C D E
11 A B C D E	25 A B C D E	39 A B C D E	53 A B C D E	67 A B C D E
12 A B C D E	26 A B C D E	40 A B C D E	54 A B C D E	68 A B C D E
13 A B C D E	27 A B C D E	41 A B C D E	55 A B C D E	69 A B C D E
14 A B C D E	28 A B C D E	42 A B C D E	56 A B C D E	70 A B C D E

Cytogenetics/Cytology

1	A B C D E	6	A B C D E	11	A B C D E	16	A B C D E	21	A B C D E
2	A B C D E	7	A B C D E	12	A B C D E	17	A B C D E	22	A B C D E
3	A B C D E	8	A B C D E	13	A B C D E	18	A B C D E	23	A B C D E
4	A B C D E	9	A B C D E	14	A B C D E	19	A B C D E	24	A B C D E
5	A B C D E	10	A B C D E	15	A B C D E	20	A B C D E	25	A B C D E

Quality Control/Laboratory Safety/Laboratory Management

1	A B C D E	17	A B C D E	33	A B C D E	49	A B C D E	65	A B C D E
2	A B C D E	18	A B C D E	34	A B C D E	50	A B C D E	66	A B C D E
3	A B C D E	19	A B C D E	35	A B C D E	51	A B C D E	67	A B C D E
4	A B C D E	20	A B C D E	36	A B C D E	52	A B C D E	68	A B C D E
5	A B C D E	21	A B C D E	37	A B C D E	53	A B C D E	69	A B C D E
6	A B C D E	22	A B C D E	38	A B C D E	54	A B C D E	70	A B C D E
7	A B C D E	23	A B C D E	39	A B C D E	55	A B C D E	71	A B C D E
8	A B C D E	24	A B C D E	40	A B C D E	56	A B C D E	72	A B C D E
9	A B C D E	25	A B C D E	41	A B C D E	57	A B C D E	73	A B C D E
10	A B C D E	26	A B C D E	42	A B C D E	58	A B C D E	74	A B C D E
11	A B C D E	27	A B C D E	43	A B C D E	59	A B C D E	75	A B C D E
12	A B C D E	28	A B C D E	44	A B C D E	60	A B C D E	76	A B C D E
13	A B C D E	29	A B C D E	45	A B C D E	61	A B C D E	77	A B C D E
14	A B C D E	30	A B C D E	46	A B C D E	62	A B C D E	78	A B C D E
15	A B C D E	31	A B C D E	47	A B C D E	63	A B C D E	79	A B C D E
16	A B C D E	32	A B C D E	48	A B C D E	64	A B C D E	80	A B C D E